Multidisciplinary Care of the Cancer Patient

Editor

GREGORY A. MASTERS

SURGICAL ONCOLOGY CLINICS OF NORTH AMERICA

www.surgonc.theclinics.com

Consulting Editor
NICHOLAS J. PETRELLI

April 2013 • Volume 22 • Number 2

ELSEVIER

1600 John F. Kennedy Boulevard • Suite 1800 • Philadelphia, Pennsylvania, 19103-2899

http://www.theclinics.com

SURGICAL ONCOLOGY CLINICS OF NORTH AMERICA Volume 22, Number 2
April 2013 ISSN 1055-3207, ISBN-13: 978-1-4557-7336-7

Editor: Jessica McCool

Surgical Oncology Clinics of North America (ISSN 1055-3207) is published quarterly by Elsevier Inc., 360 Park Avenue South, New York, NY 10010-1710. Months of publication are January, April, July, and October. Business and Editorial Offices: 1600 John F. Kennedy Blvd., Ste. 1800, Philadelphia, PA 19103-2899. Customer Service Office: 3251 Riverport Lane, Maryland Heights, MO 63043. Periodicals postage paid at New York, NY and additional mailing offices. Subscription prices are $274.00 per year (US individuals), $401.00 (US institutions) $135.00 (US student/resident), $314.00 (Canadian individuals), $498.00 (Canadian institutions), $193.00 (Canadian student/resident), $392.00 (foreign individuals), $498.00 (foreign institutions), and $193.00 (foreign student/resident). Foreign air speed delivery is included in all *Clinics* subscription prices. All prices are subject to change without notice. **POSTMASTER**: Send address changes to *Surgical Oncology Clinics of North America*, Elsevier Health Science Division, Subscription Customer Service, 3251 Riverport Lane, Maryland Heights, MO 63043. **Customer Service: 1-800-654-2452 (US and Canada). 314-447-8871 (outside U.S. and Canada). Fax: 314-447-8029. E-mail: journalscustomerservice-usa@elsevier.com** (for print support); **journalsonline support-usa@elsevier.com** (for online support).

Reprints. For copies of 100 or more, of articles in this publication, please contact the Commercial Reprints Department, Elsevier Inc., 360 Park Avenue South, New York, New York 10010-1710. Tel. 212-633-3813; Fax: 212-462-1935; E-mail: reprints@elsevier.com.

Surgical Oncology Clinics of North America is covered in *MEDLINE/PubMed (Index Medicus) and EMBASE/Excerpta Medica, Current Contents/Clinical Medicine, and ISI/BIOMED.*

Printed and bound by CPI Group (UK) Ltd, Croydon, CR0 4YY

Transferred to digital print 2012

Contributors

CONSULTING EDITOR

NICHOLAS J. PETRELLI, MD, FACS
Bank of America Endowed Medical Director, Helen F. Graham Cancer Center at Christiana Care, Newark, Delaware; Professor of Surgery, Thomas Jefferson University, Philadelphia, Pennsylvania

EDITOR

GREGORY A. MASTERS, MD
Medical Oncology Hematology Consultants, Helen F. Graham Cancer Center, Newark, Delaware; Associate Professor of Medicine, Thomas Jefferson University Medical School, Philadelphia, Pennsylvania

AUTHORS

JAY BAKER, MD
Department of Radiology, Duke Cancer Institute, Duke University School of Medicine, Durham, North Carolina

IGOR J. BARANI, MD
Assistant Professor in Residence, Clinical Research Director and Vice Chair, Department of Radiation Oncology, University of California, San Francisco, San Francisco, California

JOSEPH J. BENNETT, MD
Department of Surgery, Helen F. Graham Cancer Center, Christiana Care Hospital, Newark, Delaware

ORIN BLOCH, MD
Resident, Department of Neurological Surgery, University of California, San Francisco, San Francisco, California

SUSAN M. CHANG, MD
Professor in Residence and Lai Wan Kan Endowed Chair and Vice Chair, Department of Neurological Surgery, University of California, San Francisco, San Francisco, California

ROBERT CHIN, MD, PhD
Assistant Professor, Department of Radiation and Cellular Oncology, The University of Chicago, Chicago, Illinois

EZRA E.W. COHEN, MD
Associate Professor, Section of Hematology/Oncology, Department of Medicine, The University of Chicago, Chicago, Illinois

JORGE A. GARCIA, MD
Staff, Taussig Cancer Center, Cleveland Clinic, Cleveland, Ohio

MARK GARZOTTO, MD
Associate Professor, Departments of Urology and Radiation Medicine, Portland Veterans Administration Medical Center, Oregon Health and Science University, Portland, Oregon

JOSEPH GERADTS, MD, MA
Department of Pathology, Duke Cancer Institute, Duke University School of Medicine, Durham, North Carolina

SARAH B. GOLDBERG, MD, MPH
Assistant Professor, Department of Hematology/Oncology, Yale Cancer Center, New Haven, Connecticut

SEUNGGU J. HAN, MD
Resident, Department of Neurological Surgery, University of California, San Francisco, San Francisco, California

REBECCA S. HEIST, MD, MPH
Assistant Professor, Department of Hematology/Oncology, Massachusetts General Hospital Cancer Center, Boston, Massachusetts

JOSEPH M. HERMAN, MD, MS
Department of Radiation Oncology and Molecular Radiation Sciences, The Sidney Kimmel Comprehensive Cancer Center; Department of Oncology, The Sol Goldman Pancreatic Cancer Center, The Skip Viragh Center for Pancreatic Cancer, The Sidney Kimmel Comprehensive Cancer Center, Johns Hopkins University School of Medicine, Baltimore, Maryland

JANET HORTON, MD
Department of Radiation Oncology, Duke Cancer Institute, Duke University School of Medicine, Durham, North Carolina

TANNIE HUANG, MD
Clinical Instructor, Division of Hematology Oncology, Department of Pediatrics, University of California, San Francisco, San Francisco, California

ARTHUR Y. HUNG, MD
Assistant Professor, Department of Radiation Medicine, Oregon Health and Science University, Portland, Oregon

E. SHELLEY HWANG, MD, MPH
Department of Surgery, Duke Cancer Institute, Duke University School of Medicine, Durham, North Carolina

DORAID JARRAR, MD
Thoracic Surgery, Albert Einstein Medical Center Philadelphia, Philadelphia, Pennsylvania

KIRANPREET K. KHURANA, MD
Urology Resident, Glickman Urological and Kidney Institute, Cleveland Clinic, Cleveland, Ohio

GRETCHEN KIMMICK, MD
Department of Medicine, Duke Cancer Institute, Duke University School of Medicine, Durham, North Carolina

RACHIT KUMAR, MD
Department of Radiation Oncology and Molecular Radiation Sciences, The Sidney Kimmel Comprehensive Cancer Center, Johns Hopkins University School of Medicine, Baltimore, Maryland

ALEXANDER LANGERMAN, MD
Assistant Professor, Section of Otolaryngology – Head and Neck Surgery, Department of Surgery, The University of Chicago, Chicago, Illinois

MICHAEL J. LIPTAY, MD
Thoracic Oncology Program; Professor of Surgery, Chief, Division of Thoracic Surgery, Rush University Medical Center, Chicago, Illinois

GARY H. LYMAN, MD, MPH, FRCP(Edin)
Professor of Medicine and Director, Comparative Effectiveness and Outcomes Research Program, Department of Medicine, Duke Cancer Institute, Duke University School of Medicine, Durham, North Carolina

GREGORY A. MASTERS, MD
Medical Oncology Hematology Consultants, Helen F. Graham Cancer Center, Newark, Delaware; Associate Professor of Medicine, Thomas Jefferson University Medical School, Philadelphia, Pennsylvania

JAMAL G. MISLEH, MD
Department of Medical Oncology, Medical Oncology Hematology Consultants, Helen F. Graham Cancer Center, Christiana Care Hospital, Newark, Delaware

PRIYA MITRA, MD
Radiation Oncology, Albert Einstein Medical Center Philadelphia, Philadelphia, Pennsylvania

SABINE MUELLER, MD, PhD
Assistant Clinical Professor, Departments of Neurology, Pediatrics and Neurological Surgery, University of California, San Francisco, San Francisco, California

CHARLES R. MULLIGAN Jr, MD, FACS, FCCP
Thoracic Surgery, Helen F. Graham Cancer Center, Christiana Health Care System, Newark, Delaware; Medical Director, Thoracic Surgery and Thoracic Surgical Oncology, Centra Thoracic Surgery, Alan B. Pearson Regional Cancer Center, Centra Health, Lynchburg, Virginia

ANDREW T. PARSA, MD, PhD
Professor in Residence and Vice Chairman of Neurological Surgery, Department of Neurological Surgery, University of California, San Francisco, San Francisco, California

JEFFREY PEPPERCORN, MD
Department of Medicine, Duke Cancer Institute, Duke University School of Medicine, Durham, North Carolina

SCOTT PRUITT, MD
Department of Surgery, Duke Cancer Institute, Duke University School of Medicine, Durham, North Carolina

SONALI RUDRA, MD
Resident, Department of Radiation and Cellular Oncology, The University of Chicago, Chicago, Illinois

MARTIN J. RUTKOWSKI, MD
Resident, Department of Neurological Surgery, University of California, San Francisco, San Francisco, California

VASSILIKI SALOURA, MD
Fellow, Section of Hematology/Oncology, Department of Medicine, The University of Chicago, Chicago, Illinois

PETER SANTORO, MD
Department of Surgery, Helen F. Graham Cancer Center, Christiana Care Hospital, Newark, Delaware

ANTHONY SCARPACI, MD
Medical Oncology, Albert Einstein Medical Center Philadelphia, Philadelphia, Pennsylvania

RANDALL P. SCHERI, MD
Department of Surgery, Duke Cancer Institute, Duke University School of Medicine, Durham, North Carolina

DAVID D. SHERSHER, MD
Thoracic Oncology Program; Resident, Department of General Surgery, Rush University Medical Center, Chicago, Illinois

ANDREW J. STEPHENSON, MD
Director of Urologic Oncology, Glickman Urological and Kidney Institute, Cleveland Clinic, Cleveland, Ohio

JONATHON F. STRASSER, MD
Department of Radiation Oncology, Helen F. Graham Cancer Center, Christiana Care Hospital, Newark, Delaware

PAUL H. SUGARBAKER, MD, FACS, FRCS
Washington Cancer Institute, Washington Hospital Center, Washington, DC

RAHUL D. TENDULKAR, MD
Associate Staff, Taussig Cancer Center, Cleveland Clinic, Cleveland, Ohio

HENNING WILLERS, MD
Assistant Professor, Clark Center for Radiation Oncology, Department of Radiation Oncology, Massachusetts General Hospital Cancer Center, Boston, Massachusetts

CHRISTOPHER L. WOLFGANG, MD, PhD
Departments of Surgery, Oncology and Pathology, The Sol Goldman Pancreatic Cancer Center, The Skip Viragh Center for Pancreatic Cancer, The Sidney Kimmel Comprehensive Cancer Center, Johns Hopkins University School of Medicine, Baltimore, Maryland

LEI ZHENG, MD, PhD
Departments of Oncology and Surgery, The Sol Goldman Pancreatic Cancer Center, The Skip Viragh Center for Pancreatic Cancer, The Sidney Kimmel Comprehensive Cancer Center, Johns Hopkins University School of Medicine, Baltimore, Maryland

Contents

Foreword xi

Nicholas J. Petrelli

Preface: Multidisciplinary Care of the Cancer Patient xiii

Gregory A. Masters

Multidisciplinary Care of Patients with Brain Tumors 161

Tannie Huang, Sabine Mueller, Martin J. Rutkowski, Seunggu J. Han, Orin Bloch, Igor J. Barani, Andrew T. Parsa, and Susan M. Chang

Patients with brain tumors are some of the most complex patients in the medical system, necessitating treatment teams of multiple subspecialists for optimal care. This article examines the roles of these subspecialists, with the goal of summarizing standard-of-care practices, recent therapeutic advances, and ongoing clinical investigations within each subspecialty.

Multidisciplinary Care of the Patient with Head and Neck Cancer 179

Vassiliki Saloura, Alexander Langerman, Sonali Rudra, Robert Chin, and Ezra E.W. Cohen

Head and neck cancer is a heterogeneous group of cancers, which require a multidisciplinary approach to achieve excellent treatment results. This article focuses on current treatment guidelines and controversies in the management of head and neck cancer. It also provides insight into future directions and newest advances in the treatment of head and neck cancer.

Multidisciplinary Management of Esophageal Cancer 217

Charles R. Mulligan Jr

This article reviews the current management of esophageal cancer, including staging and treatment options, as well as providing support for using multidisciplinary teams to better manage esophageal cancer patients.

Multidisciplinary Management of Gastric Cancer 247

Jamal G. Misleh, Peter Santoro, Jonathon F. Strasser, and Joseph J. Bennett

Treatment of gastric cancer involves a multidisciplinary approach to achieve long-term outcome, including surgery, chemotherapy, and radiation therapy. Most patients present with advanced disease and are not candidates for a curative approach. Palliative chemotherapy is recommended for symptom control and for short-term advances in survival. Surgery combined with different chemotherapy and chemoradiation options improves survival. Initial studies focused on adjuvant chemoradiation and showed improved survival. More recent trials have demonstrated that perioperative chemotherapy before and after surgery provides a survival

advantage. Such an approach may also downstage marginal patients who can then be selected to undergo curative resection and complete adjuvant chemotherapy.

Multidisciplinary Management of Pancreatic Cancer 265

Rachit Kumar, Joseph M. Herman, Christopher L. Wolfgang, and Lei Zheng

Pancreatic cancer (pancreatic adenocarcinoma) remains one of the deadliest malignancies in the western hemisphere despite improved surgical technique, chemotherapy, and radiation therapy. The appropriate management of this malignancy should incorporate multiple treatment modalities for optimal opportunity for cure. Recent trials with a variety of treatment techniques confer improved survival of patients with pancreatic cancer, even in the metastatic setting. In this review, the importance of multidisciplinary management of pancreatic cancer based on disease stage is discussed.

Colorectal Cancer Metastases: A Surgical Perspective 289

Paul H. Sugarbaker

Metastases from colorectal cancer occur to the regional lymph nodes, the liver, the peritoneal surfaces, and lung. These metastases may occur synchronously or metachronously and the timing of the metastatic process is important in terms of treatment possibilities. Each anatomic site for metastatic disease has a unique management strategy. Systemic chemotherapy as an adequate management plan for all sites of colorectal metastatic disease is not compatible with a high standard of care. Formulation of an individualized plan combining surgery with regional chemotherapy and systemic chemotherapy is a necessary function of the multidisciplinary team.

Multidisciplinary Care of Patients with Early-Stage Breast Cancer 299

Gary H. Lyman, Jay Baker, Joseph Geradts, Janet Horton, Gretchen Kimmick, Jeffrey Peppercorn, Scott Pruitt, Randall P. Scheri, and E. Shelley Hwang

There is a compelling need for close coordination and integration of multiple specialties in the management of patients with early-stage breast cancer. Optimal patient care and outcomes depend on the sequential and often simultaneous participation and dialogue between specialists in imaging, pathologic and molecular diagnostic and prognostic stratification, and the therapeutic specialties of surgery, radiation oncology, and medical oncology. These are but a few of the various disciplines needed to provide modern, sophisticated management. The essential role for coordinated involvement of the entire health care team in optimal management of patients with early-stage breast cancer is likely to increase further.

Multimodality Approach to Management of Stage III Non–Small Cell Lung Cancer 319

Anthony Scarpaci, Priya Mitra, Doraid Jarrar, and Gregory A. Masters

Stage III non–small cell lung cancer represents a heterogeneous group of patients who are best managed with a multidisciplinary approach, including evaluation for surgical, radiation, and chemotherapeutic options.

Multidisciplinary Care of the Cancer Patient

SURGICAL ONCOLOGY CLINICS OF NORTH AMERICA

FORTHCOMING ISSUES

July 2013
Practical Radiation Oncology for Surgeons
Christopher G. Willett, MD, *Editor*

October 2013
Translational Cancer Research for Surgeons
William G. Cance, MD, *Editor*

January 2014
Colorectal Cancer
Nancy N. Baxter, MD and
Marcus Burnstein, MD, *Editors*

RECENT ISSUES

January 2013
Laparoscopic Approaches in Oncology
James Fleshman, MD, *Editor*

October 2012
Treatment of Peritoneal Surface Malignancies
Jesus Esquivel, MD, *Editor*

July 2012
Outcomes Research in Surgical Oncology
Clifford Y. Ko, MD, MS, MSHS, *Editor*

RELATED INTEREST

Hematology/Oncology Clinics of North America, December 2012 (Vol. 26, Issue 6)
Rare Cancers
Guy D. Eslick, MD, *Editor*
Available at: http://www.hemonc.theclinics.com/

Foreword

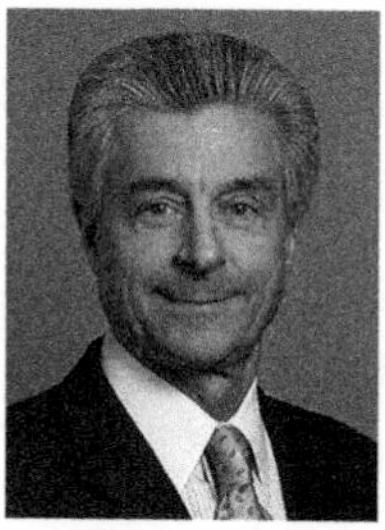

Nicholas J. Petrelli, MD, FACS
Consulting Editor

This issue of the *Surgical Oncology Clinics of North America* is entitled, "The Multidisciplinary Care of the Cancer Patient." Gregory Masters, MD, is the guest editor of this issue. Dr Masters is a medical oncology member of the Thoracic Multidisciplinary Center at the Helen F. Graham Cancer Center in Newark, Delaware. He is an Associate Professor in the Department of Medicine at Thomas Jefferson University. Dr Masters was recruited to the Helen F. Graham Cancer Center in 2003 from Northwestern University. His area of expertise is in the treatment of lung and esophageal cancer.

High-quality cancer care is extremely complex and involves coordination among multiple treatments and providers inclusive of information technology support and regular detailed communication flow between all of the multidisciplinary team members. Advances in surgical techniques, chemotherapy, targeted therapies, and radiation technology have all led to an increase in multimodality treatment, which increases the number of interfaces involving cancer specialists and subspecialists in the treatment of the cancer patient. Failure of communication between various physician specialists and care providers can lead to a delay in treatment planning, unnecessary duplication of tests, decreased patient satisfaction, and a decrease in the patient's quality of life.

Dr Masters has used his expertise to complete an outstanding edition of the *Surgical Oncology Clinics of North America*. Individual tumor sites, such as non–small-cell lung cancer and gastric cancer among others, are described in detail in the approach to the multidisciplinary care in patients who present with these and other cancers.

I thank Dr Masters and his colleagues for taking the time and effort to complete this edition of *Surgical Oncology Clinics of North America*. The topic of the multidisciplinary

Surg Oncol Clin N Am 22 (2013) xi–xii
http://dx.doi.org/10.1016/j.soc.2012.12.009
1055-3207/13/$ – see front matter

care of the cancer patient is timely in view of the fact that our Country is on the verge of health care reform.

Nicholas J. Petrelli, MD, FACS
Helen F. Graham Cancer Center at Christiana Care
4701 Ogletown-Stanton Road
Newark, DE 19713, USA

E-mail address:
npetrelli@christianacare.org

Preface

Multidisciplinary Care of the Cancer Patient

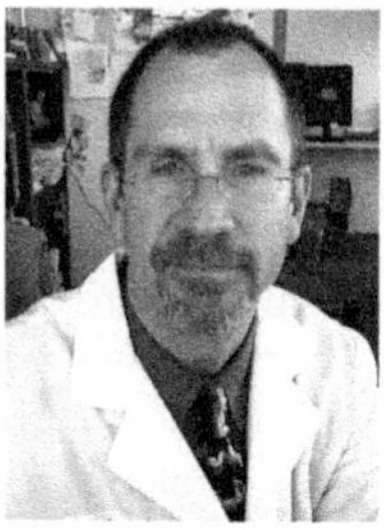

Gregory A. Masters, MD
Editor

I am excited to help bring you this most recent addition of the *Surgical Oncology Clinics of North America*, focusing on the multidisciplinary treatment of cancer patients. Ongoing clinical research demonstrates the value of a team approach to complicated cancers, especially in this age of increasing technical complexity of surgical procedures, radiation oncologic techniques, and systemic therapy, including new biologically targeted agents.

We have put together a table of contents focusing on multiple different cancer subtypes and have asked the authors to focus on the multidisciplinary approach to these patients, including ways that systemic therapy and regional radiation can be integrated with new and improved surgical techniques to offer patients the best chance for tumor control and palliation.

In these articles you will read about aggressive approaches to patients with localized disease, regionally advanced cancers, and even patients with metastatic disease who may benefit from a multimodality approach to therapy. This is an exciting time for clinicians caring for cancer patients, given the increasing armamentarium available for combating this disease. I hope this text provides you additional insight into the many ways that clinical care is advancing through clinical research. I also hope this will stimulate further enrollment of cancer patients into clinical trials investigating these new techniques.

Surg Oncol Clin N Am 22 (2013) xiii–xiv
http://dx.doi.org/10.1016/j.soc.2012.12.010
1055-3207/13/$ – see front matter © 2013 Published by Elsevier Inc.

I thank the authors and coauthors for their insight, diligence, and hard work in putting together these articles.

Gregory A. Masters, MD
Helen F. Graham Cancer Center
4701 Ogletown-Stanton Road, Suite 3400
Newark, DE 19713, USA

E-mail address:
gmasters@cbg.org

Multidisciplinary Care of Patients with Brain Tumors

Tannie Huang, MD[a], Sabine Mueller, MD, PhD[b,c,d],
Martin J. Rutkowski, MD[d], Seunggu J. Han, MD[d], Orin Bloch, MD[d],
Igor J. Barani, MD[e], Andrew T. Parsa, MD, PhD[d],
Susan M. Chang, MD[d,*]

KEYWORDS

- Multidisciplinary • Brain tumors • Neurosurgery • Radiation therapy
- Neuro-oncology • Endocrine • Psychiatry • Palliative care • Rehabilitation medicine

KEY POINTS

- Patients with brain tumors have complex medical problems that require multidisciplinary subspecialty care.
- Symptoms will vary based on tumor histology and location, necessitating individualized treatment plans.
- Medical issues can arise from the brain tumor itself or the treatment plan.

INTRODUCTION

Despite only representing about 2% of all cancer diagnoses, patients with primary brain tumors are some of the most complex patients in the medical system. Medical personnel from different disciplines, including physicians, nurses, rehabilitation therapists, family counselors, and social workers, all contribute to the care of patients with brain tumors. This clinic focuses on the roles of different physician subspecialists in the care of these patients, with the goal of summarizing standard-of-care practices, recent therapeutic advances, and ongoing clinical investigations within each subspecialty. Each patient requires an individualized treatment plan developed by a team of

---

Disclosures: Dr Barani would like to disclose that he receives research funding from BrainLab AG. The other authors have no conflicts to disclose.

[a] Division of Hematology Oncology, Department of Pediatrics, University of California, San Francisco, 505 Parnassus Avenue M649, San Francisco, CA 94143, USA; [b] Department of Neurology, University of California, San Francisco, 505 Parnassus Avenue Box 0106, San Francisco, CA 94143, USA; [c] Department of Pediatrics, University of California, San Francisco, 505 Parnassus Avenue, San Francisco, CA 94143, USA; [d] Department of Neurological Surgery, University of California, San Francisco, 505 Parnassus Avenue, San Francisco, CA 94143, USA; [e] Department of Radiation Oncology, University of California, San Francisco, 505 Parnassus Avenue, Room L-08, San Francisco, CA 94143, USA
* Corresponding author.
E-mail address: ChangS@neurosurg.ucsf.edu

Surg Oncol Clin N Am 22 (2013) 161–178
http://dx.doi.org/10.1016/j.soc.2012.12.011 surgonc.theclinics.com
1055-3207/13/$ – see front matter

these physicians in consultation with the patient, with different subspecialties playing a larger role at different points during treatment.

THE ROLE OF THE NEUROSURGEON

The identification and resection of brain tumors is often the first intervention in the treatment of patients with both benign and malignant lesions. Interval monitoring, radiation-based treatments, and chemotherapy all offer promise in the treatment of certain subpopulations of patients; but for those suffering from a high burden of disease, a mass effect from tumor expansion, the need for definitive pathologic diagnosis, or for those with intolerable presenting symptoms, surgery is a critical first-line intervention.

Preoperative Assessment

Proper neurosurgical preoperative assessment takes into consideration both patient anatomy and overall health. Assuming a patient is healthy enough to undergo an operation, the neurosurgeon must create an operative plan that takes into consideration a tumor's intrinsic anatomy; proximity to adjacent vital structures, such as cranial nerves, vessels, and motor and sensory areas; and the surgical approach with the greatest likelihood of maximizing the extent of resection and minimizing operative morbidities.

It is also important to acknowledge that goals of care may vary depending on the benign versus malignant nature of a tumor. For example, subtotal resection of a vestibular schwannoma may be enough to preserve hearing without compromising adjacent cranial nerves, such as the facial nerve, whereas the greater extent of resection for glioblastoma multiforme (GBM) has a significant effect on the length of survival. As opposed to high-grade tumors, in which the extent of resection becomes the most important predictor of survival, the treatment of benign tumors should be based on the amelioration of symptoms and comorbidities. In conjunction with other members of the treatment team, meaningful postoperative quality of life, prognosis, and the likelihood of morbidity should all be discussed at length with patients before any surgical intervention.

Biopsy and Resection

Because of the highly precise nature of tumor resection, the use of the operating microscope has greatly improved the ability of neurosurgeons to obtain more complete resections without compromising healthy brain structures. Additionally, the concomitant usage of neuro-navigation techniques, such as StealthStation (Medtronic, Minneapolis, MN) and VectorVision (Brainlab, Feldkirchen, Germany), allows for real-time correlation of intraoperative findings with magnetic resonance imaging (MRI), further facilitating resection of tumor tissues without extension beyond tumor margins.

Recently, evidence has shown a possible role for adjuvant measures that enhance the ability of neurosurgeons to obtain more extensive resection: intraoperative MRI and dyes that highlight neoplastic tissues for removal. In a randomized clinical trial, the use of intraoperative MRI led to higher rates of complete tumor resection without increasing the rate of operative neurologic complications,[1] which is a finding that match those reported in prior nonrandomized trials.[2] In a prospective, randomized controlled trial of patients assigned 5-aminolevulinic acid, a prodrug that leads to fluorescent accumulation in GBM tissues, the use of this dye led to more complete resections, in turn resulting in longer progression-free survival.[3] Both of these findings make it clear that techniques to enhance the neurosurgeon's ability to more completely resect GBM allows for better patient outcomes.

A subset of patients presents with tumors arising from or involving eloquent brain areas, including language centers, such as the Broca and Wernicke areas, the motor strip, and the sensory strip. The development of cortical mapping techniques, performed with both awake and asleep patients, has allowed for safer resection of such tumors that were previously deemed untreatable.

Practice with such techniques has allowed for better understanding of the inherent interpatient variability seen in language localization; consequently, smaller craniotomies can be performed with negative mapping strategies in which the cortex overlying tumors can be safely removed when it is shown that local depolarizing stimulation does not cause a loss of language ability.[4] Resecting at least 1 cm away from stimulation-established language sites is safest[5]; in a large series of patients who underwent dominant hemisphere tumor resection with language mapping, less than 2% of patients suffered language deficits at 6 months, demonstrating the utility of such mapping techniques in avoiding postoperative deficits.[6] Subcortical mapping and diffusion tensor imaging–based tractography have additional utility in mapping motor pathways,[4,7] whereas techniques, such as functional MRI, positron emission tomography scanning, and magnetoencephalography, remain too imprecise at present to have major surgical utility.[8,9]

Postoperative Complications

As a highly invasive intervention, neurosurgery for resection of brain tumors carries several important complications and risks, including infection, hematomas, hydrocephalus, pseudomeningocele, posterior fossa syndrome (mutism, emotional lability, difficulties initiating movement), and other focal neurologic deficits. Much of the complication profile following the resection of brain tumors arises from approach selection, tumor size, and operator skill.

Despite anecdotal reports that postoperative infection may, in fact, prolong survival, presumably because of the presence of local inflammation with antitumor effects, this remains controversial.[10,11] Hemostasis remains an important intraoperative goal to reduce the onset of hematomas, whereas cerebrospinal fluid–related complications, such as hydrocephalus and pseudomeningocele, remain rare complications.[5,12] Focal neurologic deficits can largely be avoided through the use of intraoperative mapping and a reluctance to resect tumor from vital adjacent structures, such as vessels and nerves.

Second Look Surgery

The use of second look surgery to rule out residual disease is not typically performed in the postoperative management of brain tumors. The close relationship between neurosurgeons, neuro-oncologists, and radiation oncologists typically ensures the close follow-up of patients, with interval scans being performed to document the absence or presence of either tumor recurrence or progression, which can necessitate repeat craniotomy for resection in select cases.

THE ROLE OF THE RADIATION ONCOLOGIST

Radiation therapy (RT) is an integral and a highly effective component in the multidisciplinary management of patients with brain tumors.[13] RT plans are designed and their implementation overseen by specially trained physicians, radiation oncologists. RT is a procedure whose outcome (balance between treatment benefits and side effects) depends on the skill of the treating physician. Because of this and because RT plans are specific to a treatment device, radiation treatment often cannot be easily transferred from one facility to another. This point is important for patients to understand before embarking on a treatment course so that treatment breaks and/or delays are avoided.

The choice of RT modality is determined by details of the clinical scenario, including patient factors (eg, performance status, severity of symptoms), tumor type and extent, tumor location in the brain (eg, proximity to eloquent brain areas or critical normal structures), and prior treatment history. RT comes in different forms, broadly divided into external and internal RT.

External Beam RT

External beam RT (EBRT), also known as teletherapy by its older name, is the most common form of RT. During EBRT, the patient is positioned on a flat table and immobilized in a treatment position using a thermoplastic mask to minimize movement during treatment. X rays are produced by a medical linear accelerator (linac) that can rotate and, in conjunction with the movable treatment table, can generate multiple beams that are projected at the tumor target from outside the patient. In general, multiple beams are used to treat a tumor target so that no one beam delivers all (or most) of the intended radiation; it is at the intersection of the beams where the intended radiation dose accumulates.

To calculate and control the distribution of the radiation dose, patients must complete a computed tomography (CT) simulation scan, a scan of patients in the simulated treatment position. A CT scan gives radiation oncologists information about the relative density of tissues within the patients' body and, when imported into an RT planning computer, permits accurate calculation of radiation dose distribution, a process called planning. This form of EBRT, when coupled with the ability to mimic or conform to the tumor (target) shape, is called 3-dimensional conformal RT. A more sophisticated variant of this treatment technique, intensity-modulated RT (IMRT), can also vary or modulate the intensity of each beam and deliver doses that match complex tumor shapes. Furthermore, most modern linacs are equipped with a wide array of on-board imaging tools that permit real-time or near real-time monitoring of patient setup and/or tumor (or organ) motion. When these imaging techniques are used in conjunction with IMRT delivery, terms such as *image-guided* radiotherapy or *image-guided adaptive* radiotherapy can be used to describe them.

Most EBRT treatment courses extend over several weeks and allow radiation oncologists to treat tumors that often involve or invade critical brain structures (eg, anterior optic pathways) without injuring them. This selective injury of tumor and relative preservation of normal brain structures can be achieved by delivering small doses of radiation daily (5 days per week) for several weeks until the cumulative dose known to be effective for a particular tumor type is reached. The basis of fractionation is the concept that a daily dose is insufficient to cause lethal injury in cells with intact DNA damage repair mechanisms (normal cells) but adequate to cause tumor cell death where the intracellular repair machinery is aberrant. For these reasons, fractionated EBRT is considered to be a form of nonablative therapy.

Stereotactic Radiosurgery

Stereotactic radiosurgery (SRS) is a highly precise form of RT with an application that is limited to select cases when target obliteration is desired. Unlike EBRT, radiosurgery treatments are delivered with submillimeter accuracy to high doses given over 1 to 5 days. Because high doses of radiation are delivered, a high level of precision and accuracy is mandated. This level is achieved by the application of a rigid immobilization device, like a head frame, or by using robotics to automatically adjust for any deviations in the patient's position that are seen on imaging. Both of these approaches rely on the use of a stereotactic coordinate system that is referenced to the immobilization device and/or treatment couch. For example, Gamma Knife (Elekta, Stockholm, Sweden) uses a rigid frame that is attached to the patient's skull for immobilization and localization, whereas the CyberKnife (Accuray, Sunnyvale, California) and Novalis (Varian Medical Systems Inc, Palo Alto, CA and Brainlab, Feldkirchen, Germany) (a modified radiosurgical linac) rely on the use of more rigid thermoplastic masks and imaging to adjust for deviations in the patient's position. Furthermore, SRS techniques use many beamlets, each of which does not transport much energy, that converge on the target. With this approach, the dose within the tumor is much higher than the dose in the surrounding normal brain tissue as a result of a sharp dose gradient (dose falloff) achieved by the multiple intersecting beams of radiation. Because the normal tissue interface is larger and the dose falloff is less rapid for larger lesions, increasing the exposure of the surrounding normal brain tissue, the prescribed dose is inversely proportional to the maximum tumor diameter. This physical phenomenon largely limits the application of SRS to lesions 3 cm or less in diameter.

SRS applications are generally limited to small tumor targets where obliterative, high doses can be delivered safely. The most common applications are brain metastases, benign brain tumors (eg, meningiomas, schwannomas), and select cases of recurrent malignant tumors.

Brachytherapy

Brachytherapy is a form of internal RT whereby the source of radiation is either permanently or temporarily implanted into tumor-bearing tissue. Depending on the application, different radioisotopes can be used. Most commonly, iodine-125 seeds are used for brain applications[14,15]; but increasingly, phosphorous-32–impregnated polymer film and other formulations are being used.[16] The primary rationale for brachytherapy is that it can deliver highly localized radiation over the effective life of the radioisotope to a well-defined target, thereby preserving the surrounding normal tissue from dose. Brachytherapy applications in the brain are generally limited to cases of recurrent tumors,[17,18] although different applications are actively being explored.[17]

Radiation Sensitizers

Radiation sensitizers are drugs that enhance the sensitivity of tumor cells to radiation. Many compounds demonstrated promise in preclinical studies and have also been tested in humans with disappointing results. Halogenated pyrimidines and the nitroimidazoles have been most extensively studies; but more recently, hypoxic cell sensitizers, such as tirapazamine[19] and RSR-13 (2-[4-[[(3,5-dimethylanilino)carbonyl]methyl]phenoxyl]-2-methylpropionic acid),[20] have been evaluated. Other interesting compounds include motexafin gadolinium,[21–23] which is a synthetic porphyrinlike agent that is thought to alter redox state of tumor cells. Topoisomerase inhibitors are another class of drugs that have both direct antitumor activity but additionally prevent DNA repair of radiation-induced DNA lesions.[24] Other agents are actively being investigated.

Side Effects of RT

RT effects are concentrated on the tumor and surrounding involved tissue. For this reason, side effects of RT are primarily focal and dependent on the brain location being treated and often cannot be reliably distinguished from the effects of the tumor. The impact of treatment location, dose, target volume, and technique on the expected side-effect profile must always be considered when attempting to extrapolate one patient's experience to another.

Acute side effects of EBRT include common effects (occurring in >50% of patients), such as partial alopecia, fatigue, scalp erythema, and less common effects (occurring in <20% of patients), such as otitis externa, impaired sense of taste, nausea, and headache. Early delayed and late side effects of RT may include tanning of the scalp, alopecia, hearing loss, neurocognitive decline, behavioral changes, somnolence syndrome, cataracts, and radiation necrosis. Neurocognitive effects of RT are a well-recognized phenomena; however, much of the available literature with few notable exceptions[25,26] relies on the use of a Mini-Mental State Examination that is a poor outcome measure.[27] Radiation Therapy Oncology Group and other groups have developed a brief, sensitive, repeatable, and highly standardized test battery to assess neurocognitive function.[28–30] These tests have been shown to be sensitive to the impact of tumors and the neurotoxic effects of therapy.

Acute side effects from SRS include common complications, such as pin-site soreness and headache after frame removal in the case of Gamma Knife, as well as less frequent complications (occurring in <5% of patients), such as pin-site infection, short-term exacerbation of neurologic symptoms, and seizures. Later side effects, either early delayed or late, are uncommon (<5%–10% of patients) and include brain edema, radiation necrosis, and the worsening of preexisting neurologic deficits or the development of new ones.

It is important to again note that all forms of RT are procedures and, therefore, highly dependent on the design and implementation of the treatment plan by the treating radiation oncologist and his or her team. For these reasons, side-effect profiles can vary considerably.

THE ROLE OF THE NEURO-ONCOLOGIST

The role of the neuro-oncologist varies between patients with different histology. In addition, the physician-patient relationship can change over the course of treatment. For example, the natural history of low-grade gliomas is often characterized by an initial period of slow growth. During this time, patients undergo surveillance imaging and may intermittently take chemotherapy that maintains quality of life. At some point, however, these low-grade gliomas undergo malignant transformation and begin a period of rapid growth. Chemotherapy may become more intense, and patients may have more frequent office visits and hospitalizations with complications from these treatments. Death can occur many years after the initial diagnosis; by this time, patients have undergone multiple therapies.

Chemotherapy

Ultimately, treatment plans are individualized to the patient and differ based on tumor histology, location, and goals of care. For many tumors, chemotherapy is primarily given as adjuvant therapy to surgery and radiation. An exception is germinomas, which are highly chemosensitive and the outcome is not improved by surgical resection. Chemotherapy can also provide the primary means of disease control in some patients whose tumors are unresectable and radiation is not an option. In patients with optic pathway gliomas, low-dose metronomic chemotherapy can be used to delay radiation and the resulting endocrinopathies. In patients less than 3 years of age, neuro-oncologists often use chemotherapy to avoid radiation at such a young age because of the known neurocognitive sequelae. In adults, high-dose chemotherapy followed by stem cell transplant has generally not been shown to be effective and is not well tolerated.

Not all tumors respond to chemotherapy. Controversy exists about the role of the blood-brain barrier in chemotherapy delivery in patients with brain tumors. Brain tumors interrupt the blood-brain barrier, and chemotherapy delivery can be inconsistent. Yet many chemotherapy agents do cross the blood-brain barrier, such as nitrosoureas, platinum agents, and procarbazine. Intraventricular and intrathecal chemotherapy has been tried with mixed results. Chemotherapy-impregnated wafers, such as lomustine wafers, are directly implanted into the resection bed and used for adult patients with malignant gliomas.

Regardless of its delivery, traditional chemotherapy agents are not just toxic to tumor cells but also affect healthy tissue. Although patients are primarily concerned about hair loss, nausea, and fatigue, physicians manage many other side effects. This management can be challenging in patients with brain tumors because some of the chemotherapy agents can cause neurologic symptoms that may otherwise be mistaken for tumor progression. For example, vincristine can cause neuropathic pain and foot drop leading to gait abnormalities or other neuropathies that can present as weakness. Vincristine, carboplatin, and cisplatin can cause syndrome of inappropriate antidiuretic hormone, leading to hyponatremia and seizures. Because patients with brain tumors have a lower seizure threshold, they may have seizures with even mild hyponatremia. Knowledge about these side effects and appropriate monitoring is necessary.

Novel Therapies

The forefront of cancer therapy is the development of targeted therapies against cancer cells with the goal to increase efficacy with fewer side effects. The field is rapidly changing, and the following sections are intended as an introduction to some of these therapies in various stages of development.

The rapid rate of tumor proliferation requires the tumor to form new blood vessels to bring in the necessary nutrients for growth. The development of bevacizumab, a monoclonal antibody that inhibited vascular endothelial growth factor (VEGF), was the first antiangiogenic agent. It is generally well tolerated but has been associated with an increased risk of bleeding. A significant portion of patients with glioblastoma have a 3- to 6-month survival advantage with this treatment. Unfortunately, patients will inevitably progress and relapse. Bevacizumab is now a mainstay in glioblastoma therapy, and current studies are now evaluating the efficacy of bevacizumab in combination with other agents to try to prolong survival.

Although bevacizumab attacks a ligand likely to be important in multiple tumor types as well as some healthy tissues, more targeted therapy would be desirable. Drug development is now focused on drugs that work against specific mutations in particular tumor types or subtypes. Small molecule inhibitors targeting the sonic hedgehog pathway, a signaling pathway important in cell growth in a specific subset of medulloblastomas, are now entering the clinic. One of the first published cases using such an inhibitor reported on a remarkable tumor regression in a patient with metastatic medulloblastoma; however, the tumor eventually returned because of an additional mutation that developed in the tumor cells.[31] Ongoing trials are currently testing if combination strategies with multiple agents can prevent the development of resistance and achieve sustained responses.

Despite significant advances in our understanding of the underlying molecular pathways leading to brain tumors, many patients with brain tumors will eventually progress through standard therapies and must decide if they would like to participate in clinical trials with investigational agents. Oncologists can inform patients about different trial options and consent them to study or refer them to an academic center with an open trial. However, patients who choose to participate must understand that there is limited knowledge about the efficacy and toxicity of many agents, particularly those still in early phase I trials. Furthermore, not all patients who desire to participate will be eligible. Clinical trials typically require a minimum performance score, and many trials exclude patients older than 70 years. Participation in clinical trials also varies by age, with a larger proportion of pediatric patients with brain tumors participating in at least one clinical trial during their treatment course. In a large survey of adults with malignant glioma, only 15% participated in a clinical trial.[32] Part of this may be because of increasing cognitive decline that occurs with tumor progression, making study consent challenging.

Palliative Care

With the poor prognosis of brain tumors, many times all therapeutic options are exhausted, even investigational agents. Although palliative care specialization is growing in the United States, currently many neuro-oncologists and primary care physicians are often the main directors of palliative care for their patients. End-of-life and goals-of-care discussions should be started early in patients with brain tumors with grim prognoses before tumors may have progressed to the point that the patients can no longer express their wishes. A Dutch study found that approximately half of the patients with brain tumors were not deemed competent to participate in end-of-life decisions in the last weeks of life.[33] However, the assessment of competence may be challenging. A study in patients with a recent diagnosis of malignant glioma (<6 months) found that more than 50% of patients already had markedly diminished understanding and reasoning of medical choices, although they were still able to express a treatment choice as well as controls.[34]

Overall, palliative care of patients with brain tumors focuses on symptom relief. Pain control is often the top concern for patients and their families. Patients with brain tumors often have headaches, which can be managed with nonsteroidals and opioids. Neuropathic pain can be managed with gabapentin. Corticosteroids can reduce edema around the tumor and allow further symptom relief.

Other than pain, dysphagia is the most prevalent symptom with tumor progression, and the most common end-of-life decisions concern withholding hydration.[35] Medications also have to be changed to rapidly dissolving sublingual forms or changed to transdermal or intravenous formulations.

It is important to note that family members and caregivers often have to deal with a rapidly changing neurocognitive status. Increasing neurologic impairment and dependency may increase mood fluctuations, adding further stress. Psychotherapy and support groups may be helpful in these situations.

THE ROLE OF THE ENDOCRINOLOGIST

Endocrine dysfunction is a frequent problem in patients with brain tumors either from the tumor itself or from treatment side effects. The incidence varies based on the tumor location. Patients with hypothalamic or pituitary tumors, craniopharyngiomas, optic pathway gliomas, and pineal tumors are more likely to have endocrinopathies on presentation. However, baseline screening for endocrinopathies should be done on all patients with brain tumors. One study showed that the pretreatment incidence of endocrinopathies in pediatric patients with brain tumors was already greater than 60%.[36] Many tumors were located away from the hypothalamic-pituitary axis; in this subset of patients, thyroid and corticotropin abnormalities predominated with an unclear biologic basis.

Even patients who present without endocrinopathies are at risk for developing it from side effects related to treatment. Operative interventions can lead to damage in surrounding tissues, but effects are often seen in distant areas of the brain. In a series following postsurgical patients who had neurosurgery for benign tumors away from hypothalamic-pituitary axis, De Marinis and colleagues[37] found that more than 40% developed some form of hypopituitarism. It is well known that the hypothalamus and pituitary gland are sensitive to radiation, even at lower doses, leading to postradiation endocrinopathies. These effects can take years to develop, so long-term endocrine surveillance is necessary.[38,39]

Other treatment-related toxicity can also develop from medications. Steroid-induced obesity and adrenal dysfunction is common. The syndrome of inappropriate antidiuretic hormone is a known side effect of vincristine, cisplatin, and carboplatin, all chemotherapeutic agents used in the treatment of brain tumors. Younger female patients may have premature ovarian failure and have difficulties with fertility following chemotherapy, both with traditional cytotoxic chemotherapy as well as with newer targeted agents like bevacizumab. A close relationship between oncologists and endocrinologists should be maintained.

This relationship is particularly important in deciding the timing of growth hormone replacement, which is controversial and varies with institution. Although multiple studies show that growth hormone replacement does not increase the risk of tumor recurrence,[40–42] at least one study showed an increased risk for secondary neoplasms.[43] However, the low number of patients in these studies makes the true risk difficult to assess. On the other hand, growth hormone deficiency does have long-term consequences, particularly in children, whereby untreated growth hormone deficiency is associated with an increased risk for metabolic syndrome and cardiovascular events in adulthood. Even in adults, growth hormone deficiency can cause cognitive decline, further worsening the functional abilities of patients with brain tumors. Growth hormone replacement improved subjective quality-of-life scores in patients with brain tumors with growth hormone deficiency.[44] Ultimately, endocrinologists and oncologists working in conjunction must balance whether replacement therapy is best for an individual patient.

As therapies for brain tumors improve and the population of long-term survivors increases, endocrinologists will play increasing roles in managing the sequelae of these treatment modalities. This increased role is particularly true in the treatment of pediatric brain tumors, whereby growth and development can be severely affected by the treatment, especially RT, and survivors live for many more years. For patients of any age, weight and lifestyle issues are a critical component of primary care management because long-term survivors are at an increased risk for cardiovascular disease[45] and obesity.[46] Patients with hypothalamic obesity, whereby damage to the hypothalamus either from the tumor or its treatment leads to severe weight gain and hyperinsulinemia in response to glucose, may respond to a somatostatin-agonist, octreotide.[47] Osteopenia from endocrinopathies and prolonged glucocorticoid exposure can lead to chronic pain, early fractures, and joint replacements.[48] For a more extensive list of the late effects of brain tumor treatment, please see **Table 1**.

THE ROLE OF THE NEUROLOGIST

Multidisciplinary teams caring for patients with brain tumors should include a neurologist to deal with the frequent neurologic complications seen in patients with brain tumors. Although neurologists will participate in many aspects of patient care, this section addresses the management of seizures and strokes, which are 2 common problems requiring emergent care.

Table 1
Late effects of brain tumor therapy by organ system (partial list)

Organ	Late Effect
CNS	Secondary malignancy Cataracts Cognitive impairment Peripheral neuropathy Sensorineural hearing loss Leukoencephalopathy Stroke Seizures
Endocrine	Growth hormone deficiency Hypothyroidism or hyperthyroidism Syndrome of inappropriate diuretic hormone Diabetes insipidus Precocious or delayed puberty
Cardiovascular	Dyslipidemia Coronary artery disease Heart failure
Orthopedic	Osteoporosis, osteonecrosis Scoliosis
Renal	Hematuria, renal dysfunction, Fanconi syndrome
Gastrointestinal	Hepatitis and cirrhosis Fibrosis leading to obstruction Obesity
Pulmonary	Fibrosis
Hematologic	Secondary leukemia Thrombosis
Gynecologic	Infertility Premature ovarian failure Low testosterone

Abbreviation: CNS, central nervous system.

Seizures

Depending on the location, between 20% and 40% of patients with brain tumors will present with seizures; the management of seizures can be challenging in these patients. Not surprisingly, gross total resection of the primary tumor was associated with seizure-freedom in multiple studies.[49] Patients who continue to have seizures after surgery will need long-term seizure management with antiepileptic drugs (AEDs). Unfortunately, subtherapeutic levels of AEDs are frequent in this patient population. Side effects are also more common in patients with brain tumors than in others taking AEDs, causing almost a quarter of patients to change medications.[50] Optimal seizure management needs to take these factors into account, as well as considering interactions with chemotherapy both in changing metabolism as well as potentiating the hematologic toxicities.

No single AED has been shown to be more effective than others in the treatment of seizures in patients with brain tumors.[51] However, one recent retrospective analysis showed improved survival rate in patients with glioblastoma multiforme taking temozolamide and valproic acid over other AEDs or no AEDs.[52] The biologic basis for this, if true, may be caused by changes in the bioavailability of temozolamide. Further, valproic acid is also known to act as a histone deacetylase inhibitor (HDACi). HDACis have been shown to have an anticancer property, especially in combination with other DNA-damaging agents, such as radiation. Further studies are needed to validate this finding.

Even those without seizures at presentation remain at a high seizure risk during their treatment course. However, seizure prophylaxis is not effective and is generally not recommended.[53,54] A meta-analysis of several studies looking at AED prophylaxis after craniotomy did not find a significant decrease in postsurgical seizures.[55] A survey investigating practice patterns in the management of malignant gliomas found that, despite this evidence and practice guidelines recommending against AED prophylaxis, 89% of patients were still treated with AEDs, despite only 32% presenting with seizures.[32]

Strokes

In contrast to seizures, strokes in patients with brain tumors are often undertreated and not recognized in a timely fashion. Patients with brain tumors are at a high risk of stroke for a variety of reasons. Their neurologic impairments may cause them to be less mobile, increasing the risk of thrombosis. Vessel walls can be compressed by tumor progression or disrupted from tumor invasion. In addition, RT and certain chemotherapies have been associated with an increased risk of stroke. For example, antiangiogenic chemotherapy, like the frequently used VEGF-inhibitor bevacizumab, increase the risk of ischemic stroke and intracranial hemorrhage.[56] Further, there is increasing recognition of radiation-induced vasculopathies and its long-term effects on the heightened stroke risk in patients with brain tumors (**Fig. 1**). The Childhood Cancer Survivor study has shown that pediatric brain tumor survivors have a significantly elevated stroke risk compared with a randomly selected sibling control group.[57,58] The increased atherosclerosis and dyslipidemia also seen in long-term cancer survivors may also play a role in the elevated stroke risk. However, because

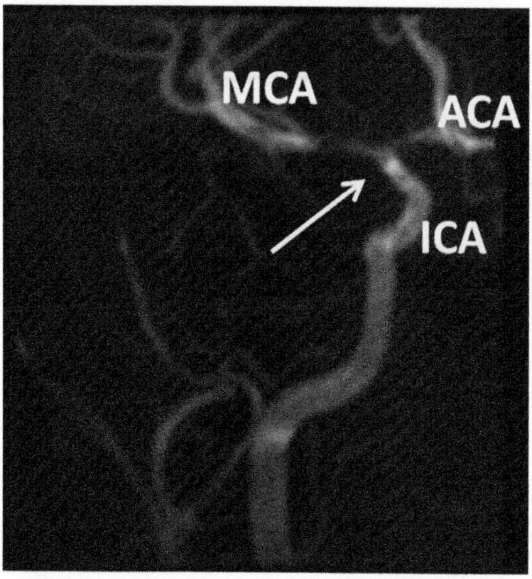

Fig. 1. Magnetic resonance angiogram of a child with ependymoma showing radiation-induced vasculopathy within 2 years after RT. Images shown here are dedicated views of right distal internal carotid artery. Arrow points to right ICA, proximal MCA, and ACA stenosis. Vascular imaging before RT was normal. ACA, anterior cerebral artery; ICA, internal carotid artery; MCA, middle cerebral artery.

patients frequently have other neurologic deficits, signs of stroke are commonly overlooked. In one single-institution series of 66 patients, stroke was the initial clinical diagnosis in only 43%.[59] The diagnosis was discovered only after imaging was obtained. Often the workup for the cause of the stroke in these patients is incomplete, especially if the prognosis of the primary brain tumor is grim. Secondary stroke prevention may not be in keeping with the goals of care. A neurologist who has been involved in the care of patients since their diagnosis can help patients navigate these decisions.

THE ROLE OF THE PSYCHIATRIST

Psychiatric changes are common in patients with brain tumors, both at presentation and subsequent treatment. The full range of psychiatric symptoms has been described in the initial presentation of brain tumors, including depression, mania, auditory and visual hallucinations, anxiety, and amnesia. Often subtle behavioral changes predate the neurologic symptoms that eventually led patients to seek medical care; for example, patients with dorsolateral lesions may have problems with organizational difficulties weeks to months before their diagnosis (**Table 2**).

Even patients without presenting psychiatric history are at a high risk for developing symptoms after diagnosis. New symptoms can arise from tumor progression or from the treatment itself. Many common preoperative and postoperative medications can cause mood disturbances; the most well known of these medications are the glucocorticoids, but many other medications, like certain antibiotics, antiepileptic agents, and isotretinoin, have also been implicated. Antiepileptic agents can also decrease the bioavailability of psychiatric medications. In contrast to other treatments, radiation-induced depressive symptoms are relatively rare. However, radiation-induced somnolence syndrome can mimic or mask some of the symptoms of depression. Psychiatric symptoms may be exacerbated by poor sleep-wake cycles in the hospital and diagnosis- or procedure-related anxiety.

Understandably, the poor prognosis of many brain tumors will often lead to emotional reactions from patients, leading to adjustment disorder or major depressive disorders. One study found that 93% of patients with a high-grade glioma had

Table 2
Range of neurologic symptoms in patients with brain tumors[a] (partial list)

Symptom	Percentage
Headache	56.0
Memory loss	35.5
Cognitive changes	34.4
Motor deficits	33.0
Language deficits	32.5
Seizure	31.9
Personality change	23.1
Visual problems	21.6
Changes in consciousness	16.2
Sensory defects	12.6

[a] Percentages derived from a survey of patients with malignant glioma, the most common form of brain tumor in adults, and do not include all reported symptoms.

Data from Chang S, Parney IF, Huang W, et al. Patterns of care for adults with newly diagnosed malignant glioma. JAMA 2005;293(5):557–64.

symptoms consistent with depression in the first 6 months after surgery. These depressive symptoms are often missed; physicians reported only a 15% rate of depression in the same group of patients, and then only some of these patients were treated with antidepressants.[60]

Depression is an important predictor of outcome. In certain diagnoses, studies have shown that depression is associated with decreased survival.[61–63] Depression has also been associated with an increased postoperative complication rate.[60]

Given the difficulty in recognizing depressive symptoms in postoperative patients, particularly those with poor neurologic examinations, early neurocognitive testing and involvement of a psychiatric consult service is recommended. Continued involvement beyond the initial hospitalization is important. Multiple studies have shown that long-term survivors of brain tumors have a decreased quality of life and more frequent depressive episodes. A Danish study found that of all patients with cancer, males with brain tumors were at the highest risk for psychiatric hospitalization in the year after their diagnosis.[64]

Because patients' signs and symptoms, tumor location, treatment modality, and response vary, the treatment needs to be tailored toward the individual patient. Early neurocognitive assessment and intervention with speech and motor therapy improves long-term functional outcome,[65] and an improved quality of life decreases depressive episodes. Psychotherapy can be beneficial to patients as well as the caregivers who often deal with family members with rapidly changing cognitive states.[66] Pharmacologic intervention is primarily based on efficacy in primary psychiatric disorders. However, small studies have promising results that methylphenidate, modafinil, and donepezil can improve cognitive function and depressive symptoms specifically in patients with brain tumors.[67–69] Further studies assessing the effect of these interventions on overall survival are still ongoing.

THE ROLE OF THE REHABILITATION PHYSICIAN

Despite being relatively rare, brain tumors have a high rate of disability, ranging from neurocognitive deficits to quadriparesis. In one series, cognitive impairment was present in as many as 80% of patients. Most patients (74.5%) had 3 or more concurrent deficits, and 38.2% had 5 or more deficits.[70] Given the enormous impact that brain tumors can have on functional ability, rehabilitation is a key component of treatment.

Early involvement (within 2 weeks) of an inpatient rehabilitation team can lead to marked improvement after initial surgery.[71] Neurocognitive, speech, language, occupational, and physical therapists all play an important role. Regardless of tumor histology, patients with brain tumors achieve similar improvements in cognitive, motor, and occupational skills as patients with other types of brain injury.[72] A close relationship between the medical and rehabilitation teams is necessary to maximize improvement because rehabilitation can be hampered by treatment side effects. For example, many patients with brain tumors are on prolonged courses of glucocorticoids, which also cause muscle wasting, bone pain, and weakness. However, overall, patients on chemotherapy or radiation during their rehabilitation therapy were able to make the same functional gains as those who were undergoing rehabilitation therapy only.[72] As expected, the best outcomes were seen in patients who had an absent or controlled primary tumor, who were less than 60 years old, and who had higher initial function scores.

Gains achieved in the inpatient setting can continue with outpatient rehabilitation. Although inpatient rehabilitation is objectively tied to improved functional outcomes, improvement in patient-perceived quality-of-life scores is seen with continued outpatient rehabilitation therapy.[73] Outpatient therapy can play a major role in helping patients and their caregivers adjust to their home routines. Regular exercise at home is correlated with improved survival.[74]

Patients who have completed therapy and are in remission still benefit from ongoing therapy, especially in mitigating the long-term neurocognitive sequelae. A multicenter trial of 161 childhood cancer survivors (with either primary brain tumors or other malignancies requiring treatment that affected the central nervous system) who were randomized to receive 25 two-hour sessions of cognitive and psychological therapy showed modest improvements in academic achievement compared with survivors with no intervention.[75] Many cognitive interventions are resource and time intensive and may limit feasibility on a larger scale. Pilot studies of cognitive interventions using computer-based cognitive exercises have shown promising results in improving memory and learning.[76]

INTEGRATING SUBSPECIALTY CARE

Over the last 20 years, the number of diagnostic and therapeutic options for patients with brain tumors has increased substantially and will likely continue to do so in the future. With all of these options, treatment plans need to be specialized for individual patients to optimize survival and quality of life. As survival improves, the medical community is also learning more about the management of long-term sequela from brain tumors and their treatment. Throughout the treatment course, a multidisciplinary approach to these complex patients is critical. Fortunately, multidisciplinary cancer conferences have become the norm in larger institutions, facilitating communication between the different subspecialty services.

REFERENCES

1. Senft C, Bink A, Franz K, et al. Intraoperative MRI guidance and extent of resection in glioma surgery: a randomised, controlled trial. Lancet Oncol 2011;12:997.
2. Kubben PL, ter Meulen KJ, Schijns OE, et al. Intraoperative MRI-guided resection of glioblastoma multiforme: a systematic review. Lancet Oncol 2011;12:1062.
3. Stummer W, Pichlmeier U, Meinel T, et al. Fluorescence-guided surgery with 5-aminolevulinic acid for resection of malignant glioma: a randomised controlled multicentre phase III trial. Lancet Oncol 2006;7:392.
4. Sanai N, Berger MS. Intraoperative stimulation techniques for functional pathway preservation and glioma resection. Neurosurg Focus 2010;28:E1.
5. Gulati S, Jakola AS, Nerland US, et al. The risk of getting worse: surgically acquired deficits, perioperative complications, and functional outcomes after primary resection of glioblastoma. World Neurosurg 2011;76:572.
6. Sanai N, Mirzadeh Z, Berger MS. Functional outcome after language mapping for glioma resection. N Engl J Med 2008;358:18.
7. Keles GE, Lundin DA, Lamborn KR, et al. Intraoperative subcortical stimulation mapping for hemispherical perirolandic gliomas located within or adjacent to the descending motor pathways: evaluation of morbidity and assessment of functional outcome in 294 patients. J Neurosurg 2004;100:369.
8. FitzGerald DB, Cosgrove GR, Ronner S, et al. Location of language in the cortex: a comparison between functional MR imaging and electrocortical stimulation. AJNR Am J Neuroradiol 1997;18(8):1529–39.
9. Herholz K, Reulen HJ, von Stockhausen HM, et al. Preoperative activation and intraoperative stimulation of language-related areas in patients with glioma. Neurosurgery 1997;41:1253.

10. Bohman LE, Gallardo J, Hankinson TC, et al. The survival impact of postoperative infection in patients with glioblastoma multiforme. Neurosurgery 2009;64:828.
11. De Bonis P, Albanese A, Lofrese G, et al. Postoperative infection may influence survival in patients with glioblastoma: simply a myth? Neurosurgery 2011;69:864.
12. Montano N, D'Alessandris QG, Bianchi F, et al. Communicating hydrocephalus following surgery and adjuvant radiochemotherapy for glioblastoma. J Neurosurg 2011;115:1126.
13. Ricard D, Idbaih A, Ducray F, et al. Primary brain tumours in adults. Lancet 2012; 379:1984–96.
14. Ruge MI, Kickingereder P, Grau S, et al. Stereotactic iodine-125 brachytherapy for brain tumors: temporary versus permanent implantation. Radiat Oncol 2012;7:94.
15. Schwarz SB, Thon N, Nikolajek K, et al. Iodine-125 brachytherapy for brain tumours–a review. Radiat Oncol 2012;7:30.
16. Folkert MR, Bilsky MH, Cohen GN, et al. Intraoperative 32P high dose rate brachytherapy of the dura for recurrent primary and metastatic intracranial and spine tumors. Neurosurgery 2012;71:1003–11.
17. Ruge MI, Kickingereder P, Grau S, et al. Stereotactic biopsy combined with stereotactic (125)iodine brachytherapy for diagnosis and treatment of locally recurrent single brain metastases. J Neurooncol 2011;105:109–18.
18. Larson DA, Suplica JM, Chang SM, et al. Permanent iodine 125 brachytherapy in patients with progressive or recurrent glioblastoma multiforme. Neuro Oncol 2004;6:119–26.
19. Shulman LN, Buswell L, Riese N, et al. Phase I trial of the hypoxic cell cytotoxin tirapazamine with concurrent radiation therapy in the treatment of refractory solid tumors. Int J Radiat Oncol Biol Phys 1999;44:349–53.
20. Stea B, Suh JH, Boyd AP, et al. Whole-brain radiotherapy with or without efaproxiral for the treatment of brain metastases: determinants of response and its prognostic value for subsequent survival. Int J Radiat Oncol Biol Phys 2006;64:1023–30.
21. Mehta MP, Rodrigus P, Terhaard CH, et al. Survival and neurologic outcomes in a randomized trial of motexafin gadolinium and whole-brain radiation therapy in brain metastases. J Clin Oncol 2003;21:2529–36.
22. Mehta MP, Shapiro WR, Glantz MJ, et al. Lead-in phase to randomized trial of motexafin gadolinium and whole-brain radiation for patients with brain metastases: centralized assessment of magnetic resonance imaging, neurocognitive, and neurologic end points. J Clin Oncol 2002;20:3445–53.
23. Mehta MP, Shapiro WR, Phan SC, et al. Motexafin gadolinium combined with prompt whole brain radiotherapy prolongs time to neurologic progression in non-small-cell lung cancer patients with brain metastases: results of a phase III trial. Int J Radiat Oncol Biol Phys 2009;73:1069–76.
24. Lamond JP, Mehta MP, Boothman DA. The potential of topoisomerase I inhibitors in the treatment of CNS malignancies: report of a synergistic effect between topotecan and radiation. J Neurooncol 2004;30:1–6.
25. Chang EL, Wefel JS, Hess KR, et al. Neurocognition in patients with brain metastases treated with radiosurgery or radiosurgery plus whole-brain irradiation: a randomised controlled trial. Lancet Oncol 2009;10:1037–44.
26. Chang EL, Wefel JS, Maor MH, et al. A pilot study of neurocognitive function in patients with one to three new brain metastases initially treated with stereotactic radiosurgery alone. Neurosurgery 2007;60:277–83 [discussion: 283–4].
27. Meyers CA, Wefel JS. The use of the mini-mental state examination to assess cognitive functioning in cancer trials: no ifs, ands, buts, or sensitivity. J Clin Oncol 2003;21:3557–8.

28. Meyers CA, Hess KR. Multifaceted end points in brain tumor clinical trials: cognitive deterioration precedes MRI progression. Neuro Oncol 2003;5:89–95.
29. Meyers CA, Hess KR, Yung WK, et al. Cognitive function as a predictor of survival in patients with recurrent malignant glioma. J Clin Oncol 2000;18:646–50.
30. Wefel JS, Kayl AE, Meyers CA. Neuropsychological dysfunction associated with cancer and cancer therapies: a conceptual review of an emerging target. Br J Cancer 2004;90:1691–6.
31. Rudin CM, Hann CL, Laterra J, et al. Treatment of medulloblastoma with hedgehog pathway inhibitor GDC-0449. N Engl J Med 2009;361(12):1173–8.
32. Chang S, Parney IF, Huang W, et al. Patterns of care for adults with newly diagnosed malignant glioma. JAMA 2005;293(5):557–64.
33. Sizoo EM, Pasman HR, Buttolo J, et al. Decision-making in the end-of-life phase of high-grade glioma patients. Eur J Cancer 2012;48(2):226–32.
34. Tribiel K, Martin RC, Nabors LB, et al. Medical decision-making capacity in patients with malignant glioma. Neurology 2009;73(24):2086–92.
35. Pace A, Di Lorenzo C, Guariglia L, et al. End of life issues in brain tumor patients. J Neurooncol 2009;91(1):39–43.
36. Merchant TE, Williams T, Smith JM, et al. Preirradiation endocrinopathies in pediatric brain tumor patients determined by dynamic tests of endocrine function. Int J Radiat Oncol Biol Phys 2002;54(1):45–50.
37. De Marinis L, Fusco A, Bianchi A, et al. Hypopituitarism findings in patients with primary brain tumors 1 year after neurosurgical treatment: preliminary report. J Endocrinol Invest 2006;29(6):516–22.
38. Sara M, Claudio F, Marco L, et al. Time course of hypothalamic-pituitary deficiency in adults receiving cranial radiotherapy for primary extrasellar brain tumors. Radiother Oncol 2011;99(1):23–8.
39. Agha A, Sherlock M, Brennan S, et al. Hypothalamic-pituitary dysfunction after irradiation of nonpituitary brain tumors in adults. J Clin Endocrinol Metab 2005; 90(12):6355–60.
40. Arslanian S, Becker DJ, Lee PA, et al. Growth hormone therapy and tumor recurrence findings in children with brain neoplasms and hypopituitarism. Arch Pediatr Adolesc Med 1985;139(4):347–50.
41. Moshang T, Rundle AC, Graves DA, et al. Brain tumor recurrence in children treated with growth hormone: the National Cooperative Growth Study experience. J Pediatr 1996;128:S4–7.
42. Packer RJ, Boyett JM, Janss AJ, et al. Growth hormone replacement therapy in children with medulloblastoma: use and effect on tumor control. J Clin Oncol 2001;19(2):480–7.
43. Ergun-Longmire B, Mertens AC, Mitby P, et al. Growth hormone treatment and risk of second neoplasms in the childhood cancer survivor. J Clin Endocrinol Metab 2006;91(9):3494–8.
44. Mukerjee A, Tolhurst-Cleaver S, Ryder WD, et al. The characteristics of quality of life impairment in adult growth hormone (GH)-deficient survivors of cancer and their response to GH replacement therapy. J Clin Endocrinol Metab 2005;90(3): 1542–9.
45. Gurney JG. Endocrine and cardiovascular late effects among adult survivors of childhood brain tumors: Childhood Cancer Survivor Study. Cancer 2003;97(3): 663–73.
46. Lustig R, Post SR, Srivannaboon K, et al. Risk factors for the development of obesity in children surviving brain tumors. J Clin Endocrinol Metab 2003;88(2): 611–6.

47. Lustig R, Rose SR, Burghen GA, et al. Hypothalamic obesity caused by cranial insult in children: altered glucose and insulin dynamics and reversal by a somatostatin agonist. J Pediatr 1999;135(2 Pt 1):162–8.
48. Barr RD, Simpson T, Webber CE, et al. Osteopenia in children surviving brain tumours. Eur J Cancer 1998;34(6):873–7.
49. Chang EF, Potts MB, Keles GE, et al. Seizure characteristics and control following resection in 332 patients with low-grade gliomas. J Neurosurg 2008;108(2):227–35.
50. Glantz MJ, Cole BF, Friedberg MH, et al. A randomized, blinded, placebo-controlled trial of divalproex sodium prophylaxis in adults with newly diagnosed brain tumors. Neurology 1996;46:985–91.
51. Kerrigan S, Grant R. Antiepileptic drugs for treating seizures in adults with brain tumours. Cochrane Database Syst Rev 2011;(8):CD008586.
52. Weller M, Gorlia T, Cairncross JG. Prolonged survival with valproic acid use in the EORTC/NCIC temozolomide trial for glioblastoma. Neurology 2011;77(12):1156–64.
53. Glantz MJ, Cole BF, Forsyth PA. Practice parameter: anticonvulsant therapy in patients with newly diagnosed brain tumors. Neurology 2000;54:1886–93.
54. Sirven JI, Wingerchuk DM, Drazkowski JF, et al. Seizure prophylaxis in patients with brain tumors: a meta-analysis. Mayo Clin Proc 2004;79(12):1489–94.
55. Kuijlen JM, Teernstra OP, Kessels AG, et al. Effectiveness of antiepileptic prophylaxis used with supratentorial craniotomies: a meta-analysis. Seizure 1996;5(4):291–8.
56. Fraum TJ, Kreisl TN, Sul J, et al. Ischemic stroke and intracranial hemorrhage in glioma patients on antiangiogenic therapy. J Neurooncol 2011;105(2):281–9.
57. Morris B, Partap S, Yeom K, et al. Cerebrovascular disease in childhood cancer survivors. Neurology 2009;73:1906–13.
58. Bowers DC, Liu Y, Leisenring W, et al. Late-occurring stroke among long-term survivors of childhood leukemia and brain tumors: a report from the Childhood Cancer Survivor Study. J Clin Oncol 2006;24(33):5277–82.
59. Kreisl T, Toothaker T, Karimi S, et al. Ischemic stroke in patients with primary brain tumors. Neurology 2008;70:2314–20.
60. Litofsky NS, Farace E, Anderson F Jr, et al. Depression in patients with high-grade glioma: results of the Glioma Outcomes Project. Neurosurgery 2004;54(2):358–66.
61. Mainio A, Hakko H, Niemelä A, et al. Depression in relation to survival among neurosurgical patients with a primary brain tumor: a 5-year follow-up study. Neurosurgery 2005;56(6):1234–41.
62. Mainio A, Tuunanen S, Hakko H, et al. Decreased quality of life and depression as predictors for shorter survival among patients with low-grade gliomas: a follow-up from 1990 to 2003. Eur Arch Psychiatry Clin Neurosci 2006;256(8):516–21.
63. Gathinji M, McGirt M, Attenello F, et al. Association of preoperative depression and survival after resection of malignant brain astrocytoma. Surg Neurol 2009;71(3):299–303.
64. Dalton SO, Laursen TM, Ross L, et al. Risk for hospitalization with depression after a cancer diagnosis: a nationwide, population-based study of cancer patients in Denmark from 1973 to 2003. J Clin Oncol 2009;27(9):1440–5.
65. Gerhring K, Sitskoorn MM, Gundy CM, et al. Cognitive rehabilitation in patients with gliomas: a randomized, controlled trial. J Clin Oncol 2009;27(22):3712–22.
66. Northhouse LL, Katapodi MC, Song L, et al. Interventions with family caregivers of cancer patients: meta-analysis of randomized trials. CA Cancer J Clin 2010;60(5):317–39.

67. Meyers CA, Weitzner MA, Valentine AD, et al. Methylphenidate therapy improves cognition, mood, and function of brain tumor patients. J Clin Oncol 1998;16(7):2522–7.
68. Shaw EG, Rosdhal R, D'Agostino RB Jr, et al. Phase II study of donepezil in irradiated brain tumor patients: effect on cognitive function, mood, and quality of life. J Clin Oncol 2006;24(9):1415–20.
69. Gehring K, Patwardhan SY, Collins R, et al. A randomized trial on the efficacy of methylphenidate and modafinil for improving cognitive functioning and symptoms in patients with a primary brain tumor. J Neurooncol 2012;107(1):165–74.
70. Mukand JA, Blackinton DD, Crincoli MG, et al. Incidence of neurologic deficits and rehabilitation of patients with brain tumors. Am J Phys Med Rehabil 2001;80:346–50.
71. Bartolo M, Zucchella C, Pace A, et al. Early rehabilitation after surgery improves functional outcome in inpatients with brain tumours. J Neurooncol 2012;107(3):537–44.
72. Marciniak CM, Sliwa JA, Heinemann AW, et al. Functional outcomes of persons with brain tumors after inpatient rehabilitation. Arch Phys Med Rehabil 2001;82:457–63.
73. Pace A, Parisi C, Di Lelio M, et al. Home rehabilitation for brain tumour patients. J Exp Clin Cancer Res 2007;26:297–300.
74. Ruden E, Reardon DA, Coan AD, et al. Exercise behavior, functional capacity, and survival in adults with malignant recurrent glioma. J Clin Oncol 2011;29(21):2918–23.
75. Butler A, Copeland DR, Fairclough DL, et al. Multicenter, randomized clinical trial of a cognitive remediation program for childhood survivors of a pediatric malignancy. J Consult Clin Psychol 2008;76(3):367–78.
76. Kesler SR, Lacayo NJ, Jo B. A pilot study of an online cognitive rehabilitation program for executive function skills in children with cancer-related brain injury. Brain Inj 2011;25(1):101–12.

Multidisciplinary Care of the Patient with Head and Neck Cancer

Vassiliki Saloura, MD[a,*], Alexander Langerman, MD[b], Sonali Rudra, MD[c], Robert Chin, MD, PhD[c], Ezra E.W. Cohen, MD[a]

KEYWORDS

- Head and neck cancer • Multidisciplinary • Robotic surgery • Altered fractionation
- Induction chemotherapy • Sequential chemotherapy • Human papilloma virus

KEY POINTS

- Squamous carcinoma of the head and neck cancer is the sixth most common cancer in the United States, with an increasing incidence largely because of a rising epidemic of human papilloma virus (HPV)-positive oropharyngeal cancer.
- Early-stage or locally advanced head and neck cancer is treated with curative intent, and management is a multidisciplinary effort, which should encompass head and neck surgeons, radiation oncologists, and medical oncologists.
- Metastatic head and neck cancer is treated with palliative intent with platinum-based or taxane-based chemotherapy regimens, such as cisplatin/5-fluorouracil and cisplatin/paclitaxel. The addition of cetuximab to this regimen has been the only progress over the past decade that has shown an increase in overall survival.
- HPV-positive head and neck cancer has a distinct pathogenesis compared with the classic HPV-negative, smoking/alcohol-induced head and neck cancer, which is caused by a stepwise accumulation of multiple mutations. HPV-positive cancers typically have a better prognosis compared with HPV-negative cancers.
- Head and neck cancer is a heterogeneous disease with distinct genetic subsets, which are under investigation.

Funding Sources: Not applicable.
Conflict of Interest: Not applicable.
[a] Section of Hematology/Oncology, Department of Medicine, The University of Chicago, 5841 South Maryland Avenue, MC2115, Chicago, IL 60637-1470, USA; [b] Section of Otolaryngology – Head and Neck Surgery, Department of Surgery, The University of Chicago, 5841 South Maryland Avenue, MC 1035, Chicago, IL 60637-1470, USA; [c] Department of Radiation and Cellular Oncology, The University of Chicago, 5841 South Maryland Avenue, MC 9006, Chicago, IL 60637-1470, USA
* Corresponding author.
E-mail address: vassiliki.saloura@uchospitals.edu

Surg Oncol Clin N Am 22 (2013) 179–215
http://dx.doi.org/10.1016/j.soc.2012.12.001 surgonc.theclinics.com
1055-3207/13/$ – see front matter

INTRODUCTION

Head and neck cancer (HNC) comprises a heterogeneous group of cancers, which primarily affect the oral cavity, oropharynx, hypopharynx, larynx, and nasopharynx. In 2010, HNC was the sixth most frequent cancer by incidence worldwide, with more than 500,000 new cases diagnosed.[1] The highest incidence rates occur in South-Central Asia and Central and Eastern Europe. In North America and Europe, oral cavity, oropharyngeal, and laryngeal cancer are the most common types, whereas nasopharyngeal cancer (NPC) is more common in the Far East and Mediterranean countries.

Classic HNC is caused by smoking and alcohol exposure, which drive a stepwise accumulation of mutations in the squamous epithelium (**Box 1**).[2–4] One of the most important developments in HNC is the discovery that human papilloma virus (HPV) subtype 16 is the causative factor in most oropharyngeal cancers (base of tongue, tonsil), especially in North America and Western Europe.[6,7] Based on several retrospective studies,[6] 40% to 60% of patients with oropharyngeal cancer in the United States are HPV-positive. As the incidence of smoking has decreased, the incidence of HPV-negative HNC has also declined, whereas the rates of HPV-positive HNC have increased, accounting for the rising incidence of HNC.[5,8,9] These cancers are usually seen in young, nonsmoker, nondrinker men, and they have a better prognosis compared with HPV-negative HNC. The pathogenesis of these cancers has been attributed to 2 viral proteins, E6 and E7, which bind and inactivate 2 tumor suppressor genes, p53 and retinoblastoma Rb, respectively. This process drives malignant transformation of the squamous epithelium. Based on these data, HNC is now classified into HPV-positive and HPV-negative HNC. Another important viral cause of HNC is the Epstein-Barr virus (EBV), which is associated with the endemic form of NPC in Asia and Africa. **Box 2** summarizes the major risk factors in the pathogenesis of HNC.

Clinically, a precursor premalignant lesion may precede HNC, such as oral leukoplakia or erythroplakia in the cheeks, gums, or tongue. Symptoms include mouth, throat, neck, and ear pain, persistent mouth sores, hoarseness, persistent unilateral nose

Box 1
Common mutations, copy number alterations, and chromosomal deletions/gains in HNC

- Mutations
  - TP53
  - CDKN2A (p16)
  - PIK3CA
  - NOTCH1
- Copy number alterations
  - EGFR
  - VEGF1
  - CCND1
  - MYC
  - CTTN
- Chromosomal deletions/gains
  - 3p, 3q, 7p, 7q, 8q, 9p, 10q, 11q, 17p, 18q

Data from Refs.[2–5]

Box 2
Risk factors for HNC

- Smoking
- Alcohol (>50 g/d)
- Previous history of HNC
- Advanced age (>50 years)
- Hereditary predisposition (rare):
  - Fanconi anemia
- Viral agents:
  - HPV (oropharyngeal cancer)
  - EBV (NPC)

bleeding or nasal obstruction, unilateral hearing loss, dysphagia, odynophagia, a persistent palpable neck mass and cranial neuropathies, especially with NPC. They usually spread by invasion of adjacent local structures and regional lymph nodes. Systemic metastasis is rare at presentation (<10%). Patients may also have other synchronous multiple primary malignancies or metachronous malignancies, such as second primary HNC, lung, or esophageal cancer, which occur in 20% of survivors. This finding reflects the exposure of the upper aerodigestive mucosa to the same carcinogens, an effect known as field cancerization.

Diagnosis is made by triple endoscopy (laryngoscopy, esophagoscopy, and bronchoscopy), which also allows for investigation of synchronous malignancies. Complete staging includes computed tomography (CT) or magnetic resonance imaging (MRI) of the head and neck, and CT of the chest to rule out pulmonary metastasis, although these are rare.

The treatment of HNC requires a highly specialized, multidisciplinary team (**Box 3**) and should ideally take place in centers of excellence in the management of this

Box 3
Multidisciplinary team in the management of patients with HNC

- Medical oncology
- Head and neck surgery
- Radiation oncology
- Plastic and reconstructive surgery
- Palliative medicine
- Psychiatry
- Ancillary services
  - Nutrition
  - Social work services
  - Tracheostomy care
  - Speech and swallow evaluation/therapy
  - Smoking and alcohol cessation counselling
  - Dental care before chemoradiation

disease. This article focuses on the mainstay approaches and most recent advances in the multidisciplinary treatment of patients with HNC. The emerging role of HPV, molecular profiling, targeted therapy, and immunotherapy are also briefly reviewed.

PRINCIPLES OF MULTIMODALITY THERAPY IN HNC

Ninety percent of patients with HNC present with early-stage (I and II) or locally advanced disease (stage III, IVA, IVB), whereas 10% of patients have metastatic (stage IVC) disease. Almost 50% of patients with HNC can be cured. Patients with early-stage disease can be cured in 80% to 90% of cases with single modality therapy, either radiotherapy (RT) or surgery. On the other hand, patients with locally advanced disease require a multimodality approach with surgery, RT, and chemotherapy and achieve cure rates of 40% to 50%. Recurrent or metastatic disease is incurable and managed with systemic chemotherapy, although 15% of patients with locally recurrent disease may have reirradiation or salvage surgery.

Based on stage, HNC can be resectable or unresectable. However, even if a tumor is curable with resection, surgery may confer significant morbidity and compromise in quality of life, because of the anatomic complexity of the head and neck structures, most importantly the nasopharynx, oropharynx, hypopharynx, and larynx. In these cases, an organ-preservation approach is favored, with RT or concurrent chemoradiotherapy (CRT). In a similar philosophy, although early-stage cancers of the oral or nasal cavity can be cured with surgery without significant functional impairment, a nonsurgical strategy with CRT is still possible with equivalent cure rates. This approach is known as surgical sparing.

Mitigation of side effects by surgery, RT, and chemotherapy is of paramount importance to avoid acute and chronic complications. Surgical techniques are evolving toward less invasive approaches, whereas reconstructive procedures are used to achieve a better functional and aesthetic outcome. Radiation therapy techniques are gravitating toward fractionation schedules and intensity-modulated radiation therapy, which focuses on the organ of interest and spares surrounding healthy tissues. Although chemotherapy remains an integral part of a multimodality strategy, research efforts are focusing on the identification of targeted agents, which could be equally or more efficacious and at the same time less toxic.

PRINCIPLES OF SURGERY

Introduction

Treatment of HNC is a careful balance between morbidity and cure. Whereas traditional open surgical approaches remain the gold standard for many advanced tumors, the last decade has seen an increasing focus on minimally invasive approaches for early and select advanced tumors. Advances in endoscopic, robotic, and laser technology have allowed use of natural orifices and have increased the feasibility of large tumor extirpation. Adoption of sentinel lymph node mapping has also begun to occur, signaling a new era of minimal neck dissections.

In addition to serving as a primary modality, surgery is an important salvage modality after RT or CRT at both the primary site and the neck. Open and even minimally invasive approaches are feasible in a previously irradiated patient, but typically with decreased functional outcomes and higher complication rates. Free flap reconstruction is commonly used in these patients and is an important part of the head and neck surgeon's armamentarium.

Transoral, Minimally Invasive Approaches

Minimally invasive or natural orifice surgery is a natural extension of the endoscopic diagnostic techniques that have been developed over decades of head and neck surgery. These approaches have usefulness for transnasal extirpation of skull base and sinus malignancies and transoral resection of laryngeal and oropharyngeal tumors. The art of the latter approaches extends beyond the elimination of external scars and lies in the maintenance of the physiologic muscular layers of the swallowing mechanism and the preservation of respiratory and phonatory function.

Minimally invasive conservation surgery for laryngeal cancer is well established for both early-stage and late-stage tumors. Local control rates for T1 tumors are reported to be 91% to 99%,[10–12] similar to results of RT.[13,14] Local control is worse with anterior commissure involvement for both modalities.[14,15] For T2 tumors, there is low-level evidence to suggest that surgery may offer a better local control[10,16,17] and a higher rate of laryngeal preservation,[16] but definitive studies have not been conducted. For T3 laryngeal disease, reports of transoral laser[18] and open[19] conservation surgery combined with adjuvant CRT show laryngeal preservation rates in the 80% to 90% range. Much like with CRT, patients after surgery for advanced laryngeal cancer should expect some degree of aspiration[20,21] and must have appropriate lung reserve to clear secretions.

For oropharyngeal cancers, minimally invasive surgery plus neck dissection has been shown in prospective cohorts to have oncologic efficacy outcomes comparable with CRT[22–25] for both HPV-positive and HPV-negative tumors,[26,27] although comparative efficacy studies are lacking. The oncologic principles of both transoral laser microsurgery (TLM) and transoral robotic surgery (TORS) are the same: precise, complete, microscopic excision of expendable portions of the pharynx through a natural orifice. For both techniques, patients also undergo neck dissection with or without postoperative adjuvant therapy based on pathologic staging. The principle difference between these techniques is that TLM relies on a microscope and laser, whereas TORS relies on the DaVinci Surgical System (Intuitive Corporation, Sunnyvale, CA). Adoption of and publications regarding TORS have increased at a faster rate than for TLM, presumably because of enthusiasm for robotic technology. However, both techniques report similar oncologic results.[22,23]

Success with TLM with or without adjuvant CRT for treatment of oropharyngeal cancer was first reported by Steiner in 2003,[28] with a report of 48 patients with mainly locally advanced base-of-tongue cancer, showing a 5-year local control rate of 85%. These data were reinforced by a multicenter study of 204 patients with advanced oropharyngeal cancer treated with TLM,[22] with a 2-year and 5-year survival rate of 89% and 78%, respectively. In one-quarter of the patients, adjuvant therapy was avoided altogether, and only 16% required combined CRT.

Functional outcomes with TLM have been favorable, with 87% of patients in the multicenter study achieving a normal or near-normal diet at last follow-up.[22] In addition, 83% of patients did not require a gastrostomy tube (G-tube) during surgical therapy and healing. Of the patients without G-tubes, 22% later required gastrostomy during adjuvant therapy, for a total of a 44% temporary G-tube rate. However, at 2 years, this rate was only 9.3% and at 5 years only 3.8%.

TORS for oropharyngeal cancer was first pioneered by Weinstein and O'Malley in 2006[29] and has been widely adopted. The bulk of the present data on TORS are for oropharyngeal cancer, primarily early T-stage (T1–T2) and often with advanced neck disease.[30] In studies with sufficient follow-up, 2-year overall survival (OS) rate has been reported in the 80% to 95% range.[23,31–33]

Similar to TLM, studies of functional outcomes for TORS have reported low G-tube dependency rates of less than 10% at 1 year.[23,31] It is unclear whether this finding is part of a philosophy of aggressive swallowing therapy and avoidance of prophylactic G-tubes or whether this low dependency rate is a salutary effect of decreased dosing or complete avoidance of RT.

Trials of both TLM[22] and TORS[31,33,34] have used postoperative adjuvant therapy based on pathologic staging, and oncologic results must be considered in light of the 70% to 80% rate of postoperative adjuvant therapy in these series. Indications for postoperative CRT are positive or close surgical margins (<2 mm), extracapsular spread in metastatic lymph nodes,[31,34] and postoperative radiation for multiple metastatic lymph nodes, lymphovascular invasion, and perineural invasion.[31] In these series, the postoperative radiation dosing was approximately 10 Gy lower compared with primary dosing, with the exception of patients with positive margins.[31,34] The degree to which specific reductions in postoperative RT affect swallowing and other functional and quality-of-life–related outcomes remains unknown.

Surgical Management of the Neck

Neck dissection has evolved from morbid, en-bloc radical neck dissections that remove the sternocleidomastoid muscle, internal jugular vein, and cranial nerve XI to an approach introduced by Bocca[35] of the selective neck dissection, using natural fascial planes to remove the lymphatic tissue but sparing normal structures. This approach necessitates certain features, such as mobile nodes or a clinically negative neck, and encompasses all of the anticipated drainage basins of a given tumor. For instance, neck dissection for oral cancer typically involves levels I to III (supraomohyoid) and for laryngeal cancer involves levels II to IV (lateral), subject to clinical findings and the presence of lymph nodes.

Selective neck dissection can also be used as salvage or to assess persistent nodes in patients who have undergone CRT. In these cases, the dissections can often be even more limited (superselective) based on radiographic workup.[36,37] CRT can restore radiographic tissue planes and make the neck anatomy more amenable to selective dissection, so operative planning should be based on posttreatment scanning and examination.[38] Routine post-CRT neck dissection has been abandoned[39] and many centers rely on positron emission tomography (PET) scanning for post-CRT assessment of neck response.[40]

Elective neck dissection in the clinically and radiographically N0 neck is performed for patients with significant risk for occult metastases, based on tumor location and depth of invasion. However, there is an inherent trade-off between the morbidity of neck dissection and the risk of subsequent development of neck disease. In patients who are observed and develop neck metastases, the morbidity of neck dissection is higher, and in some series, the success rate is lower.[41] This finding prompted investigation of an alternative approach to the N0 neck using intraoperative mapping of the drainage patterns of head and neck tumors with selective biopsy of the first-echelon (sentinel) nodes.

Sentinel lymph node biopsy (SLNB) in the head and neck was first introduced in 1992 for melanoma[42] but has been expanded in the last decade for evaluation of the clinically and radiographically N0 neck in oral and oropharyngeal squamous carcinoma. The presence of lymph node metastases is the most significant negative prognostic indicator for HNC, and SLNB offers a minimally invasive means of assessing the status of the lymphatic basins. Compared with elective neck dissection, SLNB has been shown to result in better postoperative quality of life and shoulder function, as well as decreased scar size and a lower complication rate.[43]

Several multi-institutional groups have conducted trials of SLNB for the treatment of the N0 neck, with long-term results now becoming available. The ACSOG (American College of Surgeons Oncology Group) trial reported a negative predictive value (NPV) of 96% at 5 years for SLNB with immunohistochemistry evaluation.[44] All patients were determined radiographically N0 by CT or MRI, and all surgeons underwent standardized training. Similarly, a European multicenter trial reported an NPV of 94% at 5 years.[45] However, these investigators found the NPV to be significantly worse for floor-of-mouth tumors (88%) compared with other sites (98%). Most recently, SLNB has been shown to be feasible in patients who have had previous neck surgery or irradiation,[46] with 100% regional control at a median follow-up of 22 months. This approach in previously treated patients holds promise and warrants further study.

Salvage Surgery

For patients who have recurrent or persistent disease after radiation or CRT, salvage surgery is an option for cure or palliation. Nonsmoking patients with early-stage recurrent cancers (rT1–rT2) are better candidates for curative-intent salvage surgery compared with patients with advanced-stage cancers who continue to smoke.[47] Although some patients with smaller defects can be allowed to granulate, which takes considerably longer in an irradiated field, or in a region reconstructed with local flaps, which are more tenuous than in nonirradiated patients, many of these patients require axial or free flap reconstruction.

In a prospective study, the average survival at 5 years for patients undergoing salvage surgery was 39%, and the median disease-free survival was 17.9 months.[48] In this study, higher stage was associated with shorter survival, with median survival for stage I to III of 21 to 24 months and only 9.3 months for stage IV. Patients who recurred sooner (<6 months) after previous treatment (surgery, radiation, or chemotherapy) trended a shorter mean survival of 18.3 months versus more than 21 months for patients with longer times to recurrence. In addition, lower-stage patients also had a better chance of quality-of-life improvement after surgery compared to higher-stage patients (64% for stage I vs 39% for stage IV).

Some patients are rendered cancer free but nonfunctional after CRT. Scarring, loss of sensation, and tumor-related cartilage destruction can all contribute to a suboptimal functional status. Elective laryngectomy is an appropriate option for patients with severe laryngeal dysfunction and aspiration, and has a high success rate of restoring oral intake and improving quality of life.[49] These patients can also have voice restoration with a tracheoesophageal prosthesis, but complications of these prostheses are increased in patients with previous RT.[50]

Reconstruction

Reconstruction is a critical aspect of head and neck surgery. Goals of reconstruction are to ensure a watertight seal of the digestive tract and skull base, maintain function of critical structures (eg, oral sphincter, tongue, jaw, larynx, pharyngoesophagus), and maintain cosmesis. Local flaps derived from the mucosa, nasolabial folds, and neck skin can provide good intraoral lining. Axial flaps such as the pectoralis major myocutaneous and myofascial flaps, the temporalis or temporoparietal fascial flaps, and the supraclavicular artery island flap have multiple applications for reconstruction and are reliable, although limited by their pedicle. Free tissue transfer has become routine in most major medical centers and offers healthy, nonirradiated tissue, with full freedom of inset geometry and multiple tissue types.

Plastic surgeons, and with increasing frequency, head and neck surgeons all participate in reconstructive efforts by institution basis.[51] The most common donor sites[52] are anterolateral thigh (bulk, large skin),[53] radial forearm (thin and pliable skin, bone available),[54,55] and fibula (longest bone stock, skin).[55] The subscapular system provides a variety of tissue and can be used for multiple applications,[56] but the posterior location of the donor site makes simultaneous tumor resection and flap harvest challenging.

Overall success of microvascular free flap reconstruction of head and neck defects is more than 95%, but a quarter or more of patients can expect some perioperative complication.[57] Previous RT may lower the threshold for use of free flap reconstruction but does not seem to increase the complication rate.[58,59]

PRINCIPLES OF RADIATION THERAPY

Indications

For early-stage HNC, RT can offer an alternative to surgical resection as definitive treatment. For locally advanced disease, most patients are treated either with concurrent CRT or surgery followed by adjuvant RT with or without chemotherapy. **Box 4** summarizes the indications for adjuvant RT or CRT for early and locally advanced HNC.

Altered Fractionation Radiation

Standard radiation treatments are usually given in 2-Gy fractions per day, 5 days a week, to a total dose of 60 to 70 Gy. Altered fractionation schemes that take advantage of principles of radiation biology have been investigated to try to improve local control and toxicity rates.

Hyperfractionation

Hyperfractionation involves delivering 2 to 3 fractions per day, usually in a smaller dose per fraction than 2 Gy. Treatment in this fashion is believed to decrease late toxicity by taking advantage of the fact that late-responding normal tissues are more sensitive to large doses per fraction. Therefore, multiple treatments with smaller doses should theoretically decrease late toxicity. Consequently, the total dose of treatment using hyperfractionation can often be escalated without causing unacceptable toxicity levels.

Accelerated fractionation

In accelerated fractionation schemes, the total treatment time is reduced to try to decrease the probability of tumor repopulation during treatment. In pure accelerated

Box 4
Indications for Adjuvant RT or Adjuvant CRT

Indications for Adjuvant RT[60–62]

- One lymph node greater than 3 cm
- Multiple positive nodes (no extracapsular extension)
- Lymphovascular invasion
- Perineural invasion
- pT3 or pT4 primary tumor
- Oral cavity/oropharyngeal primary with positive level IV/V nodes

Indications for Adjuvant CRT[63]

- Extracapsular extension
- Positive margins

fractionation, the total dose and dose per fraction remain the same, but more fractions may be given per week. In hybrid models, the dose is altered.

Some of the main radiation trials involving altered fractionation are listed in **Table 1**. In aggregate, these trials suggest a locoregional benefit to altered fractionation radiation. Most of the trials investigating altered fractionation compared with standard fractionation have been performed with radiation alone. The role of altered fractionation in combination with cisplatin is being investigated.[69] In RTOG 0129, 70 Gy in 2-Gy fractions with 3 cycles of cisplatin is being compared with 72 Gy delivered with a delayed concomitant boost (twice-daily radiation for the last 12 days) plus 2 cycles of cisplatin. The preliminary results of this study[70] did not show a survival or locoregional control benefit to altered fractionation compared with the standard fractionation arm.

Dose and Treatment Volumes

To define the treatment volume, findings on physical examination, examination under anesthesia (if applicable), and multimodality imaging (including CT, MRI, or PET) are used. For definitive RT, the high-dose volume includes the areas of gross disease at the primary site and nodal regions (gross tumor volume [GTV]). The GTV is then expanded based on the anatomy of spread to account for microscopic disease involvement (clinical tumor volume [CTV1]). The CTV1 is expanded by another 2.5 to 10 mm to the planning target volume (PTV1). The typical treatment dose prescribed to PTV1 is 66 to 74 Gy in 2-Gy fractions or up to 81.6 Gy in 1.2-Gy fractions.[60] One notable exception is early-stage laryngeal cancer, because these tumors are generally treated with 63 to 65.25 Gy in 2.25-Gy fractions.[71,72] The elective nodes are contoured in a separate treatment volume and are generally treated to 44 to 64 Gy.[60]

For patients receiving adjuvant RT, preoperative imaging should be used to determine the postoperative bed based on the location of the initial tumor. A CTV should be constructed to include the postoperative bed and the pathologically involved neck. An expansion should then be performed to create a PTV. The dose to this region is 63 to 66 Gy for close or positive margins[63] and 60 Gy for negative margins.[60,73]

The typical recommendations for nodal coverage are based on the T-stage, N-stage, and the primary site. For most midline tumors, bilateral elective nodal coverage is recommended. A few institutions have shown the feasibility of treating well-lateralized tonsillar tumors with ipsilateral radiation alone. Reports from the University of Florida and Princess Margaret Hospital have shown good local control rates in patients treated with ipsilateral radiation for tonsillar carcinoma, with contralateral failure rates of approximately 3% to 4%.[74,75]

Dose Constraints

The total dose of radiation therapy is limited by the surrounding normal structures. **Table 2** shows some of the common dose-limiting structures and the dose constraints that treating physicians try to achieve.

Radiation Therapy Techniques

Treatment planning for HNC is based on CT imaging at most institutions in the United States. When using CT-based planning, the target volumes (primary site/postoperative bed and elective nodes) are delineated on the CT scan at the time of simulation and then a plan is devised to deliver radiation to these target volumes via multiple beams. This type of radiation delivery is referred to as three-dimensional conformal radiation therapy (3D CRT), which delivers radiation therapy to the target and minimizes the dose to the surrounding tissues. Before the widespread use of 3D CRT,

Table 1
Clinical trials involving altered fractionation radiation

Type of RT	Trial	Tumor Type and Stage	N	RT Dose	LCR	OS	Late Toxicity
HF	EORTC 22791 (1992)[64]	T2-3N0-1 OPx			5 y	No difference (P = .08)	No difference in ≥Gr 2 (P = .72)
			159	70/1.8–2 Gy	40%		
			166	80.5/1.15 Gy twice a day	59% (P = .02)		
HF, AF	RTOG 90-03 (2000)[65]	Stage II–IV (BOT or hypopharynx) Stage II–IV (OC, OPx, and supraglottic larynx)			2 y	2 y	Late ≥grade 3:
			268	70/2 Gy	46%	46.1%	26.8%
			263	81.6/1.2 Gy twice a day	54.4% (P = .045)	54.5% (P = .13)	28%, NS
			274	67.2/1.6 Gy twice a day (split course)	47.5% (P = .55)	46.2% (P = .86)	27.6%, NS
			268	72/1.8 Gy + 1.5 Gy DACB	54.5% (P = .05)	50.9% (P = .40)	37.2% (P = .011)
HF/AF	EORTC 22851 (1997)[66]	T2-4N0-3 (no hypopharynx)			5 y	No difference (P = .96)	Late ≥grade 3:
			253	70/1.8–2 Gy	46%		4%
			247	72/1.6 Gy three times a day	59% (P = .02)		14% (P<.001)
AF	CHART (2010)[67,68]	Locally advanced HNC (no T1N0 tumors)	552	54/1.5 Gy three times a day	HR = 0.96 (P = .71)	HR = 1.05 (P = .62)	Late mucosal necrosis: 5% vs 9% (P = .02) Grade 3 xerostomia: 23% vs 31% (P = .02) Laryngeal edema: 50% vs 60% (P = .05)
			336	66/2 Gy			
AF	DAHANCA 6/7 (2003)[69]	Stage I–IV HNC[a]			5 y	No difference (P = .78)	Severe late toxicity: no difference (P = .16)
			726	66–68/5 fxn per wk	60%		
			750	66–68/6 fxn per wk	70% (P = .0005)		

Abbreviations: AF, accelerated fractionation; BOT, base of tongue; DACB, delayed accelerated concommitant boost; fxn, fraction; HF, hyperfractionation; HR, hazard ratio; NS, not significant; OC, oral cavity; OPx, oropharynx.

[a] Subset of patients received nimorazole.

Table 2
Common dose-limiting structures and relevant radiation dose constraints

Structure	Toxicity	Dose Constraint Goal
Oral cavity	Mucositis	Maximum <55 Gy or 1% cannot exceed 65 Gy
Parotid	Xerostomia	Mean <26 Gy
Larynx	Aspiration	Mean <45–48 Gy
Inferior pharyngeal constrictor muscles	Stricture/aspiration	Mean <54 Gy
Mandible	Osteoradionecrosis	Maximum <70 Gy
Brachial plexus	Brachial plexopathy	Maximum ≤60 Gy
Spinal cord	Transverse Myelitis	Maximum <45 Gy

two-dimensional (2D) radiation was planned, which involved treatment based on anatomic landmarks identified on radiograph imaging.

In an attempt to decrease radiation-induced toxicities in patients with HNC, several alternative RT modalities have been developed. Many institutions are using a newer method of radiation delivery, called intensity-modulated radiation therapy (IMRT). IMRT is similar to 3D CRT, but the intensity of radiation can be varied across each beam. IMRT uses smaller safety margins and higher dose gradients, allowing for further sparing of the surrounding normal structures and thus decreasing toxicity. Two randomized studies[76,77] have compared salivary flow and xerostomia in patients with early-stage nasopharyngeal treated with IMRT versus 2D radiation therapy. Both of these studies found that the salivary flow rates were improved with IMRT. The study by Kam and colleagues[76] showed that there was improvement in observer-rated severe xerostomia at 1 year, but there was no difference in patient-related outcomes. A third study by Nutting and colleagues[78] compared IMRT with 2D radiation in early and locally advanced pharyngeal tumors. The investigators showed an improvement in xerostomia (greater than grade 2) at 18 months in the IMRT group compared with the conventionally treated group. These studies suggest a benefit to using IMRT.

Because small changes in the patient's position can have a large impact on the estimated RT field when using IMRT, verifying the patient's position before initiation of therapy is important. For this reason, image-guided RT (IGRT) is essential during treatment. Generally with IGRT, images are taken in the treatment position before the radiation is delivered. Some of the common forms of IGRT in HNC include MV radiographs, kV radiographs, or cone-beam CT (CBCT) scans. kV images are used to assess the bony anatomy and compare the digitally reconstructed images from the initial planning simulation scan with the image in the treatment position. CBCT is a form of 3D imaging, which involves taking a CT scan using the treatment machine on the day of treatment. CBCT scans can better delineate the soft tissues in the head and neck region and can help account for rotational shifts, which is not possible with radiographic imaging.[79] Another benefit of using IGRT is that if large shifts are required on a daily basis, the physician can choose to resimulate or replan the patient.

There is interest in using proton therapy for the treatment of HNC. The benefit of proton therapy is that the energy from the beam is deposited at a particular depth (the Bragg peak) and there is rapid dose falloff beyond this point. Therefore, proton therapy can be useful to treat tumors close to critical structures and decrease the integral dose to the patient.[80] Until recently, the disadvantage of using proton therapy for head and neck tumors was that the most common technique (passive scatter) used to deliver the treatment did not deliver the radiation as conformally as in other treatment techniques, such as IMRT. However, intensity-modulated proton therapy (IMPT) has recently been used in certain centers. IMPT takes advantage of principles of both IMRT and proton therapy, in that it is able to conform to the tumor volume and minimize low dose to the surrounding structures. Clinical outcomes from IMPT are awaited, but dosimetric studies have shown that the use of IMPT can decrease dose to surrounding critical structures, such as brainstem, spinal cord, the larynx, and parotids.[81]

PRINCIPLES OF CHEMOTHERAPY

Postoperative CRT

Postoperative CRT has been shown to decrease locoregional recurrence rates in patients with high-risk pathologic features. Two phase III trials, the RTOG 9501[73] and the EORTC 22931,[63] have investigated the role of postoperative concurrent CRT in this setting. Both trials enrolled patients with high-risk pathologic features defined as the presence of positive margins, perineural invasion, lymphovascular invasion, extracapsular extension outside the involved lymph nodes and multiple positive lymph nodes.

In the RTOG 9501 trial, 459 patients were randomized to receive cisplatin 100 mg/m^2 on day 1 of each cycle every 3 weeks for a total of 3 cycles with concurrent conventional RT (66 Gy over 6.5 weeks) versus conventional RT alone. There was a significant increase in disease-free survival and a decrease in locoregional recurrence, which was the primary end point, with 2-year locoregional control rates of 82% in the concurrent cisplatin/RT group versus 72% in the RT group. There was no benefit in OS, and the incidence of acute severe adverse events was significantly higher in the combined group (77%) compared with the RT group (34%).

In the EORTC 22931 trial, 334 patients were randomized to receive conventional RT alone (66 Gy over 6.5 weeks) versus concurrent RT with cisplatin 100 mg/m^2 every 3 weeks for 3 cycles. The primary end point was 5-year progression-free survival (PFS), which was 47% in the cisplatin/RT group versus 36% in the RT group. There was also a significant decrease in locoregional recurrence rate, with 5-year recurrence at 18% versus 31%, respectively, and a significant increase in the 5-year OS at 53% versus 40%. Severe toxicities (mucositis, myelosuppression) were more frequent (41%) in the concurrent cisplatin/RT group compared with the RT group (21%), but the incidence of late adverse events was the same.

Both trials showed that adding cisplatin does not decrease the rate of distant recurrence, which was 25% with RT versus 21% with concurrent CRT in the EORTC 22931 trial. A subsequent pooled analysis 1 year later by Bernier and colleagues[62] showed that the pathologic factors most associated with survival benefit from postoperative concurrent CRT were positive margins and extracapsular extension.

Definitive or Concurrent CRT

This approach has particular significance in locally advanced oropharyngeal, hypopharyngeal, and laryngeal cancer, in which organ preservation is of paramount importance to maintain function and quality of life. The first 2 studies that addressed the feasibility of an organ-preservation approach in HNC were the Veterans Affairs Laryngeal Cancer Study Group (VA Larynx)[82] and the EORTC 24891[83] studies, which investigated an induction strategy in patients with resectable laryngeal, hypopharyngeal, and epipharyngeal cancer (**Table 3**).

Both of these studies made evident that organ preservation is feasible and gave way to the RTOG 9–111 study, which has established the standard of care in laryngeal cancer. In this study,[84,85] 547 patients with locally advanced laryngeal cancer were randomized to receive RT alone versus concurrent CRT with weekly cisplatin for 3 cycles versus induction with cisplatin/5-fluorouracil (5FU) for 2 cycles, followed by a third cycle and then RT, if response was noted. The primary end point was larynx preservation. The results of the trial are described in more detail in **Table 3**. The 2-year larynx preservation and locoregional control rates were significantly higher at 88% and 78% in the CRT group, compared with the group receiving sequential CRT or only RT. Distant metastasis developed in 22% of patients who received only RT and was significantly lower at 15% in patients on induction chemotherapy and 12% in patients on CRT, with no difference between the latter 2 chemotherapy groups. OS was unaffected in all treatment arms, probably because patients who had recurrence after an organ-preservation approach received salvage laryngectomy.

Subsequently, multiple trials were conducted to validate the feasibility of CRT with platinum-based and 5FU-based regiments in an organ-preservation setting. The study that firmly established the use of CRT in a curative, organ preservation approach in locally advanced HNC was a meta-analysis by Pignon and colleagues[93] of 87 trials including more than 16,000 patients with early-stage and locally advanced HNC of the oral cavity, oropharynx, hypopharynx, and larynx. Included patients had received locoregional therapy alone, which mostly was RT or chemotherapy. The main conclusion was that CRT increased OS by 6.5% at 5 years, whereas no clear benefit was noted from sequential or adjuvant chemotherapy. The same study concluded that cisplatin, cisplatin/5FU, and carboplatin/5FU had a similar benefit, whereas monotherapy with any other agent other than cisplatin gave inferior results. Based on this study, the use of 5FU became questionable, given the lack of added benefit to cisplatin and the higher risk for mucosal acute toxicities. Another interesting result was that CRT had a significant impact on locoregional control rates, which was not seen with induction chemotherapy, whereas induction chemotherapy had a more pronounced impact on the rate of distant metastasis, suggesting that induction and concurrent chemotherapy may need to be administered both to achieve locoregional and distant control.

Taxane-based combination chemotherapy regimens have also been investigated[87,94] in the setting of CRT. The long-term efficacy outcomes of the combination of concurrent carboplatin/paclitaxel with standard RT was investigated in a phase II trial of locally advanced HNC in 2007 by Agarwala and colleagues.[87] Fifty-five patients with locally advanced, mostly stage IV disease were treated with weekly carboplatin and paclitaxel with concurrent standard RT for 6 to 7 weeks, with reported complete response of 52%, objective response rate of 80%, 5-year PFS of 36%, and 5-year OS of 35%. Significantly, grade 3 to 4 oral mucositis was observed in only 30% of patients. This and other trials suggest that carboplatin and paclitaxel with concurrent RT is a feasible and effective regimen, with reduced acute toxicities compared with cisplatin.

Over the past 2 decades, several phase I and II trials have been conducted at the University of Chicago[95] to evaluate the combination of 5FU and hydroxyurea concurrently with RT. The rationale behind using this combination lies in preclinical in vitro and in vivo data, which support the synergistic effect of 5FU with hydroxyurea. It is postulated that hydroxyurea depletes the intracellular pool of deoxyuridine monophosphate (dUMP) and allows for the 5FU metabolite 5-FdUMP to actively bind to its target enzyme thymidylate synthase. In addition, 5FU and hydroxyurea increase the radiosensitivity of radioresistant cell lines, in that they are both antimetabolites and act in the S phase, which is the most radioresistant phase in the cell cycle.

In 1989, Vokes and colleagues[96] conducted a phase I trial of 5FU, hydroxyurea, and concurrent standard RT (5-fluorouracil, hydroxyurea, concurrent radiotherapy [FHX])

Table 3
Clinical trials in locally advanced HNC

Clinical Trial	Chemotherapy/ Radiotherapy Regimen	N	LCR	Larynx Preservation	OS	DFR	Acute Severe Toxicities
Postoperative Concurrent Chemoradiotherapy							
RTOG 9501		459	2 y	NA	NS		≥Grade 3
(2004)	Cisplatin + RT vs RT		82%				77%
LAHN[73]	(RT: standard)		72%				34%
			(P = .01)				(P<.001)
EORTC		334	5 y	NA	5 y		≥Grade 3
22931 (2004)	Cisplatin + RT vs RT		18%		53%		41%
LAHN[63]	(RT: standard)		31%		40%		21%
			(P = .007)		(P = .02)		(P = .001)
Concurrent Chemoradiotherapy							
RTOG 9111		547	2 y	2 y	2 y	5 y	≥Grade 3 toxicities (acute and chronic)
(2003)	Cisplatin + RT		78%	88%	74%	12%	82%
LA laryngeal	vs induction cisplatin/5FU + RT		61%	75%	76%	15%	81%
cancer[84,85]	vs RT (RT: standard)		56%	70%	75%	22%	61%
			(P<.05)	(cis RT c/t induction P = .005, cis/RT c/t RT P<.001, induction c/t RT NS)	(NS)	(cis RT c/t RT, P = .03)	(cis RT c/t both other modalities p<.05)

Bonner et al (2006) LAHN[97]	Cetuximab + RT vs RT (RT: standard, AF or HF)	424	3 y 47% 34% (P<.01)	NA	3 y 55% 45% (P = .05)	2 y 16% 17% (NS)	≥Grade 3 toxicities: NS except for rash with cetux
Agarwala et al (2007)[87]	Carboplatin/paclitaxel + RT (RT: standard, boost AF)	55	Not reported	NA	5 y 35%	NA	≥Grade 3 toxicities: 30%
Sequential CRT							
VA Larynx Study (1991)[82]	Induction cisplatin/5FU + RT vs surgery + RT	332	LCR recurrence: 12% 2% (P = .0005)	5 y 66%	2 y 68% 68% (P = .09)		Grade 2 mucositis 38% 24% (p-value not reported)
EORTC 24891 (1996) Laryngeal ca[83]	Induction cisplatin/5FU + RT vs surgery + RT	202	LCR recurrence: 33% 30% (P not available)	10 y >50%	10 y 13.1% 13.8% (NS)	28% 36% (P not available)	Limiting toxicities: 14%

(continued on next page)

Table 3
(continued)

Clinical Trial	Chemotherapy/ Radiotherapy Regimen	N	LCR	Larynx Preservation	OS	DFR	Acute Severe Toxicities
TAX 323 (2007) Unresectable HNC[102]	Induction docetaxel/cisplatin/ 5FU + RT vs induction cisplatin/5FU + RT (RT: standard, AF, or HF)	358	85% 81% (*p*-value not reported)	NA	3 y 37% 26% (*P* = .02)	12.9% 10% (*P* = .003)	Neutropenia: TPF: 76% vs PF: 52% (*P*<.05) Stomatitis: TPF: 4.6% vs PF: 11.2% (*P*<.05)
TAX 324 (2007) Stage III, IV[103]	Induction docetaxel/cisplatin/5FU + concurrent CRT with carboplatin vs induction cisplatin/5FU + CRT (RT: standard)	501	30% 38% (*P* = .04)	NA	3 y 62% 48% (*P* = .006)	5% 9% (NS)	Neutropenia: 83% vs 56% (*P*<.001) Mucositis: 37% vs 38% (NS)
DeCIDE (2012) Stage III, IV[104]	Induction docetaxel/cisplatin/5FU + concurrent CRT with docetaxel/hydroxyurea/5FU vs CRT (same regimen) (RT: HF)	280	3 y LCR failure Rate 9% 12% (*P* = .5)	NA	3 y 75% 73% (*P* = .7)	10% 19% (*P* = .02)	Neutropenia: 17% Dermatitis: 19% Mucositis: 45% (all arms)

Salama et al (2008) Stage III, IV[105]	Induction carbo/taxol + CRT with paclitaxell/hydroxyurea/5FU (TFHX) (RT: HF: cohorts A, B, C/C with lower RT dose, A with higher RT dose)	222	5 y LCR 91% (similar for all groups)	NA	3 y 68% (similar for all groups)	5 y DC 87% (similar for all groups)[a]	Neutropenia:41% Mucositis: 33% (all arms)
Kies et al (2010) Stage III, IV[106]	Induction carbo/taxol/cetuximab + concurrent CRT with platinum or surgery or RT (RT: IMRT or standard RT)	47	3 y 2/47: local recurrence	NA	3 y 91%	3 y 4/47: distant recurrence	Neutropenia: 21% Dermatitis: 45%

Abbreviations: AF, accelerated fractionation; c/t, compared to; Cis, cisplatin; DC, disease control; DFR, distant failure rate; HF, hyperfractionation; LAHN, locally advanced HNC; LCR, locoregional control; NA, not available; NS, nonsignificant; TTP, time to progression.

[a] TTP worse for group C.

in poor-prognosis HNC with reported promising results. RT (180–200 cGy) administered once daily on an alternate week schedule (1 week on, 1 week off) over 13 weeks was based on a study by Byfield,[97] which allowed for amelioration of radiation-induced toxicities by delivering RT over 13 weeks. Taylor and colleagues[98] had shown promising results with good locoregional control in locally advanced HNC with concurrent 5FU/cisplatin and intermittent RT. Based on these studies, the FHX regimen was scheduled to be given in an intermittent schedule rather than continuous RT, which would have been associated with intolerable toxicities. After this study, in 1999, Haraf and colleagues[99] reported a phase II trial of patients with stage II and III HNC who received primary CRT with FHX, with surgery reserved as a salvage option. Locoregional control rate and 5-year disease-specific survival were 86% and 82%, respectively. The investigators concluded that primary CRT with FHX in stage II and III HNC was feasible and yielded similar results with historical control protocols of surgery followed by adjuvant chemotherapy and RT. The problem with this trial was the prolonged duration of RT, which was 13 weeks versus 6 weeks for the postoperative setting.

The RTOG 9703 phase II trial[100] confirmed the similar efficacy of FHX with cisplatin/5FU and cisplatin/paclitaxel with standard RT. Two-year OS was 65%, 60%, and 67%, respectively, all superior to the 2-year OS of a historical control of cisplatin with RT, which was 46%. Based on these studies and after the realization that 5FU/hydroxyurea alone yielded similar results to historical locoregional failure rates, the FHX was used as a platform for several combined chemotherapy regimens in phase I and II trials of cisplatin/5FU/hydroxyurea and paclitaxel/5FU/hydroxyurea with concurrent hyperfractionated RT in locally advanced, poor-risk, stage III and IV HNC (**Box 5**).[101,102] Hyperfractionation allows for shortening of the duration of RT with administration of higher doses of RT. These regimens are administered in the inpatient setting (Sunday–Friday) to allow for closer monitoring and ensure adequate supportive care and patient convenience. Results from these trials have been promising, with high locoregional control rates and OS compared with historical controls, achieving organ preservation and tolerable acute toxicities (**Table 4**). With such aggressive regimens, the classic failure pattern is reversed and distant failure reaches 22% compared with locoregional control failure rates of 17%, underscoring the need for strategies, such as induction chemotherapy, to address distant micrometastasis at the time of diagnosis.

Cetuximab has been approved by the US Food and Drug Administration (FDA) in the first-line setting in combination with RT. A phase III trial of cetuximab with RT by Bonner and colleagues[86] randomized 424 patients with locally advanced and unresectable HNC to receive cetuximab with RT versus RT alone. Cetuximab was started 1 week before RT at 400 mg/m^2 and was continued weekly at 250 mg/m^2 throughout RT. Compared with RT alone, cetuximab increased the 3-year OS by 10% and also increased locoregional control by 32%, which was the primary end point. Cure rate was 10% higher in the cetuximab arm. This treatment also decreased the risk of death by 26%, but the 1-year and 2-year rates of distant metastasis remained the same in both groups. In terms of side effects, the cetuximab patient group had a higher incidence of infusion reactions, acneiform rash, and nail changes. This trial did not compare the efficacy of concurrent chemotherapy, cetuximab, and RT with concurrent CRT. To address this question, a phase III RTOG trial (RTOG 0522) compared CRT with cisplatin with CRT with cisplatin and cetuximab, with disease-free survival as the primary end point, and results were negative.[103] It may be more prudent to give cetuximab with RT to patients with locally advanced HNC who cannot tolerate CRT.

Overall, the optimal concurrent CRT regimen and whether the use of 2 drugs is superior to 1 still remains a subject of debate. CRT with cisplatin 100 m/m^2 every 3 weeks is considered a standard approach for the treatment of locally advanced

Box 5
FHX-based concurrent CRT regimens investigated in phase II trials at the University of Chicago

- FHX[99]:
  - 5FU 800 mg/m^2 × 5 days
  - Hydroxyurea 1 g twice a day
  - Standard RT with 200 cGy daily, total 65 to 75 Gy
  - 1 week on, 1 week off schedule (S-F inpatient)
  - Maximum of 7 cycles
- Cisplatin-FHX[101]:
  - Cisplatin 100 mg/m^2 on cycles 1,3, 5
  - 5FU 800 mg/m^2 x 5 days
  - Hydroxyurea 1 g twice a day
  - Hyperfractionated twice-daily RT with 150 cGy, total 65 to 75 Gy
  - 1 week on, 1 week off schedule (S-F inpatient)
  - Maximum of 5 cycles
  - GCSF
- T-FHX[102]:
  - Paclitaxel 100 mg/m^2 on day 1 of each cycle
  - 5FU 600 mg/m^2 x 5 days
  - Hydroxyurea 500 mg twice a day
  - Hyperfractionated twice-daily RT with 150 cGy, total 65 to 75 Gy
  - 1 week on, 1 week off schedule (S-F inpatient)
  - Maximum of 5 cycles
  - GCSF

Abbreviations: GCSF, granulocyte colony stimulating factor; RT CFHX, cisplatin, 5FU, hydroxyurea, RT; S-F inpatient, Sunday-Friday inpatient; TFHX, paclitaxel, 5FU, hydroxyurea.

Table 4
Summarized results of phase II trials with C-FHX and T-FHX

Regimen	C-FHX[101] (N = 76) (%)	T-FHX[102] (N = 90) (%)
T4	46	61
N2 or N3	75	66
Grade III or IV leukopenia	81	31
Feeding tube placement	96	77
3-year local PFS	92	84
3-year distant PFS	83	79
3-year PFS	72	62
3-year OS	55	59

HNC in an organ-preservation strategy. Because this dose is associated with frequent side effects, such as neuropathy, nausea, and vomiting, alternative regimens are lower-dose weekly cisplatin or carboplatin/paclitaxel. However, these regimens have not been compared head to head with standard-dose cisplatin. Our institutional experience strongly supports the T-FHX regimen with hyperfractionation, which is not more toxic than cisplatin with accelerated fractionation RT. In patients who have poor performance status (PS) and are predicted to have intolerable CRT-induced toxicities, the combination of cetuximab/RT is a reasonable alternative.

Sequential CRT

Sequential CRT refers to the administration of additional cycles of chemotherapy, known as induction chemotherapy, before definitive CRT in high-risk locally advanced HNC, in an attempt to decrease distant failure and further improve locoregional control rates. The rationale behind induction chemotherapy is based on the following points: (1) head and neck tumors are better vascularized before any surgical intervention, (2) nonirradiated patients tolerate chemotherapy-associated side effects better, and (3) higher doses of chemotherapy can be administered compared with the CRT setting, with better potential for eradication of micrometastatic disease.[104]

For almost 2 decades, the Wayne State University regimen[105] remained the most effective regimen in this regard; it consists of cisplatin (100 mg/m^2) and infusional 5FU (1000 $mg/m^2/d$ for 5 days). This result was confirmed in a meta-analysis by Pignon and colleagues[106] in 2000, which showed decreased distant failure rates and improved 5-year OS by 5% in patients with locally advanced, high-risk disease who receive induction cisplatin/5FU.

From several phase II trials that indicated a promising role for the addition of taxanes in this induction regimen, 2 phase III clinical trials (TAX 323[88] and TAX 324[89]) compared docetaxel/cisplatin/5FU with cisplatin/5FU in patients with unresectable locally advanced HNC. The regimen of docetaxel/cisplatin/5FU has now been approved by the FDA (mainly from these clinical trials) as induction chemotherapy in patients with poor-risk, locally advanced resectable or unresectable HNC.

The European TAX 323 trial was a randomized controlled phase III trial of 358 patients with locally advanced stage III and IV HNC who received docetaxel, cisplatin, and 5FU (TPF) versus cisplatin and 5FU (PF) given every 3 weeks for 4 cycles, followed by RT. Median PFS was the primary end point and it was significantly longer in the TPF group (11.4 months) compared with the PF group (8.3 months). The median OS was 18.6 versus 14.2 months, respectively ($P = .02$). In this trial, patients received chemotherapy only during the induction phase and not in combination with RT. The TAX 324 trial was designed in a similar way, with the exception that induction was followed by CRT with carboplatin for a maximum of 7 cycles, in an attempt to increase locoregional control, decrease distant failure rates, and improve survival. The median OS was significantly prolonged, at 71 months for the TPF group compared with 30 months for the PF group. TPF patients had better locoregional control, but distant failure rates were similar in both groups. In both trials, the investigators concluded that the TPF regimen conferred a significant improvement in OS with a better toxicity profile compared with the PF regimen.

Both of these trials asked the question whether the addition of docetaxel to cisplatin/5FU increases median OS and reduces distant failure rate, but there was no comparison of the induction approach followed by CRT with CRT alone. This comparison is addressed in ongoing phase III randomized clinical trials. Most recently, at the 2012 Annual Meeting of the American Society of Clinical Oncology, the DeCIDE trial[90] sought to answer this question and enrolled 280 patients with locally advanced HNC (N2/N3 disease), who were randomized to receive induction chemotherapy with TPF for 2 cycles followed by CRT with the same regimen versus docetaxel, 5FU, and hydroxyurea with concurrent hyperfractionated RT. Preliminary results revealed high 3-year OS of 75% versus 73%, respectively, but with no statistical difference ($P = .7$).

Taxane-based regimens have also been investigated in an induction setting. In a study conducted as 3 sequential cohorts of 222 patients with locally advanced stage III and IV HNC, Salama and colleagues[91] hypothesized that induction chemotherapy with carboplatin/paclitaxel for 3 cycles followed by CRT with paclitaxel/5FU/hydroxyurea and hyperfractionated RT would reduce the risk of distant recurrence, maintaining the same locoregional control rate. In addition, in an attempt to reduce toxicities, they divided patients into 3 cohorts (A, B, C) with decreasing RT doses, with cohort C receiving the lowest RT dose. The OS, locoregional control, and distant control rates were similar in all 3 groups, but time to progression was shorter in cohort C. The investigators concluded that induction chemotherapy with carboplatin/paclitaxel before concurrent CRT reduces distant recurrence and maintains high locoregional control, with cohort B providing the best therapeutic ratio.

Cetuximab has also been investigated in combination with taxane-based regimens in an induction setting. In a phase II trial of 47 patients with locally advanced HNC,[92] patients received induction chemotherapy with carboplatin/paclitaxel and cetuximab weekly for 6 weeks, followed by RT, CRT, or surgery. Results were promising, with 3-year PFS of 87% and 3-year OS of 91%. The treatment was well tolerated, with the most common side effects being skin rash (45%) and neutropenia (21%).

Overall, induction chemotherapy with TPF has already been approved in patients with bulky, high-risk disease to decrease distant failure rates and improve OS and locoregional control. Another potential induction regimen is carboplatin/paclitaxel with or without cetuximab, although this has not yet been validated in larger phase III trials. **Table 3** summarizes landmark clinical trials in the management of locally advanced HNC.

Chemotherapy for Metastatic Disease

Despite the aggressive treatment protocols for the treatment of locoregional disease, approximately 50% of patients relapse either with locoregional or metastatic disease. For locoregional recurrences, salvage surgery and reirradiation should be considered. For metastatic disease, systemic chemotherapy with combinations of chemotherapy agents, targeted agents alone, or in combination with chemotherapy agents, or single-agent chemotherapy confer no OS benefit, with the exception of only 1 study that has shown statistically significant prolongation in OS[107] with the addition of cetuximab to cisplatin and 5FU. Based on this study, the standard chemotherapy regimen in this setting is considered to be cisplatin/5FU/cetuximab, but options also include platinum/5FU, platinum/taxane, single-agent chemotherapy and cetuximab monotherapy. Median OS is 6 to 9 months, whereas 1-year survival is up to 40%. Thus, the goal of treatment is palliative and aims at symptom control and improvement of quality of life. Combination chemotherapies have the highest response rates (up to 81%),[108] but this comes with higher toxicities and, potentially, worse quality of life, compared with single-agent chemotherapy.

Management recommendations for patients with recurrent/metastatic (R/M) HNC are based on several factors, such as PS, comorbidities, expected toxicity profiles, and the presence of symptoms. Another important factor is platinum refractoriness, which is defined as progression on or recurrence within 6 months of treatment with platinum-based CRT. In such cases, treatment with non–cross-resistant agents, such as taxanes and cetuximab, or enrollment in a clinical trial, should be considered.

Single-agent chemotherapy

Single-agent chemotherapy can be used in patients with poor PS, although response rates range from 10% to 15%. Active agents include platinum agents (cisplatin, carboplatin), taxanes (paclitaxel, docetaxel), 5FU/capecitabine, pemetrexed, and methotrexate.[109] Generally, monotherapy is reserved for patients who are asymptomatic and have low-burden disease or in patients with poor PS and symptomatic disease, who would not be able to tolerate the toxicities related to combination chemotherapy.

Combination chemotherapy

There are 2 main categories of combination chemotherapy regimens for metastatic HNC: platinum-based regimens (such as cisplatin/5FU) and taxane-based regimens (such as paclitaxel/cisplatin). These regimens are characterized by increased response rates but also increased toxicity and no increase in OS, with the exception of the cisplatin/5FU/cetuximab combination, as mentioned earlier, which is considered to be a reasonable first-line regimen. Generally, combination chemotherapy is indicated for patients with good PS who are symptomatic from their disease and in whom a partial response would ameliorate symptoms, even at the expense of increased toxicities. The choice between a platinum-based versus a taxane-based regimen is based more on the expected toxicity profile, with gastrointestinal, renal, and hematologic toxicities more prominent with the platinum-based regimens and neurotoxicity with the taxane-based regimens.

Platinum-based regimens (cisplatin/5FU, carboplatin/5FU). A landmark phase III randomized trial treated 249 patients[110] with R/M HNC with cisplatin or 5FU monotherapy or the combination cisplatin/5FU. Response rates were 17%, 13%, and 32%, respectively, but no differences in OS were noted.

Another randomized trial of 277 patients with R/M HNC compared cisplatin/5FU versus carboplatin/5FU versus methotrexate.[111] Response rates were 32%, 21%, and 10%, respectively, and were statistically significant compared with methotrexate. The carboplatin/5FU regimen was better tolerated compared with cisplatin/5FU. The investigators concluded that the combination regimens were associated with increased response rates, but median response durations and OS were similar for all 3 groups, with the expense of increased toxicities. This study is one of the few randomized trials that have compared combination with single-agent chemotherapy in M/R HNC.

Based on the first 2 studies, cisplatin is considered to be more effective in combination with 5FU compared with alone, as well as more effective than carboplatin, in terms of producing a response rate, but neither cisplatin-based nor carboplatin-based combination regimens have been shown to improve OS compared with single-agent chemotherapy. In addition, substitution with carboplatin is frequently inevitable because of cisplatin-induced toxicities.

Taxane-based regimens (paclitaxel/cisplatin, paclitaxel/carboplatin). A phase III randomized trial of 280 patients with metastatic HNC by Gibson and colleagues[112] compared cisplatin/5FU with cisplatin/paclitaxel. Median OS was 8.7 months compared with 8.1 months and response rates were 27% versus 26%, respectively. The most frequent toxicities included myelosuppression, nausea, vomiting, stomatitis, and diarrhea. Overall, gastrointestinal, renal, and hematologic toxicities and a higher risk of infection as a result of placement of central venous catheters were more common in the cisplatin/5FU group, whereas neurotoxicity was equally common in the 2 groups. This study supported the finding that the 2 regimens were similar in efficacy, with differences only in the toxicity profiles.

In a phase II trial,[113] 27 patients with M/R HNC were treated with carboplatin/paclitaxel in a second-line setting. Median OS was 8 months and overall response and disease control rates were 26% and 51%, respectively. The most common side effects were myelosuppression and peripheral neuropathy. The investigators concluded that this regimen was safe and moderately effective in this patient population.

Overall, the paclitaxel/carboplatin regimen seems to be gaining more acceptance in the oncology practice, mainly because of the convenience of administration and the lower rates of renal toxicity, compared with cisplatin-based regimens. It is a reasonable option for patients with metastatic disease who are expected not to tolerate cisplatin-induced toxicities, although no trials have yet shown the noninferiority of paclitaxel/carboplatin compared with cisplatin/5FU.

Targeted therapy: cetuximab

Single-agent cetuximab in platinum-resistant disease in second-line setting. Cetuximab has been approved by the FDA as a single agent in the setting of platinum-refractory HNC. This was based on a phase II, open-label, multicenter trial of 103 patients with platinum-resistant M/R HNC, the results of which were published by Vermorken and colleagues[114] in 2007. Patients who had developed progressive disease after 2 to 6 cycles of platinum-based chemotherapy were enrolled to receive cetuximab (initial dose of 400 mg/m^2 followed by weekly doses of 250 mg/m^2) for more than 6 weeks, until progressive disease ensued. In patients with progressive disease, a platinum agent could be added to cetuximab until there was further disease progression. The observed response rate to cetuximab monotherapy was 13%, and the rate of disease control (complete response, partial response, and stable disease) was 46%. The median time to disease progression was 70 days, and the median OS was 5.9 months. During the combination phase, response rate was 0%, disease control rate was 26%, and time to progression was 50 days. The only adverse side effects were allergic reactions (mostly skin rash) and a treatment-related death. The investigators concluded that cetuximab monotherapy was active and well tolerated in this patient population.

Cetuximab in combination with chemotherapy in first-line setting. In a landmark phase III trial (EXTREME) by Vermorken and colleagues[107] published in 2007, 442 patients with previously untreated M/R HNC were randomized to receive weekly cetuximab with infusional 5FU (from day 1–4 of each cycle) and cisplatin or carboplatin every 3 weeks for a maximum of 6 cycles versus 5FU with cisplatin or carboplatin in the dosage mentioned earlier. Patients in the cetuximab arm had a significantly increased median OS of 10.1 months compared with 7.4 months in the noncetuximab arm. This effect seemed to be more prominent in patients younger than 65 years who received cisplatin and had a good PS. This trial represents the only study that has shown a survival advantage in M/R HNC with a platinum-based combination and has thus established the standard of care in this patient population.

Taxane-based combinations with cetuximab have not yet been established by large phase III trials, but there is evidence that the combination may achieve the higher end of median OS in M/R HNC. In a phase II trial,[115] 46 patients with previously untreated M/R HNC received paclitaxel and weekly cetuximab until there was disease progression or unacceptable toxicity. The response rate, which was the primary end point, was 54%, with 10 (22%) complete responses and 80% disease control. Median PFS and OS were 4.2 and 8.1 months, respectively.

Overall, the current standard of care in M/R HNC is considered to be a combination of cetuximab with a platinum-based regimen, such as cisplatin/5FU or carboplatin/5FU (**Table 5**).

Table 5
Clinical trials in recurrent or metastatic HNC

Clinical Trial	Chemotherapy Regimen	N	Target Population	Response Rate	Median Overall Survival (mos)
EXTREME,[107] 2007	Cisplatin/5FU/cetuximab vs cisplatin/5FU	442	First-line recurrent or metastatic	35.6 vs 19.5%	10.1 vs 7.4
Vermorken et al,[114] 2007	Cetuximab	103	Second-line platinum-resistant recurrent or metastatic	13%	6
Hitt et al,[115] 2011	Cetuximab + paclitaxel	46	First-line recurrent or metastatic	54%	8.1
Jacobs et al,[110] 1992	Cisplatin vs 5FU vs Cisplatin/5FU	243	First-line recurrent or metastatic	17% 13% 32%	5.7 (NS)
Forastiere et al,[111] 1992	Cisplatin/5FU vs carboplatin/5FU vs MTX	261	First-line recurrent or metastatic	32% ($P<.001$ c/t MTX) 21% ($P = .05$ c/t MTX) 10%	6.6 5 5.6 (NS)
Gibson et al,[112] 2005	Cisplatin/5FU vs cisplatin/paclitaxel	280	First-line recurrent or metastatic	27% 26% (NS)	8.7 8.1 (NS)
Ferrari et al,[113] 2009	Carboplatin/paclitaxel	27	Second-line recurrent or metastatic	26%	8

Abbreviations: c/t, compared to; MTX, methotrexate; NS, not significant.

BIOMARKERS

Although HNC comprises a wide variety of tumors with different biologic behaviors, prognosis, and response to treatment, its classification is based mainly on histopathologic criteria. Under this light, attempts have been made to identify biomarkers that could help with prediction of response to treatments. The most validated predictive biomarker in HNC is HPV status, which predicts better responses to both chemotherapy and RT, and is analytically discussed in the section on future directions. Other extensively studied predictive biomarkers are epidermal growth factor receptor (EGFR), ERCC-1/XPF (excision repair cross-complementing group 1/xenoderma pigmentosum), and hypoxia-inducible factor 1a (HIF-1a). Although EGFR overexpression by immunohistochemistry, as well as increased EGFR copy number by fluorescence in situ hybridization have been shown to correlate with poor prognosis in patients with early-stage and locally advanced HNC, the same markers have been found not to be predictive of response to cetuximab.[116]

HIF-1a is a transcription factor that mediates the response of the cell to hypoxia andtranscribes vascular endothelial growth factor, glucose-transporter 1, and carbonic anhydrase genes, all involved in angiogenesis and anaerobic metabolism. Overexpression of HIF-1a by immunohistochemistry has been shown to correlate with resistance to carboplatin CRT,[117] but this has not been validated in prospective trials.

ERCC-1 forms a complex with XPF that incises damaged DNA. Because cisplatin causes the formation of DNA adducts with interstrand and intrastrand cross-linking, increased levels of the DNA repair enzymes ERCC-1/XPF are postulated to provide a resistance mechanism to its cytotoxic effect. Although some retrospective studies have shown that ERCC-1 may be a useful predictive marker of response to concurrent platinum-based RT, a comprehensive retrospective analysis of 73 tissue samples from locally advanced HNC patients who received induction with carboplatin/taxane followed by 5FU/hydroxyurea and RT[118] showed that low levels of XPF were significantly associated with good response to induction platinum-based chemotherapy ($P = .039$), whereas ERCC-1 was not correlated with OS ($P = .085$).

FUTURE DIRECTIONS

HNC is a biologically heterogeneous group of tumors that are currently treated homogeneously. Median survival of M/R HNC is less than 1 year with the use of current chemotherapy and cetuximab and 5-year OS of all stages is 40% to 50%. It is thus evident that new therapeutic approaches are needed.

To this purpose and over the past few years, different pathways have been targeted in M/R HNC, including the EGFR, VEGFR, MET, IGFR, and the Src kinase pathways. Several tyrosine kinase inhibitors as well as antibodies have been investigated as monotherapies in phase I/II trials, but results have invariably been modest. Although the analysis of these trials overrides the scope of this review, **Table 6** summarizes the inhibitors and antibodies already tested and under investigation thus far. The PI3K/Akt/mTOR, dual HER1/2, and paninhibition of HER1/2/3/4 pathways have shown more promise, with several phase III trials under way. A possible reason for these modest results is the presence of multiple driver pathways, which underscores the molecular heterogeneity of this disease and thus the need for more personalized approaches, which could tailor an inhibitor, chemotherapeutic agent, or immunotherapeutic strategy (or a cocktail of these) to specific patients. In this direction, genomic expression analysis studies are under way and have already identified distinct subtypes with differences in recurrence-free survival and OS. In a study by Chung et al,[119] these subtypes included a subtype with a possible EGFR-pathway signature,

Table 6
Clinical Trials with targeted agents in M/R Head and Neck Cancer

Clinical Trial	Phase	Line	Intervention	No	ORR	Median survival (mos)	Median\PFS (mos)
EGFR-inhibition							
Vermorken[129] 2010 (SPECTRUM)	III	1st or 2nd	Cis/5FU/panitumumab vs Cis/5FU	657	36% vs 25% (P = .007)	11.1 vs 9 (P = .14)	5.8 vs 4.8 (P = .004)
Machiels[130] 2011 (ZALUTE)	III	2nd	Zalutumumab vs BSC ± MTX	286	NA	6.7 vs 5.2 (P = .06)	9.9 vs 8.4 wks (P = .012)
Soulieres[131] 2004	II	2nd	Single agent erlotinib	115	4%	6	2.2
Stewart[132] 2009	III	2nd	Gefitinib vs MTX	466	7.6% vs 3.9% (NS)	6 vs 6.7 (NS)	NA
Seiwert[133] 2010	II	2nd	Afatinib vs Cetuximab	124	8.1% vs 9.7%	NA	13 wk vs 15 wk (P = .05)
de Souza[134] 2012	II	2nd	Single agent Lapatinib	42	0%	NA	1.6-1.7
Le Tourneau[135] 2010	II	1st	Single agent PF00299804	35	7%	NA	3.1
VEGFR-inhibition							
Gibson[136] 2009	II	1st or 2nd	Bev/Cetux	48	18% DCR = 73%	7.6	2.8
Cohen[137] 2009	I/II	1st or 2nd	Bev/Erlotinib	48	15%	7.1	4.1

Argiris[138] 2011	II	1st or 2nd	Bev/Pem	40	30% DCR: 86%	11.5	4.9
Machiels[139] 2010	II	2nd	Single agent sunitinib	38	3% DCR = 50%	3.4	2
Choong[140] 2010	II	1st, 2nd, 3rd	Single agent sunitinib	22 (PS0-1 = 15 PS 2 = 7)	PS = 0-1: RR = 8%, DCR = 33% PS = 2: RR = 0% DCR = 29%	4.9 4.4	1.8 4
Elser[141] 2007	II	1st, 2nd	Single agent sorafenib	27	3.7% DCR: 41%	4.2	1.8
Williamson[142] 2010	II	1st	Single agent sorafenib	41	2% DCR: 51%	9	4

PI3K/Akt/mTOR-inhibition

Clinical Trial	Phase	Location/Sponsor	Primary Endpoint
Temsirolimus with or without cetuximab NCT01256385	II	University of Chicago	PFS
Cis or carboplatin+cetuximab+everolimus NCT01009346	I/II	Hopkins	PFS
Everolimus+ erlotinib NCT00942734	II	MD Anderson	ORR
Cisplatin+cetuximab+temsirolimus NCT01015664	I/II	University of Tennessee	PFS
Temsirolimus+erlotinib NCT01009203	II	New Mexico Cancer Care Alliance	ORR

Abbreviations: Bev, bevacizumab; BSC, best supportive care; DCR, disease control rate; NA, not available; pem, pemetrexed; RR, response rate.

a mesenchymal-enriched subtype, a normal epitheliumlike subtype, and a subtype with high levels of antioxidant enzymes. Incorporation of these subtypes into clinical practice and guidance in decision making should be the next step in a personalized strategy.

A significant discovery in HNC was that HPV-16 is a major causative factor of oropharyngeal cancer. Several retrospective studies and case series[120,121] have already shown that HPV-positive cancers have better response to chemotherapy and radiotherapy and a significantly better OS. A landmark retrospective study by Ang and colleagues[122] in 2010 showed that HPV-positive status is an independent good prognostic factor of increased OS, irrespective of nodal status, smoking history, tumor stage, and treatment assignment. The biologic explanation of the better prognosis of HPV-positive oropharyngeal cancers is still elusive. Speculative hypotheses include the absence of the field cancerization effect by smoking and alcohol exposure and the presence of immune-surveillance mechanisms to HPV viral antigens. Several studies have also reported and validated an inverse relationship between HPV positivity and p53 mutational status, in that HPV-positive tumors tend to have a lower rate of p53 mutations.[123] Thus, the observed chemotherapy and radiation sensitivity may be caused by intact p53 tumor suppressor pathways. HPV status has not yet been incorporated in guidelines of clinical decision. Thus, HPV status should always be assessed in future clinical trial design. Treatment de-escalation and less intensive multimodality treatment of HPV-positive patients with oropharhyngeal cancer could be envisioned, sparing these patients from acute and long-term treatment-related complications with the same treatment outcome. In addition, because the incidence of HPV-positive oropharyngeal cancers is increasing, HPV vaccination is a reasonable preventive strategy, especially in younger, sexually active populations.

Over the past few years, immunotherapy strategies have been gaining more momentum as potential therapeutic approaches in HNC, more so in HPV-positive HNC.[124–126] A report at the 2012 American Society of Clinical Oncology Meeting by Lyford-Pike and colleagues[127] suggested that the PD-1:PD-L1 pathway may play a significant role in immune evasion in HPV-positive HNC. These investigators found that most tumor-infiltrating lymphocytes expressed the PD-1 coinhibitory molecule and that its ligand PD-L1 was also expressed on tumor cells and tumor-infiltrating macrophages, suggesting a therapeutic role of inhibition of this pathway with the relevant antibodies.

Finally, the fact that 8%[128] of patients with HNC develop and die of a second primary tumor highlights the importance of developing secondary screening and chemoprevention strategies.

SUMMARY

Median survival of M/R HNC with current treatment modalities is poor and thus new therapeutic approaches are urgent. Most of the biologic agents that have been tested as monotherapies show modest efficacy in M/R HNC. A possible reason is the presence of multiple driver pathways. Personalization is needed both for the agent or cocktail of agents to be used, as well as for the dosing/frequency of each agent. Standardized, cost-effective, and clinically applicable methods for molecular genomic or proteomic profiling are anticipated to define specific molecular phenotypes that are amenable to specific chemotherapeutic or targeted agents. Multimodality therapy with RT, conventional chemotherapy, and surgery will probably still remain the backbone of future therapy strategies, with the potential addition of biologics and immune interventions.

Studies have shown that patients with HNC have a significant mortality risk from causes other than their primary cancer, including acute or late treatment-related toxicities, cardiopulmonary comorbidities, and second primary tumors. Eight percent develop and die of a second primary tumor, such as lung or esophageal cancer or a second HNC. This highlights the importance of managing acute and long-term toxicities and developing secondary screening and chemoprevention strategies for these patients.

REFERENCES

1. Jemal A, Bray F, Center MM, et al. Global cancer statistics. CA Cancer J Clin 2011;61(2):69–90.
2. Braakhuis BJ, Tabor MP, Kummer JA, et al. A genetic explanation of Slaughter's concept of field cancerization: evidence and clinical implications. Cancer Res 2003;63:1727–30.
3. Leemans CR, Braakhuis BJ, Brakenhoff RH. The molecular biology of head and neck cancer. Nat Rev Cancer 2011;11(1):9–22.
4. Gasco M, Crook T. The p53 network in head and neck cancer. Oral Oncol 2003; 39:222–31.
5. Haddad RI, Shin DM. Recent advances in head and neck cancer. N Engl J Med 2008;359(11):1143–54.
6. D'Souza G, Kreimer AR, Viscidi R, et al. Case-control study of human papillomavirus and oropharyngeal cancer. N Engl J Med 2007;356(19):1944.
7. Gillison ML, Lowy DR. A causal role for human papillomavirus in head and neck cancer. Lancet 2004;363(9420):1488.
8. Sturgis EM, Cinciripini PM. Trends in head and neck cancer incidence in relation to smoking prevalence: an emerging epidemic of human papillomavirus-associated cancers? Cancer 2007;110(7):1429–35.
9. Siegel R, Ward E, Brawley O, et al. Cancer statistics, 2011. CA Cancer J Clin 2011;61(4):212–36.
10. Peretti G, Piazza C, Cocco D, et al. Transoral CO(2) laser treatment for T(is)-T(3) glottic cancer: the University of Brescia experience on 595 patients. Head Neck 2010;32:977–83.
11. Gallo A, de Vincentis M, Manciocco V, et al. CO2 laser cordectomy for early stage glottic carcinoma: a long-term follow-up of 156 cases. Laryngoscope 2002;112:370–4.
12. Hartl DM, de Mones E, Hans S, et al. Treatment of early-stage glottic cancer by transoral laser resection. Ann Otol Rhinol Laryngol 2007;116:832–6.
13. Smee RI, Meagher NS, Williams JR, et al. Role of radiotherapy in early glottic carcinoma. Head Neck 2010;32:850–9.
14. Cellai E, Frata P, Magrini SM, et al. Radical radiotherapy for early glottic cancer: results in a series of 1087 patients from two Italian radiation oncology centers. I. The case of T1N0 disease. Int J Radiat Oncol Biol Phys 2005;63:1378–86.
15. Chone CT, Yonehara E, Martins JE, et al. Importance of anterior commissure involvement in recurrence of early glottic cancer after laser endoscopic resections. Arch Otolaryngol Head Neck Surg 2007;133:882–7.
16. Stoeckli SJ, Schnieper I, Huguenin P, et al. Early glottic carcinoma: treatment according patient's preference? Head Neck 2003;25:1051–6.
17. Frata P, Cellai E, Magrini SM, et al. Radical radiotherapy for early glottic cancer: results in a series of 1087 patients from two Italian radiation oncology centers. II. The case of T2N0 disease. Int J Radiat Oncol Biol Phys 2005;63:1387–94.

18. Grant DG, Salassa JR, Hinni ML, et al. Transoral laser microsurgery for carcinoma of the supraglottic larynx. Otolaryngol Head Neck Surg 2007;136:900–5.
19. Laccourreye O, Salzer SJ, Brasnu D, et al. Glottic carcinoma with a fixed true vocal cord: outcomes after neoadjuvant chemotherapy and supracricoid partial laryngectomy with cricohyoidoepiglottopexy. Otolaryngol Head Neck Surg 1996;114:400–6.
20. Webster KT, Samlan RA, Jones B, et al. Supracricoid partial laryngectomy: swallowing, voice and speech outcomes. Ann Otol Rhinol Laryngol 2010;119:10–6.
21. Simonelli M, Ruoppolo G, de Vincentis M, et al. Swallowing ability and chronic aspiration after supracricoid partial laryngectomy. Otolaryngol Head Neck Surg 2010;142:873–8.
22. Haughey BH, Hinni ML, Salassa JR, et al. Transoral laser microsurgery as primary treatment for advanced-stage oropharyngeal cancer: a United States multicenter study. Head Neck 2011;33:1683–94.
23. Weinstein GS, O'Malley BW Jr, Cohen MA, et al. Transoral robotic surgery for advanced oropharyngeal carcinoma. Arch Otolaryngol Head Neck Surg 2010;136:1079–85.
24. Rusthoven KE, Raben D, Ballonoff A, et al. Effect of radiation techniques in treatment of oropharynx cancer. Laryngoscope 2008;118:635–9.
25. Lee NY, de Arruda FF, Puri DR, et al. A comparison of intensity-modulated radiation therapy and concomitant boost radiotherapy in the setting of concurrent chemotherapy for locally advanced oropharyngeal carcinoma. Int J Radiat Oncol Biol Phys 2006;66:966–74.
26. Rich JT, Milov S, Lewis JS Jr, et al. Transoral laser microsurgery (TLM) +/- adjuvant therapy for advanced stage oropharyngeal cancer: outcomes and prognostic factors. Laryngoscope 2009;119:1709–19.
27. Cohen MA, Weinstein GS, O'Malley BW Jr, et al. Transoral robotic surgery and human papillomavirus status: oncologic results. Head Neck 2011;33:573–80.
28. Steiner W, Fierek O, Ambrosch P, et al. Transoral laser microsurgery of the base of tongue. Arch Otolaryngol Head Neck Surg 2003;129:36–43.
29. O'Malley BW Jr, Weinstein GS, Snyder W, et al. Transoral robotic surgery (TORS) for base of tongue neoplasms. Laryngoscope 2006;116:1465–72.
30. De Almeida JR, Genden EM. Robotic surgery for oropharynx cancer: promise, challenges, and future directions. Curr Oncol Rep 2012;14:148–57.
31. Genden EM, Kotz T, Tong CCL, et al. Transoral robotic resection and reconstruction for head and neck cancer. Laryngoscope 2011;121:1668–74.
32. White HN, Moore EJ, Rosenthal EL, et al. Transoral robotic-assisted surgery for head and neck squamous cell carcinoma: one and 2-year survival analysis. Arch Otolaryngol Head Neck Surg 2010;136:1248–52.
33. Moore EJ, Olsen SM, LaBorde RR, et al. Long term functional and oncologic results of transoral robotic surgery for oropharyngeal squamous cell carcinoma. Mayo Clin Proc 2012;87:219–25.
34. Weinstein GS, Quon H, O'Malley BW Jr, et al. Selective neck dissection and deintensified postoperative radiation and chemotherapy for oropharyngeal cancer: a subset analysis of the University of Pennsylvania transoral robotic surgery trial. Laryngoscope 2010;120:1749–55.
35. Bocca E. Conservative neck dissection. Laryngoscope 1975;85:1511–5.
36. Robbins KT, Shannon K, Vieira F. Superselective neck dissection after chemoradiation: feasibility based on clinical and pathologic comparisons. Arch Otolaryngol Head Neck Surg 2007;133:486–9.

37. Langerman A, Plein C, Vokes EE, et al. Neck response to chemoradiotherapy: complete radiographic response correlates with pathologic complete response in locoregionally advanced head and neck cancer. Arch Otolaryngol Head Neck Surg 2009;135:1133–6.
38. Langerman A, Plein C, Vokes EE, et al. Neck dissection planning based on post-chemoradiation computed tomography in patients with head and neck cancer. Arch Otolaryngol Head Neck Surg 2009;135:876–80.
39. Ferlito A, Corry J, Silver CE, et al. Planned neck dissection for patients with complete response to chemoradiotherapy: a concept approaching obsolescence. Head Neck 2010;32:253–61.
40. de Bree R, van den Putten L, Brouwer J, et al. Detection of locoregional recurrent head and neck cancer after (chemo)radiotherapy using modern imaging. Oral Oncol 2009;45:386–93.
41. Nieuwenhuis EJ, Castelijns JA, Pijpers R, et al. Wait-and-see policy for the N0 neck in early stage oral and oropharyngeal squamous cell carcinoma using ultrasound-guided cytology: is there a role for identification of the sentinel node? Head Neck 2002;24:282–9.
42. Morton DL, Wen DR, Wong JH, et al. Technical details of intraoperative lymphatic mapping for early stage melanoma. Arch Surg 1992;127:392–9.
43. Murer K, Huber GF, Haile SR, et al. Comparison of morbidity between sentinel node biopsy and elective neck dissection for treatment of the N0 neck in patients with oral squamous cell carcinoma. Head Neck 2011;33:1260–4.
44. Civantos FJ, Zitsch RP, Schuller DE, et al. Sentinel lymph node biopsy accurately stages the regional lymph nodes for T1-T2 oral squamous cell carcinomas: results of a prospective multi-institutional trial. J Clin Oncol 2010;28: 1395–400.
45. Alkureishi LW, Ross GL, Shoaib T, et al. Sentinel node biopsy in head and neck squamous cell cancer: 5-year follow-up of European multicenter trial. Ann Surg Oncol 2010;17:2459–64.
46. Flach GB, Broglie MA, van Schie A, et al. Sentinel node biopsy for oral and oropharyngeal squamous cell carcinoma in the previously treated neck. Oral Oncol 2012;48:85–9.
47. Kim AJ, Suh JD, Sercarz JA, et al. Salvage surgery with free flap reconstruction: factors affecting outcome after treatment of recurrent head and neck squamous carcinoma. Laryngoscope 2007;117:1019–23.
48. Goodwin WJ. Salvage surgery for patients with recurrent squamous cell carcinoma of the upper aerodigestive tract: when do the ends justify the means? Laryngoscope 2000;110:1–18.
49. Hutcheson KA, Alvarez CP, Barringer DA, et al. Outcomes of elective total laryngectomy for laryngopharyngeal dysfunction in disease-free head and neck cancer survivors. Otolaryngol Head Neck Surg 2012;146:585–90.
50. Starmer HM, Agrawal N, Koch W, et al. Does prosthesis diameter matter? The relationship between voice prosthesis diameter and complications. Otolaryngol Head Neck Surg 2011;144:740–6.
51. Spiegel JH, Polat JK. Microvascular flap reconstruction by otolaryngologists: prevalence, postoperative care, and monitoring techniques. Laryngoscope 2007;117:485–90.
52. Lutz BS, Wei FC. Microsurgical workhorse flaps in head and neck reconstruction. Clin Plast Surg 2005;32:421–30.
53. Park CW, Miles BA. The expanding role of the anterolateral thigh free flap in head and neck reconstruction. Curr Opin Otolaryngol Head Neck Surg 2011;19:263–8.

54. Kruse AL, Bredell MG, Lubbers HT, et al. Clinical reliability of radial forearm free-flap procedure in reconstructive head and neck surgery. J Craniofac Surg 2011;22:822–5.
55. Dean NR, Wax MK, Virgin FW, et al. Free flap reconstruction of lateral mandibular defects: indications and outcomes. Otolaryngol Head Neck Surg 2012;146:547–52.
56. Moukarbel RV, White JB, Fung K, et al. The scapular free flap: when versatility is needed in head and neck reconstruction. J Otolaryngol Head Neck Surg 2010;39:572–8.
57. Genden EM, Rinaldo A, Suarez C, et al. Complications of free flap transfers for head and neck reconstruction following cancer resection. Oral Oncol 2004;40:979–84.
58. Arce K, Bell RB, Potter JK, et al. Vascularized free tissue transfer for reconstruction of ablative defects in oral and oropharyngeal cancer patients undergoing salvage surgery following concomitant chemoradiation. Int J Oral Maxillofac Surg 2012;41:733–8.
59. Choi S, Schwartz DL, Farwell DG, et al. Radiation therapy does not impact local complications rates after free flap reconstruction for head and neck cancer. Arch Otolaryngol Head Neck Surg 2004;130:1308–12.
60. Pfister DG, Ang KK, Brizel D, et al, National Comprehensive Cancer Network Clinical Practice Guidelines in Oncology. Head and neck cancers. J Natl Compr Canc Netw 2011;9(6):596–650.
61. Ang KK, Trotti A, Brown BW, et al. Randomized trial addressing risk features and time factors of surgery plus radiotherapy in advanced head-and-neck cancer. Int J Radiat Oncol Biol Phys 2001;51(3):571–8.
62. Bernier J, Cooper JS, Pajak TF, et al. Defining risk levels in locally advanced head and neck cancers: a comparative analysis of concurrent postoperative radiation plus chemotherapy trials of the EORTC (#22931) and RTOG (# 9501). Head Neck 2005;27(10):843–50.
63. Bernier J, Domenge C, Ozsahin M, et al. Postoperative irradiation with or without concomitant chemotherapy for locally advanced head and neck cancer. N Engl J Med 2004;350(19):1945–52.
64. Horiot JC, Le Fur R, N'Guyen T, et al. Hyperfractionation versus conventional fractionation in oropharyngeal carcinoma: final analysis of a randomized trial of the EORTC cooperative group of radiotherapy. Radiother Oncol 1992;25(4):231–41.
65. Fu KK, Pajak TF, Trotti A, et al. A Radiation Therapy Oncology Group (RTOG) phase III randomized study to compare hyperfractionation and two variants of accelerated fractionation to standard fractionation radiotherapy for head and neck squamous cell carcinomas: first report of RTOG 9003. Int J Radiat Oncol Biol Phys 2000;48(1):7–16.
66. Horiot JC, Bontemps P, van den Bogaert W, et al. Accelerated fractionation (AF) compared to conventional fractionation (CF) improves loco-regional control in the radiotherapy of advanced head and neck cancers: results of the EORTC 22851 randomized trial. Radiother Oncol 1997;44(2):111–21.
67. Saunders MI, Rojas AM, Parmar MK, et al. Mature results of a randomized trial of accelerated hyperfractionated versus conventional radiotherapy in head-and-neck cancer. Int J Radiat Oncol Biol Phys 2010;77(1):3–8.
68. Dische S, Saunders M, Barrett A, et al. A randomised multicentre trial of CHART versus conventional radiotherapy in head and neck cancer. Radiother Oncol 1997;44(2):123–36.

69. Overgaard J, Hansen HS, Specht L, et al. Five compared with six fractions per week of conventional radiotherapy of squamous-cell carcinoma of head and neck: DAHANCA 6 and 7 randomised controlled trial. Lancet 2003;362(9388):933–40.
70. Ang KK, Wheeler RH, Rosenthal DI, et al. A phase III trial to test accelerated versus standard fractionation in combination with concurrent cisplatin for head and neck carcinomas (RTOG 0129): report of efficacy and toxicity. Int J Radiat Oncol Biol Phys 2010;77(1):1–2.
71. Yamazaki H, Nishiyama K, Tanaka E, et al. Radiotherapy for early glottic carcinoma (T1N0M0): results of prospective randomized study of radiation fraction size and overall treatment time. Int J Radiat Oncol Biol Phys 2006;64(1):77–82.
72. Le QT, Fu KK, Kroll S, et al. Influence of fraction size, total dose, and overall time on local control of T1-T2 glottic carcinoma. Int J Radiat Oncol Biol Phys 1997; 39(1):115–26.
73. Cooper JS, Pajak TF, Forastiere AA, et al. Postoperative concurrent radiotherapy and chemotherapy for high-risk squamous-cell carcinoma of the head and neck. N Engl J Med 2004;350(19):1937–44.
74. O'Sullivan B, Warde P, Grice B, et al. The benefits and pitfalls of ipsilateral radiotherapy in carcinoma of the tonsillar region. Int J Radiat Oncol Biol Phys 2001; 51(2):332–43.
75. Mendenhall WM, Morris CG, Amdur RJ, et al. Definitive radiotherapy for tonsillar squamous cell carcinoma. Am J Clin Oncol 2006;29(3):290–7.
76. Kam MK, Leung SF, Zee B, et al. Prospective randomized study of intensity-modulated radiotherapy on salivary gland function in early-stage nasopharyngeal carcinoma patients. J Clin Oncol 2007;25(31):4873–9.
77. Pow EH, Kwong DL, McMillan AS, et al. Xerostomia and quality of life after intensity-modulated radiotherapy vs. conventional radiotherapy for early-stage nasopharyngeal carcinoma: initial report on a randomized controlled clinical trial. Int J Radiat Oncol Biol Phys 2006;66(4):981–91.
78. Nutting C, A'Hern R, Rogers MS, et al. First results of a phase III multicenter randomized controlled trial of intensity modulated (IMRT) versus conventional radiotherapy (RT) in head and neck cancer (PARSPORT: ISRCTN48243537; CRUK/03/005) [abstract LBA6006]. J Clin Oncol 2009;27(suppl):18s.
79. Parvathaneni U, Laramore GE, Liao JJ. Technical advances and pitfalls in head and neck radiotherapy. J Oncol 2012;2012:597467.
80. Mendenhall NP, Malyapa RS, Su Z, et al. Proton therapy for head and neck cancer: rationale, potential indications, practical considerations, and current clinical evidence. Acta Oncol 2011;50(6):763–71.
81. Simone CB 2nd, Ly D, Dan TD, et al. Comparison of intensity-modulated radiotherapy, adaptive radiotherapy, proton radiotherapy, and adaptive proton radiotherapy for treatment of locally advanced head and neck cancer. Radiother Oncol 2011;101(3):376–82.
82. [No authors listed] Induction chemotherapy plus radiation compared with surgery plus radiation in patients with advanced laryngeal cancer. The Department of Veterans Affairs Laryngeal Cancer Study Group. N Engl J Med 1991; 324(24):1685–90.
83. Lefebvre JL, Andry G, Chevalier D, et al. Laryngeal preservation with induction chemotherapy for hypopharyngeal squamous cell carcinoma: 10-year results of EORTC trial 24891. Ann Oncol 2012;23(10):2708–14.
84. Forastiere AA, Goepfert H, Maor M, et al. Concurrent chemotherapy and radiotherapy for organ preservation in advanced laryngeal cancer. N Engl J Med 2003;349(22):2091–8.

85. Forastiere AA, Maor M, Weber RS, et al. Long-term results of Intergroup RTOG 91-11: a phase III trial to preserve the larynx–induction cisplatin/5-FU and radiation therapy versus concurrent cisplatin and radiation therapy versus radiation therapy. Journal of Clinical Oncology, 2006 ASCO Annual Meeting Proceedings Part I. Vol. 24, No. 18S (June 20 Supplement). 2006. p. 5517.
86. Bonner JA, Harari PM, Giralt J, et al. Radiotherapy plus cetuximab for squamous-cell carcinoma of the head and neck. N Engl J Med 2006;354(6):567–78.
87. Agarwala SS, Cano E, Heron DE, et al. Long-term outcomes with concurrent carboplatin, paclitaxel and radiation therapy for locally advanced, inoperable head and neck cancer. Ann Oncol 2007;18(7):1224–9.
88. Vermorken JB, Remenar E, van Herpen C, et al, EORTC 24971/TAX 323 Study Group. Cisplatin, fluorouracil, and docetaxel in unresectable head and neck cancer. N Engl J Med 2007;357(17):1695–704.
89. Posner MR, Hershock DM, Blajman CR, et al, TAX 324 Study Group. Cisplatin and fluorouracil alone or with docetaxel in head and neck cancer. N Engl J Med 2007;357(17):1705–15.
90. Cohen EE, Karrison T, Kocherginsky M, et al. DeCIDE: a phase III randomized trial of docetaxel (D), cisplatin (P), 5-fluorouracil (F) (TPF) induction chemotherapy (IC) in patients with N2/N3 locally advanced squamous cell carcinoma of the head and neck (SCCHN). 2012 ASCO Annual Meeting [abstract 5500]. J Clin Oncol 2012;30(suppl).
91. Salama JK, Stenson KM, Kistner EO, et al. Induction chemotherapy and concurrent chemoradiotherapy for locoregionally advanced head and neck cancer: a multi-institutional phase II trial investigating three radiotherapy dose levels. Ann Oncol 2008;19(10):1787–94.
92. Kies MS, Holsinger FC, Lee JJ, et al. Induction chemotherapy and cetuximab for locally advanced squamous cell carcinoma of the head and neck: results from a phase II prospective trial. J Clin Oncol 2010;28(1):8–14.
93. Pignon JP, le Maître A, Maillard E, et al. Meta-analysis of chemotherapy in head and neck cancer (MACH-NC): an update on 93 randomised trials and 17,346 patients. Radiother Oncol 2009;92(1):4–14.
94. Chougule PB, Akhtar MS, Akerley W, et al. Chemoradiotherapy for advanced inoperable head and neck cancer: a phase II study. Semin Radiat Oncol 1999;9:58–63.
95. Argiris A, Haraf DJ, Kies MS, et al. Intensive concurrent chemoradiotherapy for head and neck cancer with 5-fluorouracil- and hydroxyurea-based regimens: reversing a pattern of failure. Oncologist 2003;8:350–60.
96. Vokes EE, Panje WR, Schilsky RL, et al. Hydroxyurea, fluorouracil and concomitant radiotherapy in poor prognosis head and neck cancer: a phase I-II study. J Clin Oncol 1989;7:761–8.
97. Byfield JE, Sharp TR, Frankel SS, et al. Phase I and II trial of five-day infused 5-fluorouracil and radiation in advanced cancer of the head and neck. J Clin Oncol 1984;2(5):406–13.
98. Taylor SG 4th, Murthy AK, Showel JL, et al. Improved control in advanced head and neck cancer with simultaneous radiation and cisplatin/5-FU chemotherapy. Cancer Treat Rep 1985;69(9):933–9.
99. Haraf DJ, Kies M, Rademaker AW, et al. Radiation therapy with concomitant hydroxyurea and fluorouracil in stage II and III head and neck cancer. J Clin Oncol 1999;17:638–44.
100. Garden AS, Pajak TF, Vokes E et al. Preliminary results of RTOG 9703- a phase II randomized trial of concurrent radiation (RT) and chemotherapy for advanced

squamous cell carcinomas (SCC) of the head and neck. 2001 ASCO Annual Meeting. Proc Am Soc Clin Oncol 2001:20. [abstract 891].
101. Haraf DJ, Vokes EE, Weichselbaum RR, et al. Concomitant chemoradiotherapy with cisplatin, 5-fluorouracil and hydroxyurea in poor prognosis head and neck cancer. Laryngoscope 1992;102:630–6.
102. Vokes EE, Haraf DJ, Brockstein BE, et al. Paclitaxel, 5-fluorouracil, hydroxyurea, and concomitant radiation therapy for poor-prognosis head and neck cancer. Semin Radiat Oncol 1999;9(2 Suppl 1):70–6.
103. Ang KK, Zhang QE, Rosenthal DI, et al. A randomized phase III trial (RTOG 0522) of concurrent accelerated radiation plus cisplatin with or without cetuximab for stage III-IV head and neck squamous cell carcinomas (HNC) [abstract 5500]. J Clin Oncol 2011;29(suppl).
104. Posner MR, Haddad RI, Wirth L, et al. Induction chemotherapy in locally advanced squamous cell cancer of the head and neck: evolution of the sequential treatment approach. Semin Oncol 2004;31:778–85.
105. Rooney M, Kish J, Jacobs J, et al. Improved complete response rate and survival in advanced head and neck cancer after three-course induction therapy with 120-hour 5-FU infusion and cisplatin. Cancer 1985;55:1123–8.
106. Pignon JP, Bourhis J, Domenge C, et al. Chemotherapy added to locoregional treatment for head and neck squamous-cell carcinoma: three metaanalyses of updated individual data. Lancet 2000;355:949–55.
107. Vermorken JB, Mesia R, Rivera F, et al. Platinum-based chemotherapy plus cetuximab in head and neck cancer. N Engl J Med 2008;359(11):1116–27.
108. Colevas AD. Chemotherapy options for patients with metastatic or recurrent squamous cell carcinoma of the head and neck. J Clin Oncol 2006;24(17): 2644–52.
109. Urba SG, Forastiere AA. Systemic therapy of head and neck cancer: most effective agents, areas of promise. Oncology (Williston Park) 1989;3(4):79–88 [discussion: 88, 90, 97–8].
110. Jacobs C, Lyman G, Velez-Garcia E, et al. A phase III randomized study comparing cisplatin and fluorouracil as single agents and in combination for advanced squamous cell carcinoma of the head and neck. J Clin Oncol 1992;10:257–63.
111. Forastiere AA, Metch B, Schuller DE, et al. Randomized comparison of cisplatin plus fluorouracil and carboplatin plus fluorouracil versus methotrexate in advanced squamous-cell carcinoma of the head and neck: a Southwest Oncology Group study. J Clin Oncol 1992;10(8):1245–51.
112. Gibson MK, Li Y, Murphy B, et al. Randomized phase III evaluation of cisplatin plus fluorouracil versus cisplatin plus paclitaxel in advanced head and neck cancer (E1395): an intergroup trial of the Eastern Cooperative Oncology Group. J Clin Oncol 2005;23:3562–7.
113. Ferrari D, Fiore J, Codecà C, et al. A phase II study of carboplatin and paclitaxel for recurrent or metastatic head and neck cancer. Anticancer Drugs 2009;20(3): 185–90.
114. Vermorken JB, Trigo J, Hitt R, et al. Open-label, uncontrolled, multicenter phase II study to evaluate the efficacy and toxicity of cetuximab as a single agent in patients with recurrent and/or metastatic squamous cell carcinoma of the head and neck who failed to respond to platinum-based therapy. J Clin Oncol 2007;25(16):2171–7.
115. Hitt R, Irigoyen A, Cortes-Funes H, et al. Phase II study of the combination of cetuximab and weekly paclitaxel in the first-line treatment of patients with

recurrent and/or metastatic squamous cell carcinoma of head and neck. Spanish Head and Neck Cancer Cooperative Group (TTCC). Ann Oncol 2012;23(4):1016–22.
116. Licitra L, Mesia R, Rivera F, et al. Evaluation of EGFR gene copy number as a predictive biomarker for the efficacy of cetuximab in combination with chemotherapy in the first-line treatment of recurrent and/or metastatic squamous cell carcinoma of the head and neck: EXTREME study. Ann Oncol 2011;22(5):1078–87.
117. Koukourakis MI, Giatromanolaki A, Sivridis E, et al. Hypoxia-inducible factor (HIF1A and HIF2A), angiogenesis, and chemoradiotherapy outcome of squamous cell head-and-neck cancer. Int J Radiat Oncol Biol Phys 2002;53(5):1192–202.
118. Jun HJ, Ahn MJ, Kim HS, et al. ERCC1 expression as a predictive marker of squamous cell carcinoma of the head and neck treated with cisplatin-based concurrent chemoradiation. Br J Cancer 2008;99(1):167–72.
119. Chung CH, Parker JS, Karaca G, et al. Molecular classification of head and neck squamous cell carcinomas using patterns of gene expression. Cancer Cell 2004;5:489–500.
120. Mellin Dahlstrand H, Lindquist D, Bjornestal L, et al. P16(INK4a) correlates to human papillomavirus presence, response to radiotherapy and clinical outcome in tonsillar carcinoma. Anticancer Res 2005;25(6C):4375–83.
121. Lindel K, Beer KT, Laissue J, et al. Human papillomavirus positive squamous cell carcinoma of the oropharynx: a radiosensitive subgroup of head and neck carcinoma. Cancer 2001;92(4):805–13.
122. Ang KK, Harris J, Wheeler R, et al. Human papillomavirus and survival of patients with oropharyngeal cancer. N Engl J Med 2010;363(1):24–35.
123. Westra WH, Taube JM, Poeta ML, et al. Inverse relationship between human papillomavirus-16 infection and disruptive p53 gene mutations in squamous cell carcinoma of the head and neck. Clin Cancer Res 2008;14:366–9.
124. Tong CC, Kao J, Sikora AG, et al. Recognizing and reversing the immunosuppressive tumor microenvironment of head and neck cancer. Immunol Res 2012;54(1–3):266–74.
125. Ferris RL, Hunt JL, Ferrone S. Human leukocyte antigen (HLA) class I defects in head and neck cancer: molecular mechanisms and clinical significance. Immunol Res 2005;33(2):113–33.
126. De Costa AM, Young MR. Immunotherapy for head and neck cancer: advances and deficiencies. Anticancer Drugs 2011;22(7):674–81.
127. Lyford-Pike S, Peng S, Taube JM, et al. PD-1:PD-L1(B7-H1) pathway in adaptive resistance: a novel mechanism for tumor immune escape in human papillomavirus-related head and neck cancers. Oral Abstract Session, Head and Neck Cancer [abstract 5506]. J Clin Oncol 2012;30(suppl).
128. Argiris A, Brockstein BE, Haraf DJ, et al. Competing causes of death and second primary tumors in patients with locoregionally advanced head and neck cancer treated with chemoradiotherapy. Clin Cancer Res 2004;10(6):1956–62.
129. Vermorken JB, Stöhlmacher J, Davidenko I, et al. An analysis of safety in patients (pts) with recurrent and/or metastatic squamous cell carcinoma of the head and neck (R/M SCCHN) receiving chemotherapy (CT) with or without panitumumab (pmab) in a phase III clinical trial (SPECTRUM). J Clin Oncol 2009;27(Suppl 15):313s [abstract 6050].
130. Machiels JP, Subramanian S, Ruzsa A, et al. Zalutumumab plus best supportive care versus best supportive care alone in patients with recurrent or metastatic

squamous-cell carcinoma of the head and neck after failure of platinum-based chemotherapy: an open-label, randomised phase 3 trial. Lancet Oncol 2011; 12(4):333–43.
131. Soulieres D, Senzer NN, Vokes EE, et al. Multicenter phase II study of erlotinib, an oral epidermal growth factor receptor tyrosine kinase inhibitor, in patients with recurrent or metastatic squamous cell cancer of the head and neck. J Clin Oncol 2004;22(1):77–85.
132. Stewart JS, Cohen EE, Licitra L. Phase III study of gefitinib compared with intravenous methotrexate for recurrent squamous cell carcinoma of the head and neck [corrected]. J Clin Oncol 2009;27(11):1864–71.
133. Seiwert TY, Clement PM, Cupissol D, et al. BIBW 2992 versus cetuximab in patients with metastatic or recurrent head and neck cancer (SCCHN) after failure of platinum-containing therapy with a cross-over period for progressing patients: preliminary results of a randomized, open-label phase II study. J Clin Oncol 2010;28 [abstract 5501].
134. de Souza JA, Davis DW, Zhang Y. A phase II study of lapatinib in recurrent/metastatic squamous cell carcinoma of the head and neck. Clin. Cancer Res. 2012;18(8):2336–43.
135. Le Tourneau C, Winquist E, Hottes SJ, et al. Phase II trial of the irreversible oral pan-HER inhibitor PF-00299804 (PF) as first-line treatment in recurrent and/or metastatic (RM) squamous cell carcinoma of the head and neck (SCCHN). J Clin Oncol 2010;28:15s [Suppl; abstract 5531].
136. Gibson MK, Kies M, Kim S, et al. Cetuximab (C) and bevacizumab (B) in patients with recurrent or metastatic head and neck squamous cell carcinoma: An updated report. J Clin Oncol 2009;27:15s [Suppl; abstract 6049].
137. Cohen EE, Davis DW, Karrison TG, et al. Erlotinib and bevacizumab in patients with recurrent or metastatic squamous-cell carcinoma of the head and neck: a phase I/II study. Lancet Oncol 2009;10(3):247–57.
138. Argiris A, Karamouzis MV, Gooding WE, et al. Phase II trial of pemetrexed and bevacizumab in patients with recurrent or metastatic head and neck cancer. J Clin Oncol 2011;29(9):1140–5.
139. Machiels JP, Henry S, Zanetta S, et al. Phase II study of sunitinib in recurrent or metastatic squamous cell carcinoma of the head and neck: GORTEC 2006-01. J Clin Oncol 2010;28(1):21–8.
140. Choong NW, Kozloff M, Taber D, et al. Phase II study of sunitinib malate in head and neck squamous cell carcinoma. Invest New Drugs 2010;28(5):677–83.
141. Elser C, Siu LL, Winquist E, et al. Phase II trial of sorafenib in patients with recurrent or metastatic squamous cell carcinoma of the head and neck or nasopharyngeal carcinoma. J Clin Oncol 2007;25(24):3766–73.
142. Williamson SK, Moon J, Huang CH, et al. Phase II evaluation of sorafenib in advanced and metastatic squamous cell carcinoma of the head and neck: Southwest Oncology Group Study S0420. J Clin Oncol 2010;28(20):3330–5.

Multidisciplinary Management of Esophageal Cancer

Charles R. Mulligan Jr, MD[a,b,*]

KEYWORDS

• Esophageal cancer • Clinical staging • Endoscopic ultrasound
• Multidisciplinary teams

KEY POINTS

- Accurate clinical staging using fused positron emission tomography (PET)-CT scans and endoscopic ultrasound (EUS) is imperative to formulate an optimal treatment plan for patients with esophageal cancer.
- Surgery provides optimal treatment of suitable patients with stage I or IIA cancer.
- Multimodality therapy is the cornerstone of treatment of advanced-stage esophageal cancer.
- Palliative therapies for esophageal are varied and depend on patients' performance status.

Esophageal cancer was diagnosed in approximately 17,460 patients in 2012 and 15,070 succumbed to their disease in the United States.[1] Esophageal cancer is a difficult disease to cure and generally requires the input of multiple disciplines to optimize overall results. Gastroenterologists, medical oncologists, radiation oncologists, and thoracic surgical oncologists as well as nutritionists, clinical psychologists, and nurse navigators all play a part in the decision making and execution of treatment plans. Additional roles for physical therapy and speech pathology are needed at various times.

The optimum treatment depends on patient comorbidities and clinical stage at presentation. Many patients have lost significant weight and are malnourished at presentation. Risk stratification for esophageal cancer has changed over the past 30 years as adenocarcinoma has increased in incidence. Esophageal adenocarcinomas risk factors include gastroesophageal reflux disease, Barrett esophagus, and tobacco abuse.[2] Reflux disease is exacerbated by obesity, dietary habits, and medications.[3]

[a] Thoracic Surgery, Helen F. Graham Cancer Center, Christiana Health Care System, Newark, DE 19713, USA; [b] Centra Thoracic Surgery, Alan B. Pearson Regional Cancer Center, Centra Health, 1701 Thomson Drive, Lynchburg, VA 24501, USA
* Centra Thoracic Surgery, Alan B. Pearson Regional Cancer Center, Centra Health, 1701 Thomson Drive, Lynchburg, VA 24501.
E-mail address: crmulli@msn.com

Surg Oncol Clin N Am 22 (2013) 217–246
http://dx.doi.org/10.1016/j.soc.2012.12.006 surgonc.theclinics.com

Multidisciplinary tumor boards and teams have been shown to improve outcomes in treatment of esophageal cancer. By meeting and discussing each patient in a prospective fashion, a consensus on a treatment plan can be made and implemented. The improved outcomes in treatment, especially in surgically resected patients, are related to an inherent selection bias of the group decision. This bias is based on better preclinical staging by appropriate imaging studies and improved patient risk stratification obtained using clinical practice guidelines.[4,5] Stephens and colleagues[6] found a reduction in perioperative morbidity and mortality and improved survival in a patient cohort using a multidisciplinary team approach. Low and colleagues[7] similarly reported outstanding morbidity and mortality results in resected patients. They credited clinical pathways and tumor board evaluation for improved patient selection leading to better outcomes. This article reviews the multidisciplinary management of esophageal cancer.

DIAGNOSIS

Gastroenterologists typically are the gatekeepers of the esophageal cancer patients. Upper endoscopy is indicated for symptoms as well as evaluation of abnormal radiographs.[8,9] It is also used in surveillance and biopsy in Barrett esophagus. Endoscopists define the location of the tumor, screen for skip lesions, and obtain the tissue for diagnosis.

The clinical staging of esophageal cancer entails defining the extent of disease. Tumor depth of invasion and length, nodal status, and distant disease are defined by imaging studies and endoscopy. CT and PET scans are the mainstay of excluding distant disease. They provide anatomic location and can visualize potential nodal disease and define distant metastasis. EUS provides more accurate definition of the depth of invasion and nodal status; however, malignant strictures may not be passable in 10% to 38% of the cases necessitating dilation to complete.[10] Neck and abdominal ultrasound and selected MRI can be used as adjuncts to confirm or exclude metastatic disease of the liver, adrenal gland, and cervical nodal disease.

STAGING

The 7th edition of the American Joint Committee on Cancer (AJCC)/International Union Against Cancer *Cancer Staging Manual* has defined new stage categories for adenocarcinoma and squamous cell carcinoma of the esophagus, driven by surgical resected patient data.[11] It is more complex than the TNM system of the past. Now nonanatomic factors play a role, including histopathologic cell type and grade (G) as well as location. **Table 1** provides new definitions and **Tables 2** and **3** present the stage breakdown for adenocarcinoma and squamous cell carcinoma. A pictorial matrix is shown in **Figs. 1** and **2**. In adenocarcinoma, the grade affects stages IA, IB, and IIA, whereas, grade and location affect stage distribution in squamous cell carcinoma. Several groups have already begun publishing supporting case series evaluating the new stage system and they seem to support the new nodal stratification but not necessarily the grade stratification; however, the data that drove the new system were based on surgically resected disease without neoadjuvant or adjuvant therapy.[12,13] Future directions may look to the past, when tumor length was part of the staging system. Yendamuri and colleagues[14] and Gaur and colleagues[15] have demonstrated the prognostic significance of postresection tumor length and endoscopic tumor length as predictors of survival, respectively, which may play a role in future staging.

The significance of the new staging system is the impact on pretreatment clinical staging. It is imperative to try and delineate the nodal status based on the number of clinically suspicious nodes. Fused PET-CT scan and EUS will be the mechanisms by which

Table 1
7th Edition AJCC *Cancer Staging Manual* TNM definitions

Tis	Carcinoma in situ/high-grade dysplasia
T1	
T1a	Lamina propria or muscularis mucosae
T1b	Submucosa
T2	Muscularis propria
T3	Adventitia
T4	
T4a	Pleura, pericardium, diaphragm, or adjacent peritoneum
T4b	Other adjacent structures: aorta, vertebral body, trachea
N0	No regional nodes
N1	1–2 Node metastases
N2	3–6 Node metastases
N3	>6 Node metastases
M0	No distant disease
M1	Distant metastasis

these nodes are quantitated. CT node criteria of mediastinal nodes of 1 cm or greater size in short axis and paraesophageal, perigastric, and celiac nodes greater than 0.7 cm are concerning for metastatic disease, especially when coupled with increased standard uptake value (SUV) greater than 3 and number of PET abnormalities noted.[16,17] EUS can define pathologic nodes based on sonographic (greater than 1 cm, round, and hypoechoic) characteristics but can be difficult to discern the total number of suspicious nodes.[18]

Table 2
7th Edition AJCC *Cancer Staging Manual* adenocarcinoma stage stratification

Stage	T	N	M	G
0	Tis	0	0	1
IA	1	0	0	1–2
IB	1	0	0	3
	2	0	0	1–2
IIA	2	0	0	3
IIB	3	0	0	Any
	1–2	1	0	Any
IIIA	1–2	2	0	Any
	3	1	0	Any
	4a	0	0	Any
IIIB	3	2	0	Any
IIIC	4a	1–2	0	Any
	4b	Any	0	Any
	Any	3	0	Any
IV	Any	Any	1	Any

Abbreviations: G, grade of tumor; M, metastasis; N, nodal status; T, tumor size; 1, well; 2, moderate; 3, poor differentiation.

Table 3
7th Edition AJCC *Cancer Staging Manual* squamous cell carcinoma stage stratification

Stage	T	N	M	G	Location
0	Tis	0	0	1	Any
IA	1	0	0	1	Any
IB	1	0	0	2–3	Any
	2–3	0	0	1	Lower
IIA	2–3	0	0	1	Upper Middle
	2–3	0	0	2–3	Lower
IIB	2–3	0	0	2–3	Upper Middle
	1–2	1	0	Any	Any
IIIA	1–2	2	0	Any	Any
	3	1	0	Any	Any
	4a	0	0	Any	Any
IIIB	3	2	0	Any	Any
IIIC	4a	1–2	0	Any	Any
	4b	Any	0	Any	Any
	Any	3	0	Any	Any
IV	Any	Any	1	Any	Any

ASSESSMENT

All esophageal cancer patients should be discussed in a multidisciplinary tumor board in a prospective fashion. Ideally, they should be seen and examined by all appropriate specialties. In so doing, a tailored treatment plan for each patient can be developed based on stage, comorbid conditions, and patient desires. Blazeby and colleagues[19] demonstrated a 15% discordant treatment from their original multidisciplinary team

	N0	N1	N2	N3
T1G1	IA	IIB	IIIA	IIIC
T1G2	IA	IIB	IIIA	IIIC
T1G3	IB	IIB	IIIA	IIIC
T2G1	IB	IIB	IIIA	IIIC
T2G2	IB	IIB	IIIA	IIIC
T2G3	IIA	IIB	IIIA	IIIC
T3	IIB	IIIA	IIIB	IIIC
T4a	IIIA	IIIC	IIIC	IIIC
T4B	IIIC	IIIC	IIIC	IIIC

Fig. 1. Adenocarcinoma stage matrix.

	N0	N1	N2	N3
T1G1	IA	IIB	IIIA	IIIC
T1G2	IB	IIB	IIIA	IIIC
T1G3	IB	IIB	IIIA	IIIC
T2G1Lower	IB	IIB	IIIA	IIIC
T2G2lower	IIA	IIB	IIIA	IIIC
T2G3lower	IIA	IIB	IIIA	IIIC
T2G1middle/upper	IIA	IIB	IIIA	IIIC
T2G2middle/upper	IIB	IIB	IIIA	IIIC
T2G3middle/upper	IIB	IIB	IIIA	IIIC
T3G1lower	IB	IIIA	IIIB	IIIC
T3G2lower	IIA	IIIA	IIIB	IIIC
T3G3lower	IIA	IIIA	IIIB	IIIC
T3G1middle/upper	IIA	IIIA	IIIB	IIIC
T3G2middle/upper	IIB	IIIA	IIIB	IIIC
T3G3middle/upper	IIB	IIIA	IIIB	IIIC
T4a	IIIA	IIIC	IIIC	IIIC
T4b	IIIC	IIIC	IIIC	IIIC

Fig. 2. Squamous cell carcinoma stage matrix.

plan because of lack of this patient information. To aide in this endeavor, a specialized dedicated esophageal nurse navigator can help the patient and family navigate this evaluation more easily. All appropriate staging studies can be obtained as needed for their plan of treatment and the treatment expedited.

A thorough history and physical examination assess patient performance status and nutritional status. Minimal laboratory evaluation should include complete blood cell count and complete metabolic panel to evaluate nutritional status. Subjective global assessment uses focused history evaluating weight change, dietary intake, gastrointestinal symptoms, and associated comorbidities having an impact on metabolic demand and physical findings, including loss of subcutaneous fat, muscle wasting, edema, and ascites, to subjectively help evaluate nutrition status. Other concerning findings are weight loss greater than or equal to 10%, body mass index less than 20 kg/m^2, prognostic nutrition index greater than or equal to 50, severe dysphagia, albumin less than 3.5 g/dL, and prealbumin less than 10 mg/dL.[20] A formal nutrition consult is advised for all patients to help maintain their nutrition during their treatment and thereafter by providing patients a better understanding of calorie intake required to maintain adequate nutrition.

Comorbidities should be closely evaluated, especially underlying cardiovascular disease and respiratory issues. Pulmonary function test should be ordered on patients considered for surgery and cardiac stress test as indicated by history and physical examination. Patients should stop tobacco products and alcohol products. A functional assessment should be performed and either Karnofsky score or Eastern Cooperative Oncology Group (ECOG) performance status recorded (**Table 4**). Risk stratification models have been championed by different groups. Edinburgh Clinical Risk Score evaluates patients based on clinical stage, performance status, rate of weight loss, and C-reactive protein level to assess risk of dying from gastroesophageal cancer.[21] Modified Glasgow prognostic score is another mechanism used to prognosticate, using a combination of C-reactive protein and albumin levels. Crumley and colleagues[22] demonstrated, in a retrospective case

Table 4
Performance status grading

Definition		Karnofsky Score		ECOG Performance Status
Normal activity and work, no special need	100	No complaint	0	Asymptomatic (fully active, able to carry on all predisease activities without restriction)
	90	Minor signs and symptoms disease	1	Symptomatic but completely ambulatory (restricted in physically strenuous activity but ambulatory and able to carry out work of light or sedentary nature)
	80	Normal activity with effort some signs and symptoms of disease		
Unable to work; able to live at home and care for most personal needs; varying amount of assistance needed	70	Cares for self; unable to carry on normal activity or to do active work	2	Symptomatic, <50% in bed during the day (ambulatory and capable of all self-care but unable to carry out any work activities, up and about more than 50% of waking hours)
	60	Requires occasional assistance but is able to care for most of his personal needs		
	50	Requires considerable assistance and frequent medical care		
Unable to care for self; requires equivalent of institutional or hospice care; disease may be progressing rapidly	40	Disabled; requires special care and assistance	3	Symptomatic, >50% in bed, but not bedbound (capable of only limited self-care, confined to bed or chair 50% or more of waking hours)
	30	Severely disabled; hospital admission is indicated although death not imminent.	4	Bedbound (completely disabled, cannot carry on any self-care, totally confined to bed or chair)
	20	Very sick; hospital admission necessary; active supportive treatment necessary		
	10	Moribund; fatal processes progressing rapidly		
	0	Dead	5	Death

series review, that the modified Glasgow prognostic score was a significant predictor of cancer specific survival.

ENDOSCOPIC THERAPY

Barrett esophagus is a premalignant mucosal abnormality in the esophagus related to acid or, more likely, bile reflux damage, resulting in dysplastic changes at the squamocolumnar junction. Despite proton pump inhibitors and even fundoplication, Barrett esophagus can be resilient. New endoscopic therapies are available to treat dysplastic changes in the esophageal mucosa. The risk of cancer is increased and may be as low as 0.6% per year in low-grade dysplasia and up to 5% per year in high-grade dysplasia.[23] A routine surveillance program is recommended for Barrett esophagus with surveillance endoscopy with biopsies using Seattle protocol or other biopsy protocols on a regular basis.[24,25]

Argon plasma coagulation (APC) was one of the first therapies for mucosal ablations. It is used in both treatment of premalignant disease and palliation of advanced cancer. Complete eradication of dysplasia and early cancers is seen in 68% of the patients.[26] Complications occur in approximately 24% of the procedures, most of which are self-limited, such as pain, bleeding, ulceration, and stricture. There is also a finite risk of developing buried glands; exact risk is uncertain.

Photodynamic therapy has demonstrated efficacy in eradicating both premalignant and early-stage tumors. Used in combination with proton pump inhibitors, a 77% complete response is noted in high-grade dysplasia and stage I carcinomas.[26] The main drawbacks are the photosensitivity and an increased stricture rate. Buried glands have been noted in 24% to 44% of the patients and recurrent cancers have been seen in 10%.[27]

Radiofrequency ablation (RFA) is an effective treatment of Barrett esophagus. Shaheen and colleagues,[28] in a randomized trial, demonstrated 81% complete response in high-grade dysplasia and there was less progression of disease and fewer cancers noted in follow-up. The main side effect was chest pain and the stricture rate of 6%. RFA is good for flat Barrett mucosa but not as effective for lumpy-bumpy (nodular) disease because of loss of probe contact.

Cryotherapy uses low-pressure liquid nitrogen spray delivered during endoscopy with a vented stomach. Greenwald and colleagues,[29] in a multi-institutional study, demonstrated the efficacy of cryotherapy in high-grade dysplasia and intramucosal carcinoma. Dumot and coworkers[30] demonstrated a 90% response rate and their 2-year results showed 68% downgrade of high-grade dysplasia and an 80% complete response in intramucosal cancer. Multiple procedures are required for complete eradication; and side effects included mild pain and minor strictures. It is better suited for lumpy-bumpy Barrett esophagus.

Unlike the previously described endoscopic procedures, endoscopic mucosal resection (EMR) provides a pathologic specimen for review. Several techniques have been used, including submucosal injection with snare polypectomy, cap-assisted mucosal resection, and band ligator-assisted mucosal resection. In case series, Barrett esophagus was completely eradicated in 75% to 96% of the patients and dysplasia or cancer complete response in 85% to 100%.[31] Complications include bleeding and stricture. Ideal lesions are less than 2 cm in diameter, involve less than one-third of the circumference, and are confined to the mucosa.[32]

SURGERY

Surgery has been the cornerstone of curative treatment of esophageal cancer for the past several decades. The overall surgical outcomes have been improving, with most recent data demonstrating surgical mortality rates between 0.3% and 7.2% and rates of morbidity between 30% and 68% (**Table 5**).[7,12,33–42] Population-based studies, however, reflect more disparate outcomes compared to these case series. Kohn and colleagues,[43] using the Nationwide Inpatient Sample in 2007, found the esophagectomy mortality rate was 7% and pointed to improved outcomes in higher-volume centers. Ra and colleagues[44] at the University of Pennsylvania, during approximately the same time period, using Survival, Epidemiology and End Results Program data, found a mortality rate of 14%, and risk factors included advancing age, comorbidities, and hospital volume. The bottom line is that proper patient selection leads to better outcomes and, hence, the disparity of results seen in case series where selection bias may occur.

Approximately one-third of the patients who present with esophageal cancer are resection candidates. Overall cure rates with surgical resection are between 25% and 35% at 5 years. The new 7th edition AJCC staging classification was based purely on patient outcomes from surgically resected patients—all pathologically proven disease. Five-year survival rates for each of the adenocarcinoma stages are stage IA, 78%; stage IB, 64%; stage IIA, 50%; stage IIB, 39%; stage IIIA, 25%; stage IIIB, 17%; and stage IIIC, 14%.

Ivor Lewis esophagogastrectomy is the most common procedure performed for esophageal cancer. It involves laparotomy with mobilization of the stomach based on the right gastroepiploic artery. A right thoracotomy is then performed and the thoracic esophagus and its surrounding nodes mobilized. The gastric conduit is brought into the chest and then an esophagogastrectomy performed with 8-cm proximal and 5-cm distal margins. An intrathoracic anastomosis is then performed and the chest widely drained. This approach provides the optimum exposure of the esophagus and its nodal basins. It, however, is a big insult on patients already debilitated by the underlying disease. The morbidity of the procedure is higher but overall survival rates seem better from a cancer standpoint.

Transhiatal esophagectomy is the next most common procedure performed. It involves a similar laparotomy but a neck incision is performed in lieu of thoracotomy. The intrathoracic esophagus is bluntly and at times blindly mobilized. The proximal esophagus is divided in the neck and the specimen brought back into the abdomen and the esophagogastrectomy performed. The gastric conduit is then brought up to the neck, generally in the orthotopic position, and cervical anastomosis performed. This approach resects more esophagus but at the expense of oncologic node dissection. The morbidity of the operation in most studies is less and seems better tolerated by marginal surgical candidates. The anastomosis, however, is under more tension and tends to leak more often.

The McKeown 3-incision esophagectomy optimizes the benefits of both the approaches described previously. It is the optimal approach for treating upper thoracic esophageal cancers in the middle to upper third. The modified procedure is started with a right thoracotomy where the esophagus is mobilized en bloc along with a thorough lymph node dissection. The chest is drained widely and closed and the patient repositioned supine. A laparotomy is performed and the gastric conduit mobilized in a similar fashion, with a lymph node dissection. A left lateral neck incision is performed and the cervical esophagus mobilized, the proximal margin determined, and the esophagus transected. As in the transhiatal esophagectomy, the specimen is brought back into the abdomen, the distal margin determined, and gastric conduit fashioned. The conduit is brought up into neck in the orthotopic position and a cervical anastomosis performed. This approach allows for a 3-field lymphadenectomy to be performed along with the benefits of a neck anastomosis.

Left thoracotomy with phrenotomy approach for esophagectomy was first championed by Churchill and Sweet, in 1942,[45,46] when they published a case series of 11

Table 5
Esophagectomy case series articles

Study	N	Sex (M/F)	Stage I	Stage II	Stage III	Stage IV	Median Survival (Mo)	5-Y (%)	% Neoadjuvant RC	% Hospital Morbidity	% Hospital Mortality
Atkins et al,[36] 2004	379%	307/72	NR 22.1%	NR 51.7%	NR 18.8%	NR 5.1%	NR	NR	44.1	64	5.8
Mariette et al,[38] 2004	386%	347/39	51 13.2%	133 34.5%	169 43.8%	0 0	28.9	31	50.2	36.3	3.6
Portale et al,[33] 2006	263%	215/48	97 36.8%	63 23.9%	93 35.4%	10 3.8%	>48	46.5	18	62	4.5
Omloo et al,[34] 2007	205%	178/27	NR 26.9%[a]	NR	NR 73.1%	0		THE—34% TTE—36%	0	NR	3
Low et al,[7] 2007	340%	241/99	87 25.6%	133 39.1%	94 27.6%	9 2.6%	NR	NR	43	45	0.3
Adams et al,[40] 2007	330%	224/106	NR 1.8%	NR 29%	NR 56%	NR 11%	22	26	27.6	30.7	7.2
Sundelof et al,[41] 2008	232%	193/39	52 22%	61 26%	70 30%	38 16%	NR	25	23.0	33.2	3.9
Malin et al,[35] 2009	221%	191/30	24 10.8%	77 34.8%	66 29.9%	4 1.8%	NR	33	42.1	41.6	2.3
Wouters et al,[37] 2009	214%[b]	159/54	31 14.5%	82 36.3%	74 34.6%	15 7%	22	NR	25.2	66.8	4.7
Hsu et al,[12] 2010	392%	374/18	42 10.7%	151 38.5%	116 29.6%	83 21.2%	20	27.1	0	NR	NR
Cijs et al,[39] 2010	1061%	795/266	17 1.6%	573 54.0%	306 28.8%	116 10.9%	20.5	27	38.6	39	<70:5.4 >70:11.6
Pultram et al,[42] 2010	234%	196/38	28 12.0%	87 37.1%	105 44.9%	14 6.0%	26	33	0	61	6.2

Abbreviations: NR, not reported; RC, combined radiation chemotherapy; THE, transhiatal esophagectomy; TTE, trans thoracic esophagectomy.
[a] Omloo's pathologic combined stage I–II.
[b] Wouters' 2000–2004 cohort data.

patients. This approach entails a left thoracotomy for exposure through the 6th or 7th interspace. The diaphragm is then opened in a radial fashion exposing the abdominal contents. The gastric conduit is mobilized along with the distal esophagus. The tumor is resected and an intrathoracic anastomosis completed. The downside of this incision is the limited abdominal exposure and inability to place feeding access. Also, margins of resection may be compromised or at least limited by this procedure.

A left thoracoabdominal esophagogastrectomy with left neck incision is another approach that provides excellent exposure for cardia and gastroesophageal juncture tumors. A left thoracoabdominal incision is made along left chest extending into the abdomen via an oblique incision. The costal arch is divided and diaphragm is opened radially exposing the gastroesophageal juncture. The short gastrics are easily controlled and divided and the stomach mobilized along with the distal esophagus. A radical lymph node dissection is performed. An oblique left neck incision is performed and the cervical esophagus exposed and mobilized with blunt and sharp dissection. The esophagogastrectomy is performed and a cervical anastomosis created.

Minimally invasive esophagectomy (MIE) was first performed in the mid 1990s. It has been slow to gain a foothold with surgeons. It is a challenging procedure that can be performed via different approaches, most are modifications of the standard open procedures (described previously). Laparoscopy with thoracoscopy (Ivor Lewis), thoracoscopy with laparoscopy and left neck incision (McKeown esophagectomy), and laparoscopy with neck incision (transhiatal) are a few of the common procedures. Luketich and coworkers[47] published one of the largest series of MIE, 222 patients. MIE was successfully performed in 92.8% with an operative mortality of 1.4%, demonstrating the safety, feasibility, and equivalent outcomes of open techniques. Butler and colleagues[48] did an extensive review of the current literature on MIE and demonstrated comparable results from the oncologic standpoint and comparable morbidity and mortality to standard open procedures. It has, however, yet to be proved to offer improved outcomes. It is a technique all thoracic surgeons should have in their armamentarium but the learning curve is steep.

RADIATION THERAPY

Radiation therapy is another means of locally treating esophageal cancer. The gross tumor volume (GTV) can be delineated by using CT scan, PET scan, and endoscopic localization. It is the main tumor and involved nodes. The planned tumor volume (PTV) is the GTV plus a 5-cm craniocaudal margin along with a 2-cm radial margin. Addition of a 4-D CT scan helps determine and adjust for amount of organ/tumor motion. The normal surrounding structures, such as lungs, heart, and spinal cord, are delineated and the prescription dose is then evaluated by the physicist to limit exposure of the vital structures while maximizing delivery to the cancer. The current dose is generally 50.4 Gy given in 1.8-Gy fractions over 5 weeks.

3-D conformal planning is the current standard of care. 30 Gy are given using opposed anterior and posterior fields. The next 20 Gy are then given using 1 or 2 posterior oblique fields to get to the prescribed dose. An additional boost can then be given to the tumor with a 2-cm craniocaudal and radial margin.[49] Hsu and colleagues[50] investigated extending the radiation to elective nodal irradiation of supraclavicular nodes for upper third tumor and celiac axis nodes for lower third lesion and demonstrated decreased nodal failures in these former metastatic nodal regions without improvement in survival. The most common complications of radiation therapy, acutely, are radiation pneumonitis and esophagitis. Late complications include radiation pneumonitis, esophageal stricture, and cardiac complications.

Intensity-modulated radiotherapy (IMRT) improves doses delivered to the tumor while decreasing doses to normal tissue.[51] IMRT uses computer-controlled linear accelerators and multiple beams to get higher PTV doses into the tumor while limiting adjacent tissue exposure. Martin and colleagues[52] demonstrated improved therapeutic ratio of increased PTV dose with reduced cardiac and pulmonary exposure in 8 patients, using IMRT and Arc technique.

Image-guided radiotherapy techniques allow for daily treatment adjustments based on images obtained just before daily treatment.[53] This adjustment decreases cardiac doses, and may diminish late complications.

Proton beam therapy allows the GTV dose to be escalated while further sparing adjacent tissues. Protons have limited penetration and, thereby, increased doses can be focused in the PTV without changing doses to the lung or heart. Sugagara and colleagues[54] using proton beam therapy were able to increase treatment doses (69 Gy and 87 Gy), resulting in complete response in 87% of their cohort and a 34% 5-year survival rate with an acceptable morbidity (11% grade 3 or higher toxicity).

Brachytherapy results in higher doses being delivered to the tumor with sparing of normal surrounding tissue. Muijs and colleagues[55] studied 62 patients combining brachytherapy and external beam radiation 11% 5-year survival but at the expense of grade 3 or higher toxicity in 16%, predominantly related to esophageal complications.

CHEMOTHERAPY

Esophageal cancer generally presents with advanced disease. Systemic therapy is the mainstay of treatment of these patients. Chemotherapy is delivered throughout the body and treats both local and systemic sites of disease as opposed to the local therapies of surgery and radiation. It is usually given in doublet and sometime triplet therapy.

Cisplatin and 5-fluorouracil (5-FU) is one of the most common doublets used in esophageal cancer.[56] The response rate ranges from 35% to 40%. Cisplatin is given at a dose 75 mg/m^2 to 100 mg/m^2 and the 5-FU dose from 700 mg/m^2/d to 1000 mg/m^2/d by continuous infusion for 5 days. Toxicities include mucositis and myelosuppression.

Carboplatin and paclitaxel have been demonstrated in the chemoradiotherapy for oesophageal cancer followed by surgery study (CROSS) trial to be effective in esophageal and junctional cancers in neoadjuvant multimodality therapy. Weekly doses of carboplatin were targeted at an area under the curve of 2 mg/mL/min and paclitaxel was given at a dose of 50 mg/m^2. There was a 29% complete response rate in the chemoradiotherapy (CRT) arm and 92% of the patients had an R0 resection. Treatments were well tolerated, with 92% of the patients completing the appropriate cycles and only 13% suffering grade 3 or higher toxicity.[57]

Oxaliplatin has demonstrated good response in the metastatic setting and may be even more efficacious than cisplatin.[58,59] The Randomized ECF for Advanced and Locally Advanced Esophagogastric (REAL)-2 study demonstrated the combination therapy for epirubicin, oxaliplatin, and capecitabine improved survival over historical controls with less grades 3 and 4 hematologic toxicities. The REAL-3 study demonstrated the optimum dosing was epirubicin 50 mg/m^2, oxaliplatin 100 mg/m^2, capecitabine 100 mg/m^2/d, and panitumumab 9 mg/kg every 3 weeks.[60]

Docetaxel is a taxane that has shown good efficacy in esophageal and gastric carcinoma. Homann and colleagues[61] used a combination of oxaliplatin (85 mg/m^2), leucovorin (200 mg/m^2), and docetaxel (50 mg/m^2) followed by intravenous infusion of 5-FU (2600 mg/m^2) as a continuous infusion over 3 to 4 preoperative cycles followed by 4 additional postoperative cycles. The results demonstrated a complete response in 17.4%, a subtotal response in 21.7%, and a partial response in 23.9% manifested by T down staging; 95% of the patients had an R0 resection and 76.1% were able to complete all postoperative cycles of chemotherapy.

Paclitaxel is another taxane that has shown efficacy in esophageal squamous cell carcinoma. Radiotherapy in combination with cisplatin (20 mg/m^2/d continuous infusion over 24 hours for 3 days), and paclitaxel (135 mg/m^2) was given either preoperatively or postoperatively. Both multimodality arms demonstrated a 12% improvement in progression-free survival compared with surgery alone.[62] Overall survival was also improved, demonstrating the efficacy of taxane therapy in squamous cell carcinoma.

TARGETED THERAPIES

Molecular targets are being evaluated for their efficacy in esophagogastric cancer.[63] HER2/NEU, a HER tyrosine kinase receptor, has been shown to be a marker for more advanced disease gastroesophageal junction tumors and gastric cancer, and overexpression is noted in up to 43% of the advanced tumors. Trastuzumab (anti-HER2), in a phase II study in gastric cancer, had a 35% response rate in conjunction with cisplatin-based chemotherapy and, in the presence of positive receptor, 55% response. It is currently being investigated in an RTOG 1010.

Cetuximab is an epidermal growth factor receptor inhibitor. The Cancer and Leukemia Group B, in a phase II trial,[64] demonstrated a 40% response rate when cetuximab was used in combination with epirubicin/cisplatin/5-FU or with FOLFOX. Cetuximab, dosed at week 1 with 400 mg/m^2 followed by 250 mg/m^2, currently is being investigated in RTOG 0436.

Erlotinib is another epidermal growth factor receptor inhibitor that has shown promise in esophagogastric adenocarcinoma. Wainberg and associates[65] published their trial on treatment of esophagogastric tumors located within 5 cm of the gastroesophageal junction. Erlotinib was dosed at 150 mg/d in conjunction with oxaliplatin (85 mg/m^2), 5-FU (400 mg/m^2), and leucovorin (400 mg/m^2) on day 1 followed by 5-FU (2400 mg/m^2) continuous infusion for 48 hours. A complete response was noted on 6% and a partial response in 45% with acceptable toxicities. The progression-free survival was 5.5 months and overall survival was 11 months.

Bevacizumab is a vascular endothelial growth factor inhibitor. Shah and colleagues[66] published their phase II trial results using bevacizumab (10 mg/kg), docetaxel (2400 mg/m^2), leucovorin (400 mg/m^2), and 5-FU (400 mg/m^2) on day 1 and continuous infusion of 5-FU (1000 mg/m^2) for 2 days followed by cisplatin (40 mg/m^2) on day 3 repeated every 2 weeks, with 1 cycle equaling 6 weeks. Median 6-month progression-free survival was 12 months and overall survival was 16.8 months; 67% of the patients responded to therapy and 31% had stable disease.

TREATMENT

Clinical stage dictates treatment strategies. Patient factors determine which plan is implemented. In general terms, all stage I and stage IIA middle, lower, and junction esophageal cancers (T1 or T2 N0M0) should be considered for upfront surgical therapy as the mainstay of their treatment if they are deemed adequate candidates. Stage IIB and higher should be evaluated for multimodality treatment whereas stage IV disease is evaluated for best palliative treatment.

Surgery's 5-year survival rates are 34.4% for localized disease, 17.1% for locally advanced disease, and 2.8% for metastatic disease.[67] When stages I and IIA disease are examined, the cures rate are approximately 70% and 49%, respectively (**Tables 6 and 7**).[33,34,38] Unfortunately, clinical staging can overestimate or underestimate stage of disease. Eloubeidi and coworkers[68] found a false-negative rate of EUS in T1 disease

Table 6
Current case series using 7th Edition AJCC *Cancer Staging Manual* staging with esophagectomy stage-specific survival

			Patients Per Stage (5-Y Survival)						
Reference	**Years**	**Patients**	**Stage IA**	**Stage IB**	**Stage IIA**	**Stage IIB**	**Stage IIIA**	**Stage IIIB**	**Stage IIIC**
Hsu et al[12]	1995–2006	SCC—311	11 (80%)	38 (58%)	29 (37%)	108 (33%)	81 (18%)	46 (0)	61 (10%)
Gertler et al[13]	1982–2007	S—1731	NR (78%)	NR (53%)	NR (42%)	NR (52%)	NR (25%)	NR (20%)	NR (11%)
		NA—1189	646 (71%)	294 (52%)	333 (42%)	187 (48%)	380 (27%)	256 (22%)	444 (11%)
Reeh et al[100]	1992–2009	SCC – 296 Adeno—309	117(32.8%)	49 (23.4%)	72 (14.1%)	54 (19.2%)	105 (5.2%)	81 (3.8%)	112 (1.2%)

Abbreviations: Adeno, adenocarcinoma; NA, neoadjuvant treatment followed by surgery; NR, not reported; S, surgery alone; SCC, squamous cell carcinoma.

Table 7
Surgical case series survival using 6th Edition AJCC *Cancer Staging Manual* staging with esophagectomy stage-specific survival

				5-Y Survival					
Reference	**Years**	**Patients**	**pCR**	**Stage 0**	**Stage I**	**Stage II**	**Stage IIA**	**Stage IIB**	**Stage III**
Malin et al[35]	1990–2007	S—128 CRT/S—88	NA 31.8%	87% 53%	70% NR	NR	20% 36%	33% 13%	15% 0
Low et al[7]	1991–2006	S—184 CRT/S—88 C/S—51	NA 18%	NR	92.4%	57.1%	NR	NR	34.5%
Portale et al[33]	1992–2002	S—215 NA/S—48	NR	NR	81%	51%	NR	NR	14%

Abbreviations: C/S, neoadjuvant chemotherapy followed by surgery; CRT/S, neoadjuvant chemoradiation followed by surgery; NA, not applicable; NR, not reported; S, surgery alone.

of 6%; and it is uncertain what the rate would have been for T2 disease because of treatment with neoadjuvant therapy. Patients whose nodal status is understaged because evaluable nodes were EUS negative still do better than EUS-positive patients. Eloubeidi and colleagues[69] reported a 30% 5-year survival in clinical EUS node-negative patients versus 13% in clinically positive nodes.

Multimodality therapy is used for more advanced stages and is based on randomized trials performed over the past 30 years. The Radiation Therapy Oncology Group (RTOG) 85-01 demonstrated the superiority of CRT to radiation alone, with 5-year survival of 27% compared with 0, and improved local-regional control as well as less distant failures.[44,70,71] INT 0123 (RTOG 94-05) looked at radiation dose escalation in multimodality esophageal cancer treatment and failed to show any survival benefit, establishing a standard radiation dose at 50.4 Gy (**Table 8**).[72]

Walsh and colleagues[73] were the first to show the benefit of neoadjuvant CRT; however, the results have been plagued by the less than stellar surgical cure rates of 6% (**Table 9**). Urba and coworkers[74] demonstrated an insignificant improved survival 30% versus 16% at 3 years with neoadjuvant therapy. Multiple meta-analyses have been conducted on this topic and concluded with pooled data that CRT provides a survival benefit and improved local control in advanced esophageal cancer.[75–77] The CROSS Group recently reported significant improved survival (5-y survival 47% vs 34%) with preoperative CRT without increased postoperative morbidity.[55]

Preoperative chemotherapy also has been demonstrated to improve survival (**Table 10**). The Medical Research Council Oesophageal Cancer Working Group (MRC) in 2002[78] reported 94% compliance with 2 cycles of preoperative chemotherapy and 3% died before surgery. The neoadjuvant arm demonstrated smaller tumors, less nodal involvement, and overall 2-year survival of 43% versus 34% as well as improved disease-free survival. Based on this trial, many European countries moved away from preoperative CRT to chemotherapy regimens. The medical research council adjuvant gastric infusional chemotherapy (MAGIC) Trial also reported an improved survival at 5 years 36.3 versus 23% in the neoadjuvant chemotherapy arm using epirubicin (50 mg/m^2), cisplatin (60 mg/m^2), and continuous infusion 5-FU (200 mg/m^2/d).[79] With preoperative chemotherapy, there are improved overall outcomes in terms of survival and control but less complete responses.

The unresectable or inoperable patients' options are narrow and depends on overall patient condition and performance status. In poor performance status patients, definitive radiotherapy may be an option for control of local disease and improved quality of

Table 8
Radiation therapy compared with chemoradiotherapy

Reference	Year	Patients	Completed Therapy	Morbidity/Grade 3–4 Toxicity	Mortality	R0	CR	Median Survival	2-Y Survival
Shirai et al[82]	1993–2006	XRT—12	12	NR	0%	NA	33%	NR	24%
		CRT—8	8	NR	0%	NA	87%	NR	58%
Cooper et al[71] (RTOG 85-01)	1986–1990	XRT—62	58	2%[a]	0%	NA	NR	9.3	5-Y: 0
		CRT—61	36	8%	2%	NA	NR	14.1	5-Y: 26%
		nCRT—69	50	4%	0%	NA	NR	16.7	5-Y: 14%
Minsky et al[72] (INT 0123)	1995–1999	CRT (50.4 Gy)—109	NR	28%	2%	NA	NR	18.1	40%
		CRT (64.8 Gy)—109		30%	9%	NA	NR	13	31%

Abbreviations: CRT, chemotherapy combined with radiation therapy; NA, not applicable; nCRT, nonrandomized treatment; NR, not reported; XRT, radiation therapy.

[a] Grade 4 toxicity only.

Table 9
Neoadjuvant chemoradiotherapy trials

Reference	Year	Patients	Resected	Morbidity	Mortality	R0	pCR	Median Survival	5-y Survival
Kesler et al[101]	1993–2002	S—91	NR	22.7%	3.3%	92.3%	NA	16.8 Mo	26%
		CRT/S—85		26.9%	7.1%	97.6%	29.4%	15.6 Mo	37%
Urba et al[74]	1989–1994	S—50	100%	NR	4.0%	90%	NA	17.6 Mo	3-Y: 16%
		CRT/S—50	94%		2.1%	95.7%	28%	16.9 Mo	3-Y: 30%
Walsh et al[73]	1990–1995	S—55	100%	58.2%	3.6%	NR	NA	11 Mo	3-Y: 6%
		CRT/S—58	87.9	54.9%	5.8%		25%	16 Mo	3-Y: 32%
Kim et al[102]	1993–2005	CRT/S—132	73.3%	45%	7.8%	93.9%	45%	NR	44.3%
		CRT—48			2.0%				14.8%
Van Hagen et al[57]	2004–2008	S—186	86.5%	46%	4.3%	69%	NA	24 Mo	34%
		CRT/S—178	90.4%	44%	3.6%	92%	29.1%	49.4 Mo	47%

Abbreviations: CRT, chemoradiation therapy; CRT/S, chemoradiation followed by surgery; NA, not applicable; NR, not reported; pCR, pathologic complete response; S, surgery alone.

Table 10
Neoadjuvant chemotherapy trails

Reference	Year	Patients	Resected	Morbidity	Mortality	R0	Clinical Response	Median Survival	5-Y Survival
MRC[78]	1992–1998	S—386	86%	42%	10%	54%	37%	13.3 Mo	2-Y: 34%
		C/S—344	95%	41%	10%	60%		16.8 Mo	2-Y: 43%
Cunningham et al[79]	1994–2002	S—244	83.2%	45.3%	5.9%	66.4%	NR	NR	23.0%
		C/S—250	86.8%	45.7%	5.6%	69.3%			36.3%
Ando et al[103]	2000–2006	S—162	97.6%	NR	0.6%	90.7%	38%	NR	43%
		C/S—164	96.8%		0.6%	95.4%			55%

Abbreviations: C/S, chemotherapy followed by surgery; NR, not reported; S, surgery alone.

life. Semrau and colleagues[80] recently reported a case series on elderly patients with inoperable esophageal cancer and found median progression-free survival of 9.5 months and 2-year overall survival of 16.7%. As discussed previously, Muijs and colleagues had improved results by adding brachytherapy to their regime with 2-year survival of 34%.[55] Concurrent or sequential CRT can also be used as definitive treatment. Sgourakis and coworkers[81] from Germany, using a multidisciplinary team's decision in inoperable patients, reported mean survival of 6.9 months using esophageal stent only, 7.8 months with chemotherapy alone (predominantly adenocarcinoma patients), 8.6 months with radiation alone, and 13.5 months with CRT. The combination of chemotherapy and radiation improves chance for complete response rate, improves survival, and delays disease progression. In a small case series, Shirai and colleagues[82] reported a 55% complete response in adenocarcinoma patients using CRT and 2-year overall survival of 58% compared with 24% with radiation alone.

Clinical T1aN0M0 Tumors

Tumors confined to the mucosa are generally found during screening endoscopy, typically for Barrett esophagus. The likelihood of nodal involvement is low, approximately 2% to 5%. Choi and colleagues[83] retrospectively examined previously resected T1 squamous cell cancers and found a 20.5% incidence of lymph node metastasis; however, when T1a lesions were evaluated, superficial mucosal lesion had no lymph nodes involved but, as the mucosa was penetrated deeper, nodal involvement increased. EMR in conjunction with an ablative therapy, such as cryotherapy, photodynamic, or RFA, can adequately treat mucosal cancers. Pech and cowokers,[84] in Wiesbaden, Germany, reported the 5-year survival data for their case series of 288 Barrett cancers and 61 high-grade dysplasia patients treated with EMR and/or photodynamic therapy: 98% disease-specific survival, 84% overall survival, and need for esophagectomy in 3.7%. These patients need extensive follow-up imaging and endoscopy. EMR is indicated for mucosal lesions that are less than 2 cm in size, are well differentiated, and involve less than a third of the esophageal circumference. If the deep margin is involved, the tumor is upstaged to T1b tumor.

Clinical T1bN0M0 Tumors

As depth of penetration of the cancer into the lymphatic rich submucosa occurs, the incidence of lymph node metastasis rises 20%. These patients are best served with esophagectomy for best long-term results. This option definitively determines the true stage of the cancer with excellent margins. A retrospective case study, comparing resection and definitive CRT for clinical stage I carcinoma from Japan, reported similar overall survival at 3 years (81.9% vs 83.5%) but significantly decreased progression-free survival (81.9% vs 70.1%).[85] An important aside of this study was accuracy of preoperative T staging of 96% and N staging of 81% determined by surgical resection. The complication profiles were similar with operative morbidity of 34% and a grade 3 or higher toxicity in CRT of 44%. The results using definitive CRT seem better for squamous cell carcinoma as opposed to adenocarcinoma.

Clinical T2-3N0M0 Tumors

The risk of undetected pathologic nodes increases as tumor depth of invasion increases; 20% to 60% have nodal involvement. Stiles and coworkers[86] reported 55% cT2 and 78% cT3 were node positive. Despite neoadjuvant therapy, 71.8% of the cT3 cancers had persistent lymph node metastasis at surgery; however, that may reflect a stage migration because of the extent of lymphadenectomy performed. Their 5-year survival was 56.2% for neoadjuvant therapy compared with 44.2% for surgery alone. A similar study from Johns Hopkins reported a 50% nodal involvement in cT2 tumors.[87] The 5-year survival of the surgery versus neoadjuvant group was 49% versus 53.8%. Based on these data, I would still recommend primary surgical resection for T2 patients and neoadjuvant CRT for T3 patients. For nonoperative patients, definite CRT can provide better local control, symptom relief, and survival compared with lesser treatments.

Clinical T1-3N1-3M0 Tumors

Locally advanced esophageal cancers are best treated with multimodality treatment (discussed previously). Different combinations of preoperative chemotherapy or CRT can be used with good results. Luu and colleagues[88] retrospectively reviewed their series comparing neoadjuvant CRT to neoadjuvant chemotherapy and reported similar overall 5-year survival (41% vs 40%) and similar disease-free survival (31% vs 21%) rates. The complete response was significantly improved in the CRT group (17% vs 11%). Definitive CRT is also an option (**Table 11**). Gujral and colleagues[89] evaluated induction chemotherapy followed by concurrent CRT: 39% responded to induction therapy with only 8.6% progressing. Initial data evaluation found a 39% 2-year survival and median time to progression of 12 months from the start of radiation therapy. RTOG 0246 expounded on this approach, evaluating the feasibility of selective surgical salvage. Forty-three patients were enrolled and 56% were believed to have complete response after induction chemotherapy followed by definitive CRT therapy and followed. Of these patients, 3 (13%) failed during follow-up (5–15 months) and were resected. The overall 1-year survival of the cohort was 71%.[90]

With studies as such, response monitoring becomes critical. The standard has been CT scans and evaluation using Response Evaluation Criteria in Solid Tumors (RECIST) criteria (see **Table 11**).[91] New imaging, PET scan, and fused PET-CT scan allow monitoring metabolic response. The problem is the inflammatory response incited by the treatment. MD Anderson retrospectively evaluated a series of advanced-stage esophageal cancers treated with definitive CRT and correlated initial PET scan SUV with survival; SUV less than 6 was associated with increased overall survival and progression-free survival.[92] Song and coworkers evaluated change in SUV value as a predictor to response to neoadjuvant chemotherapy. In the patients with baseline SUV greater than or equal to 4, pathologic complete response correlated with greater decrease in SUV (87% vs 68.4%).[93] The Metabolic Response Evaluation for Individualization of Neoadjuvant Chemotherapy in Esophageal and Esophagogastric Adenocarcinoma II trial evaluated interval PET scan to determine response to induction chemotherapy, with nonresponders completing CRT followed by surgery and the responders (decreased SUV by ≥35%) completing 2 cycles of chemotherapy before surgery.[94] Major response defined as less than 10% viable tumor was seen in 36% of the responders and only 26% of the nonresponders; relapse occurred in 39% of the responders compared with 65% of the nonresponders. EUS has been less effective in predicting response after neoadjuvant therapy. Pathologic T tends to be overstaged because of the inflammatory response to treatment. Misra and colleagues[95] were able to accurately stage 23.6% of their cohort, with an accurate T stage in 39.1% and N stage in 58.2%.

PALLIATIVE THERAPY

Palliative therapy comes in many forms and depends on the condition of patients. Chemotherapy, radiation therapy, and CRT can be viable options. In addition, local therapies, such as argon beam coagulation, cryotherapy, and photodynamic therapy, may have a role. Stenting also may provide some quality of life.

Table 11
Surgery and neoadjuvant chemoradiation followed by surgery compared with definitive chemoradiation with or without induction chemotherapy

Reference	Year	Patients	Completed Therapy	Morbidity/Grade 3–4 Toxicity	Mortality	R0	CR	Median Survival	2-Y Survival
Bedenne et al[104]	1993–2000	CRT/S—129	110	59%	9.0%	75%	9.9%	17.7	37.1%
		CRT—130	126		1.0%	NA	10.6%	19.3	36.5%
Yamamoto et al[85]	1995–2008	CRT/S—116	116	34.0%	NR	100%	100%	NR	3-Y: 85.5%
		CRT—54	54	44.4%	1.8%	NA	98.2%		3-Y: 88.7%
Yamashita et al[105]	2000–2008	S—56	56	47%	5.3%	NR	NR	NR	4-Y: 55%
		CRT—72	72	58%	1.4%				4-Y: 29%
Stahl et al[106]	1994–2002	C/CRT/S—86	57	70%	11.3%	82%	35%	16.4	39.9%
		C/CRT—85	77	NR	2.3%	NR	NR	14.9	35.4%

Abbreviations: C/CRT, induction chemotherapy followed by definitive chemoradiation therapy; C/CRT/S, induction chemotherapy followed by chemoradiation and then surgery; CRT, chemoradiation therapy; CRT/S, chemoradiation followed by surgery; NR, not reported; S, surgery alone.

Table 12
RECIST criteria for tumor response

Response	Definition
CR	Disappearance of all disease compared with pretreatment studies
PR	Reduction in the sum of the greatest lengths (≤10 lesions, ≤5 organs) by at least 30% compared with baseline and maintained for 28 d without new disease
SD	Stable appearance of disease (<30% size reduction, <20% increase size, and no new disease)
PD	Increase in total length of all measurable lesions >20% compared with the smallest sum of lesions or appearance of new disease

Abbreviations: CR, complete response; PD, progression of disease; PR, partial response; SD, stable disease.

Ikeda and colleagues[96] retrospectively evaluated CRT as palliation for stage IV esophageal cancer using cisplatin (70 mg/m^2) on days 1 and 29 in conjunction with continuous infusion 5-FU (700 mg/m^2) on days 1 to 4 and 29 to 32 and 40 Gy delivered over 4 weeks; 30% had complete response in the primary lesion whereas 65% had either intermediate response or stable disease; 75% had improvement in their dysphagia scores. Patients who were able to maintain oral nutrition at start of treatment had nutrition support–free survival for 10 months and median survival of 13.7 months. In the patients who required nutritional support before treatment, 85% were able to wean off nutrition support within an average of 43 days and maintained nutrition support–free survival for 4.6 months.

Rupinski and coworkers,[97] in Poland, performed a randomized trial evaluating the efficacy of a combination of local therapies to palliate advanced-stage esophageal cancer dysphagia. APC was used for the initial canalization and then the patients were randomized to brachytherapy versus photodynamic therapy. Brachytherapy using iridium Ir 192 was used within 4 days of APC and was calculated to single 12-Gy dose at a distance of 1 cm from the axis of the esophagus. Photodynamic therapy was done using Photosan-3 (2–2.5 mg/kg) and a 630-nm laser light (250 J/cm). The combination of brachytherapy and APC resulted in a significant dysphagia-free period of 88 days compared with 59 days with photodynamic therapy and 35 in the control. The price of these results was an average of 7.5 procedures post treatment with brachytheapy versus 5.8 procedures with photodynamic therapy and 6.9 procedures in the control group.

Self-expanding esophageal stents can provide palliation of dysphagia caused by malignant stricture. Stewart and colleagues[98] reported their 10-year experience with stents: 138 patients underwent 250 endoscopic examinations and placement of 156 self-expanding metal stents for relief of dysphagia; 90% of the patients had improved dysphagia score (**Table 12**). Tumor overgrowth occurred in 12% and stent food impaction occurred in 7%, all requiring reinterventions. Hanna and coworkers[99] compared

Table 13
Dysphagia score

Dysphagia Score	Definition
0	No dysphagia
1	Dysphagia to solids
2	Dysphagia to semisolids
3	Dysphagia to liquids
4	Dysphagia to own saliva

Table 14
Treatment of the elderly patient with esophageal cancer case series

Reference	Year	Patients	Completed Therapy	Morbidity/Grade 3–4 Toxicity	Mortality	R0	CR	Median Survival	2-Y Survival
Kosugi et al[107]	1992–2003	S—40	40	65%	7.5%	90%	90%	22.3	3-Y: 37.3%
		CRT—24	24	66.7%	8.3%	NA	41.7%	12.8	3-Y: 17.4%
Tougeron et al[108]	1994–2007	CRT—109	80%	56.9%	2.2%	NA	57.8%	15.2	35.8%
Pultrum et al[42]	1991–2007	S—64[a]	64	69%	11%	NR	NA	NR	5-Y: 33%
Cijs et al[39]	1985–2005	Total—250[a] S – 179 RT/S—58 C/S—12 CRT/S—1	83%	55%	11%	NR	NA	20.2	5-Y: 26%

Abbreviations: C/S, chemotherapy followed by surgery; CR, complete response; CRT, chemoradiation therapy; CRT/S, chemoradiation therapy followed by surgery; NA, not applicable; NR, not reported; RT/S, radiation followed by surgery; S, surgery alone.

[a] Older age subgroup: patients ≥70 y old.

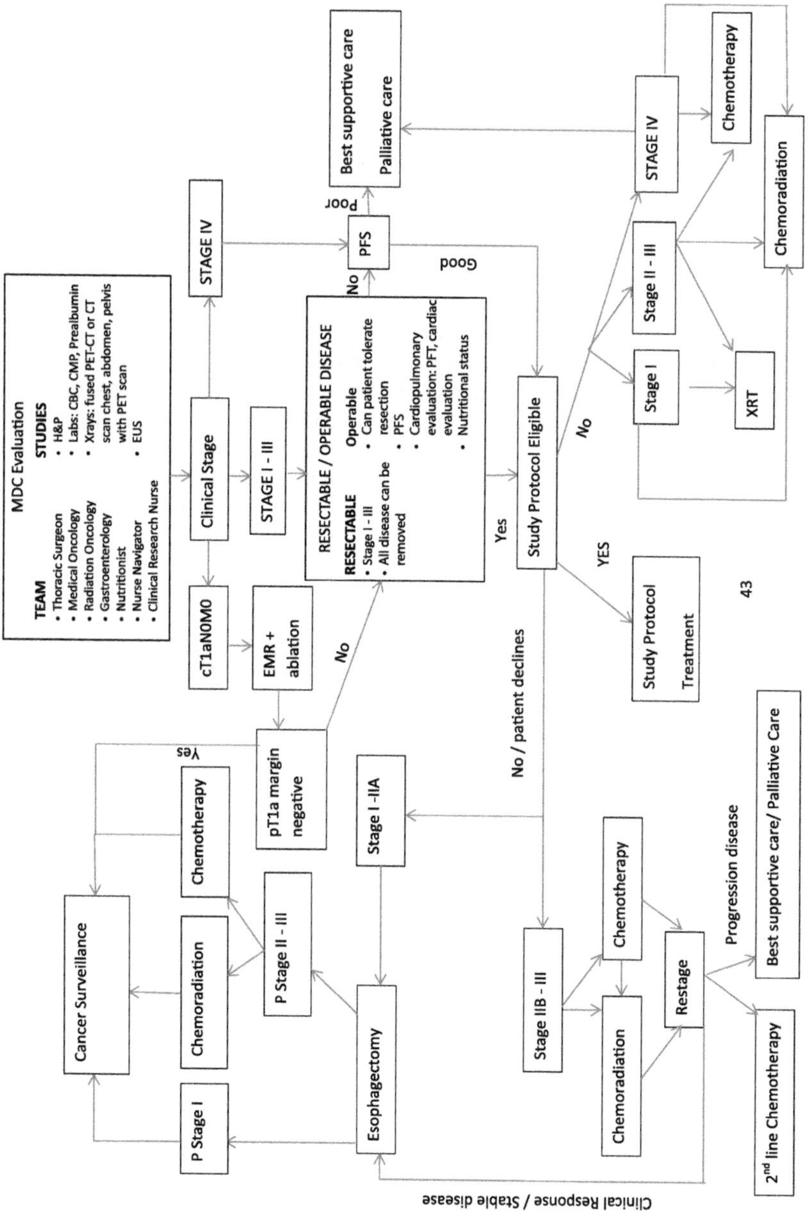

Fig. 3. Clinical flow diagram.

stenting and radiation for palliation. Stents were placed within an average of 22 days and radiation started on average within 52 days. Stent treatment required 1 day of treatment as opposed to 40 days for radiation. Palliation was adequate in 61% of the stent patients with the remaining crossed over to radiation therapy. Dysphagia scores improved more rapidly in the stent group but over 8 to 10 weeks gradually declined from initial improvement. Radiation results lagged behind, requiring up to 10 weeks for an improvement in dysphagia score of 0 to 1; however, their results were more durable.

SPECIAL CONSIDERATIONS

Treatment of elderly patients (≥75 years old) with esophageal cancer can be challenging. The initial assessment of overall patient condition is imperative. Some of these patients may be good candidates for multimodality therapy but most can only tolerate either surgical resection or definitive CRT, whereas others may only be eligible for definitive radiation or palliative treatments. Several case series have demonstrated the efficacy of both approaches (**Table 13**). Five-year survival in surgical series ranged from 26% to 33%; whereas, definitive CRT results in up to 36% 2-year survival. No randomized trials looked at this issue and only case series are reported (**Table 14**).

Clinical trials are the other special consideration. A large portion of how esophageal cancer currently is treated has come from trials. Enrollment in clinical trials appropriate for patients' stage and condition is imperative in helping determine the future treatment of esophageal cancer. Part of each patient's initial assessment should include clinical trial eligibility review by a research nurse and the doctors involved in the multidisciplinary team.

SUMMARY

The incidence of esophageal and junction carcinomas is rising. Patients typically present with more-advanced disease. This article reviews the various treatment modalities available. **Tables 6–11** give a synopsis of different treatment options and outcomes from various trials and case series that have been reported. Multidisciplinary teams can insure appropriate staging and diagnostic procedures are performed in a timely manner. Using the expertise of each subspecialty, an optimum individualized treatment plan can be formulated and executed (**Fig. 3**). The result will be improved patient care and, ultimately, improved outcomes.

REFERENCES

1. Available at: http://www.cancer.gov/cancertopics/types/esophageal. Accessed May 1, 2012.
2. Tougeron D, Richer JP, Sivain C. Management of esophageal adenocarcinoma. J Visc Surg 2011;148:e161–70.
3. Enzinger PC, Mayer RJ. Medical progress esophageal cancer. N Engl J Med 2003;349:2241–52.
4. Viklund P, Lagergren J. A care pathway for patients with oesophageal cancer. Eur J Cancer Care 2007;16:533–8.
5. Freeman RK, Woerkom JM, Vyverberg A, et al. The effect of a multidisciplinary thoracic malignancy conference on the treatment of patients with esophageal cancer. Ann Thorac Surg 2011;92:1239–43.
6. Stephens MR, Lewis WG, Brewster AE, et al. Multidisciplinary team management is associated with improved outcomes after surgery for esophageal cancer. Dis Esophagus 2006;19:164–71.

7. Low DE, Kunz S, Schembre D, et al. Esophagectomy- it's not just about mortality anymore: standardized perioperative clinical pathways improve outcomes in patients with esophageal cancer. J Gastrointest Surg 2007;11:1395–402.
8. Coehn J, Safdi MA, Deal SE, et al. Quality indicators for esophagogastroduodenoscopy. Am J Gastroenterol 2006;101:886–91.
9. ASGE Standards of Practice Committee. The role of endoscopy in dyspepsia. Gastrointest Endosc 2007;66:1071–5.
10. Hancock SM, Gopal DV, Frick TJ, et al. Dilation of malignant strictures in endoscopic ultrasound staging of esophageal cancer and metastatic spread of disease. Diagn Ther Endosc 2011;2011:3566538.
11. Rice TW, Rusch VW, Ishwaran H, et al. Cancer of the esophagus and esophagogastric junction. Cancer 2010;116:3763–73.
12. Hsu PK, Wu YC, Chou TY, et al. Comparison of the 6th and 7th editions of the American Joint Committee on cancer tumor-node-metastasis staging system in patients with resected esophageal carcinoma. Ann Thorac Surg 2010;89:1024–31.
13. Gertler R, Stein HJ, Langer R, et al. Long-term outcome of 2920 patients with cancers of the esophagus and esophagogastric junction: evaluation of the new union Internationale Contre Le Cancer/American Joint Cancer Committee staging system. Ann Surg 2011;253(4):689–98.
14. Yendamuri S, Swisher SG, Correa AM, et al. Esophageal tumor length is independently associated with long term survival. Cancer 2009;115:508–16.
15. Gaur P, Sepesi B, Hofstetter WL, et al. Endoscopic esophageal tumor length a prognostic factor for patients with esophageal cancer. Cancer 2011;117(1):63–9.
16. Okada M, Murakami T, Kumano M, et al. Integrated FDG-PET/CT compared with intravenous contrast enhanced CT for evaluation of metastatic regional lymph nodes in patients with resettable early stage esophageal cancer. Ann Nucl Med 2009;23:73–80.
17. Hsu PK, Lin KH, Wang SJ, et al. Preoperative positron emission tomography/computed tomography predicts advanced lymph node metastasis in esophageal squamous cell carcinoma patents. World J Surg 2011;35:1321–6.
18. Schreurs LM, Janssens AC, Groen H, et al. Value of EUS in determining curative resectability in reference to CT and FDG-PET: the optimal sequence in preoperative staging of esophageal cancer. Ann Surg Oncol 2011. [Epub ahead of print].
19. Blazeby JM, Wilson L, Metcalfe C, et al. Analysis of clinical decision-making in multi-disciplinary cancer teams. Ann Oncol 2006;17:457–60.
20. Bower MR, Martin RC. Nutritional management during neoadjuvant therapy for esophageal cancer. J Surg Oncol 2009;100:82–7.
21. Deans DA, Wigmore SJ, deBeaux AC, et al. Clinical prognostic scoring system to aid decision making in gastro-oesphageal cancer. Br J Surg 2007;94(12):1501–8.
22. Crumley AB, Stuart RC, Mckearnan M, et al. Comparison of pre-treatment clinical prognostic factors in patients with gastro-oesophageal cancer and proposal of a new staging system. J Gastrointest Surg 2010;14:781–7.
23. Wani S, Puli SR, Shaheen NJ, et al. Esophageal adenocarcinoma in Barrett's esophagus after ablative therapy: a meta-analysis and systematic review. Am J Gastroenterol 2009;104:502–13.
24. Fernando HC, Murthy SC, Hofstetter W, et al. The Society of Thoracic Surgeons practice guidelines for the management of Barrett's esophagus with high grade dysplasia. Ann Thorac Surg 2009;87:1993–2002.
25. American Society for Gastrointestinal Endoscopy. ASGE guideline: the role of endoscopy in the surveillance of premalignant conditions of the upper GI tract. Gastrointest Endosc 2006;63(4):570–80.

26. Gan S, Watson DI. New endoscopic and surgical treatment options for early esophageal adenocarcinoma. J Gastroenterol Hepatol 2010;50:1478–84.
27. Corti L, Skarlatos J, Boso C, et al. Outcome of patients receiving photodynamic therapy for early esophageal cancer. Int J Radiat Oncol Biol Phys 2000;47(2): 419–24.
28. Shaheen NJ, Sharma P, Overholt BF, et al. Radiofrequency ablation in Barrett's esophagus with dysplasia. N Engl J Med 2009;360:2277–88.
29. Greenwald BD, Dumot JA, Horwhat JD, et al. Safety, tolerability, and efficacy of endoscopic low-pressure liquid nitrogen cryotherapy in the esophagus. Dis Esophagus 2010;23(1):13–9.
30. Dumot JA, Vargo JJ, Falk GW, et al. An open-label, prospective trial of cryospray ablation for Barrett's esophagus, high-grade dysplasia and early esophageal cancer in high-risk patients. Gastrointest Endosc 2009;70:635–44.
31. Gerke H, Siddiqui J, Nasr I, et al. Efficacy and safety of EMR to completely remove Barrett's esophagus: experience in 41 patients. Gastrointest Endosc 2011;74:761–71.
32. Chandrasekhara V, Ginsberg GG. Endoscopic mucosal resection: not your father's polypectomy anymore. Gastroenterology 2011;141:42–9.
33. Portale G, Hagen JA, Peters JH, et al. Modern 5-year survival of resectable esophageal adenocarcinoma: single institution experience with 263 patients. J Am Coll Surg 2006;202:588–96.
34. Omloo JM, Lagarde SM, Hulscher JB, et al. Extended transthoracic resection compared with limited transhiatal resection for adenocarcinoma of the mid/distal esophagus: five-year survival of a randomized clinical trial. Ann Surg 2007; 246(6):992–1000 [discussion: 1000–1].
35. Malin E, Kiernan PD, Sheridan MJ, et al. Multimodality treatment for esophageal malignancy: the roles of surgery and neoadjuvant therapy. Am Surg 2009;75: 489–97.
36. Atkins BZ, Shah AS, Hutcheson KA, et al. Reducing hospital morbidity and mortality following esophagectomy. Ann Thorac Surg 2004;78:1170–6.
37. Wouters MW, Karim-Kos HE, le Cessie S, et al. Centralization of esophageal cancer surgery: does it improve clinical outcome? Ann Surg Oncol 2009;16:1789–98.
38. Mariette C, Tailler G, Seuningen IV, et al. Factors affecting postoperative course and survival after en bloc resection for esophageal carcinoma. Ann Thorac Surg 2004;78:1177–83.
39. Cijs TM, Verhoef C, Steyerberg EW, et al. Outcome of esophagectomy for cancer in elderly patients. Ann Thorac Surg 2010;90:900–7.
40. Adams R, Morgan M, Mukherjee S, et al. A prospective comparison of oesophageal cancer with curative intent in a UK cancer network. Eur J Surg Oncol 2007; 33:307–13.
41. Sundelof M, Lagergren J, Ye W. Surgical factors influencing outcomes in patients resected for cancer of the esophagus or gastric cardia. World J Surg 2008;32:2357–65.
42. Pultrum BB, Bosch DJ, Nijsten MW, et al. Extended esophagectomy in elderly patients with esophageal cancer: minor effect of age alone in determining the postoperative course and survival. Ann Surg Oncol 2010;17:1572–80.
43. Kohn GP, Galanko JA, Myers MO, et al. National trends in esophageal surgery—are outcomes as good as we believe. J Gastrointest Surg 2009;13:1900–12.
44. Ra J, Paulson EC, Kucharczuk J, et al. Postoperative mortality after esophagectomy for cancer: development of a preoperative risk prediction model. Ann Surg Oncol 2008;15(6):1577–84.

45. Churchill ED, Sweet RH. Transthoracic resection of tumors of the esophagus and stomach. Ann Surg 1942;115(6):897–920.
46. Churchill ED, Sweet RH. Transthoracic resection of tumors of the esophagus and stomach part II. Ann Surg 1942;116(4):566–73.
47. Luketich JD, Alvelo-Rivera M, Buenaventura PO, et al. Minimally invasive esophagectomy: outcomes in 222 patients. Ann Surg 2003;238(4):486–94 [discussion: 494–5].
48. Butler N, Collins S, Memon B, et al. Minimally invasive oesophagectomy: current status and future direction. Surg Endosc 2011;25(7):2071–83.
49. Berger B, Belka C. Evidence-based radiation oncology: oesophagus. Radiother Oncol 2009;92:276–90.
50. Hsu FM, Ling JM, Huang PM, et al. Retrospective analysis of outcome differences in preoperative concurrent chemoradiation with and without elective nodal irradiation for squamous cell carcinoma. Int J Radiat Oncol Biol Phys 2011;81(4):e593–9.
51. Vosmik M, Petera J, Sirak I, et al. Technologic advances in radiotherapy for esophageal cancer. World J Gastroenterol 2010;16(44):5555–64.
52. Martin S, Chen JZ, Dar AR, et al. Dosimetric comparison of helical tomography, RapidArc, and a novel IMRT & Arc technique for esophageal carcinoma. Radiother Oncol 2011;101:431–7.
53. Nguyen NP, Krafft SP, Vinh-Hung V, et al. Feasibility of tomotherapy to reduce normal lung and cardiac toxicity for distal esophageal cancer compred to three-dimensional radiotherapy. Radiother Oncol 2011;101:438–42.
54. Sugahara S, Tikuuye K, Okumura T, et al. Clinical results of proton beam therapy for cancer of the esophagus. Int J Radiat Oncol Biol Phys 2005;61(1):76–84.
55. Muijs C, Beukema JC, Mul VE, et al. External beam radiotherapy combined with intraluminal brachytherapy in esophageal carcinoma. Radiother Oncol 2012; 102:303–8.
56. Ilson DH, Minsky BD. Chemoptherapy and radiotherapy as primary treatment of esophageal cancer. Pearson's Thoracic and Esophageal Surgery 2008;2:509–26.
57. Van Hagen P, Hulshof MC, van Lanschot JJ, et al. Preoperative chemoradiotherapy for esophageal and junctional tumors. N Engl J Med 2012;366(22):2074–84.
58. McNamara MJ, Adelstein DJ. Current developments in management of locally advanced esophageal cancer. Curr Oncol Rep 2012;14(4):342–9.
59. Suntharalingam M. Definitive chemoradiation in management of locally esophageal cancer. Semin Radiat Oncol 2006;17:22–8.
60. Okines AF, Ashley ES, Cunningham D, et al. Epirubicin, oxaliplatin, and capecitabine with or without panitumumab for advanced esophagogastric cancer: dose-finding study for the prospective multicenter, randomized, phase II/III REAL-3 trial. J Clin Oncol 2010;28(25):3945–50.
61. Homann N, Pauligk C, Luley K, et al. Pathologic complete remission in patients with oesophagogastric cancer receiving preoperative 5-fluorouracil, oxaliplatin, and docetaxel. Int J Cancer 2012;130:1706–13.
62. Lv J, Cao XF, Zhu B, et al. Long-term efficacy of perioperative chemoradiotherapy on esophageal squamous cell carcinoma. World J Gastroenterol 2010; 16(13):1649–54.
63. Reddy D, Wainberg ZA. Targeted therapies for metastatic esophagogastric cancer. Curr Treat Options Oncol 2011;12(1):46–60.
64. Enzinger PC, Burtness B, Hollis D, et al. CALGB 80403/ECOG 1206: a randomized phase II study of three standard chemotherapy regimens (ECF, IC, FOLFOX) plus cetuximab in metastatic esophageal and GE junction cancer. J Clin Oncol 2010;28:4006 abstract.

65. Wainberg ZA, Lin LS, DiCarlo B, et al. Phase II trial of modified FOLFOX6 and erlotinib in patients with metastatic or advanced adenocarcinoma of the oesophagus and gastro-oesophageal junction. Br J Cancer 2011;105(6):760–5.
66. Shah MA, Jhawer M, Ilson DH, et al. Phase II study of modified docetaxel, cisplatin, and fluorouracil with bevacizumab in patients with metastatic gastroesophageal adenocarcinoma. J Clin Oncol 2011;29(7):868–74.
67. Tomaszek S, Cassivi S. Esophagectomy for the treatment of esophageal cancer. Gastroenterol Clin North Am 2009;38:169–81.
68. Eloubeidi MA, Cerfolio RJ, Bryant AS, et al. Efficacy of endoscopic ultrasound in patients with esophageal cancer predicted to have N0 disease. Eur J Cardiothorac Surg 2011;40:636–41.
69. Eloubeidi MA, Wallace MB, Hoffman BJ, et al. Predictors of survival for esophageal cancer patients with and without celiac axis lymphadenopathy: impact of staging endosonography. Ann Thorac Surg 2001;72:212–20.
70. Herskovic A, Martz K, Al-Sarraf M, et al. Combined Chemotherapy and radiotherapy compared with radiotherapy alone in patients with cancer of the esophagus. N Engl J Med 1992;326:1593–8.
71. Cooper JS, Guo MD, Herskovic A, et al. Chemoradiotherapy of locally advanced esophageal cancer: long term follow-up of a prospective randomized trial (RTOG 85-01). JAMA 1999;281(17):1623–7.
72. Minsky BD, Pajak TF, Ginsberg RJ, et al. INT 0123 (Radiation Therapy Oncology Group 94-05) phase III trial of combined-modality therapy for esophageal cancer: high-dose versus standard-standard dose radiation therapy. J Clin Oncol 2002;20:1167–74.
73. Walsh TN, Noonan N, Hollywood D, et al. A comparison of multimodality therapy and surgery for esophageal adenocarcinoma. N Engl J Med 1996;335(7):462–7.
74. Urba SG, Orringer MB, Turrisi A, et al. Randomized trial of preoperative chemoradiation versus surgery alone in patients with locoregional esophageal carcinoma. J Clin Oncol 2001;19:305–13.
75. Urschel JD, Vasan H. A meta-analysis of randomized controlled trials that compare neoadjuvant chemoradiation and surgery to surgery alone for resectable esophageal cancer. Am J Surg 2003;185:538–43.
76. Fiorica F, Di Bona D, Schepis F, et al. Preoperative chemoradiotherapy for oesophageal cancer: a systematic review and meta-analysis. Gut 2004;53:925–30.
77. Sjoquist KM, Burmeister BH, Smithers BM, et al. Survival after neoadjuvant chemotherapy or chemoradiation for resectable oesophageal carcinoma: an updated meta-analysis. Lancet Oncol 2011;12:681–92.
78. Medical Research Council Oesophageal Cancer Working Group. Surgical resection with and without preoperative chemotherapy in oesophageal cancer: a randomized controlled trial. Lancet 2002;359(9319):1727–33.
79. Cunningham D, Allum WH, Stenning SP, et al. Perioperative chemotherapy versus surgery alone for resectable gastroesophageal cancer. N Engl J Med 2006;355:11–20.
80. Semrau R, Herzog SL, Vallböhmer D, et al. Radiotherapy in elderly patients with inoperable esophageal cancer. Is there a benefit? Strahlenther Onkol 2012;188(3):226–32.
81. Sgourakis G, Gockel I, Karaliotas C, et al. Survival after chemotherapy and/or radiotherapy versus self-expanding metal stent insertion in the setting of inoperable esophageal cancer: a case-control study. BMC Cancer 2012;12:70.
82. Shirai K, Tamaki Y, Kitamoto Y, et al. Comparison of chemoradiotherapy with radiotherapy alone in patients with esophageal adenocarcinoma. J Radiat Res 2011;52(3):264–9.

83. Choi JY, Park YS, Jung HY, et al. Feasibility of endoscopic resection in superficial squamous cell carcinoma. Gastrointest Endosc 2011;73:881–9.
84. Pech O, Behrens A, May A, et al. Long-term results and risk factor analysis for recurrence after curative endoscopic therapy in 349 patients with high-grade intraepithelial neoplasia and mucosal adenocarcinoma in Barrett's oesophagus. Gut 2008;57(9):1200–6.
85. Yamamoto S, Ishihara R, Motoori M, et al. Comparison between definitive chemoradiotherapy and esophagectomy in patients with clinical stage I esophageal squamous cell carcinoma. Am J Gastroenterol 2011;106(6):1048–54.
86. Stiles BM, Mirza F, Coppolino A, et al. Clinical T2-T3N0M0 esophageal cancer: the risk of node positive disease. Ann Thorac Surg 2011;92(2):491–6 [discussion: 496–8].
87. Zhang JQ, Hooker CM, Brock MV, et al. Neoadjuvant chemoradiation therapy is beneficial for clinical stage T2 N0 esophageal cancer patients due to inaccurate preoperative staging. Ann Thorac Surg 2012;93(2):429–35 [discussion: 436–7].
88. Luu TD, Gaur P, Force SD, et al. Neoadjuvant chemoradiation versus chemotherapy for patients undergoing esophagectomy for esophageal cancer. Ann Thorac Surg 2008;85(4):1217–23 [discussion: 1223–4].
89. Gujral DM, Hawkins MA, Leonulli BG, et al. Nonsurgical management of esophageal adenocarcinoma. Clin Colorectal Cancer 2011;10(3):165–70.
90. Swisher SG, Winter KA, Komaki RU, et al. A Phase II study of a paclitaxel-based chemoradiation regimen with selective surgical salvage for resectable locoregionally advanced esophageal cancer: initial reporting of RTOG 0246. Int J Radiat Oncol Biol Phys 2012;82(5):1967–72.
91. Gwyther SJ. Current standards for response evaluation by imaging techniques. Eur J Nucl Med Mol Imaging 2006;33(Suppl 1):11–5.
92. Suzuki A, Xiao L, Hayashi Y, et al. Prognostic significance of baseline positron emission tomography and importance of clinical complete response in patients with esophageal or gastroesophageal junction cancer treated with definitive chemoradiotherapy. Cancer 2011;117(21):4823–33.
93. Song SY, Kim JH, Ryu JS, et al. FDG-PET in the prediction of pathologic response after neoadjuvant chemoradiotherapy in locally advanced, resectable esophageal cancer. Int J Radiat Oncol Biol Phys 2005;63(4):1053–9.
94. zum Büschenfelde CM, Herrmann K, Schuster T, et al. (18)F-FDG PET-guided salvage neoadjuvant radiochemotherapy of adenocarcinoma of the esophagogastric junction: the MUNICON II trial. J Nucl Med 2011;52(8):1189–96.
95. Misra S, Choi M, Livingstone AS, et al. The role of endoscopic ultrasound in assessing tumor response and staging after neoadjuvant chemotherapy for esophageal cancer. Surg Endosc 2012;26:518–22.
96. Ikeda E, Kojima T, Kaneko K, et al. Efficacy of concurrent chemoradiotherapy as a palliative treatment in stage IVB esophageal cancer patients with dysphagia. Jpn J Clin Oncol 2011;41(8):964–72.
97. Rupinski M, Zagorowicz E, Regula J, et al. Randomized comparison of three palliative regimens including brachytherapy, photodynamic therapy, and APC in patients with malignant dysphagia (CONSORT 1a) (Revised II). Am J Gastroenterol 2011;106(9):1612–20.
98. Stewart DJ, Balamurugan R, Everitt NJ, et al. Ten-year experience of esophageal self-expanding metal stent insertion at a single institution. Dis Esophagus 2012. [Epub ahead of print]. http://dx.doi.org/10.1111/j.1442-2050.2012.01364.x.
99. Hanna WC, Sudarshan M, Roberge D, et al. What is the optimal management of dysphagia in metastatic esophageal cancer? Curr Oncol 2012;19(2):e60–6.

100. Reeh M, Nentwich MF, von Loga K, et al. An attempt at validation of the Seventh edition of the classification by the International Union Against Cancer for esophageal carcinoma. Ann Thorac Surg 2012;93(3):890–6.
101. Kesler KA, Helft PR, Werner EA, et al. A retrospective analysis of locally advanced esophageal cancer patients treated with neoadjuvant chemoradiation therapy followed by surgery or surgery alone. Ann Thorac Surg 2005;79(4):1116–21.
102. Kim MK, Kim SB, Ahn JH, et al. Treatment outcome and recursive partitioning analysis-based prognostic factors in patients with esophageal squamous cell carcinoma receiving preoperative chemoradiotherapy. Int J Radiat Oncol Biol Phys 2008;71(3):725–34.
103. Ando N, Kato H, Igaki H, et al. A randomized trial comparing postoperative adjuvant chemotherapy with cisplatin and 5-fluorouracil versus preoperative chemotherapy for localized advanced squamous cell carcinoma of the thoracic esophagus (JCOG9907). Ann Surg Oncol 2012;19(1):68–74.
104. Bedenne L, Michel P, Bouché O, et al. Chemoradiation followed by surgery compared with chemoradiation alone in squamous cancer of the esophagus: FFCD 9102. J Clin Oncol 2007;25(10):1160–8.
105. Yamashita H, Okuma K, Seto Y, et al. A retrospective comparison of clinical outcomes and quality of life measures between definitive chemoradiation alone and radical surgery for clinical stage II-III esophageal carcinoma. J Surg Oncol 2009;100(6):435–41.
106. Stahl M, Stuschke M, Lehmann N, et al. Chemoradiation with and without surgery in patients with locally advanced squamous cell carcinoma of the esophagus. J Clin Oncol 2005;23(10):2310–7.
107. Kosugi S, Sasamoto R, Kanda T, et al. Retrospective review of surgery and definitive chemoradiotherapy in patients with squamous cell carcinoma of the thoracic esophagus aged 75 years or older. Jpn J Clin Oncol 2009;39(6):360–6.
108. Tougeron D, Di Fiore F, Thureau S, et al. Safety and outcome of definitive chemoradiotherapy in elderly patients with oesophageal cancer. Br J Cancer 2008;99(10):1586–92.

Multidisciplinary Management of Gastric Cancer

Jamal G. Misleh, MD[a], Peter Santoro, MD[b],
Jonathon F. Strasser, MD[c], Joseph J. Bennett, MD[b,*]

KEYWORDS

• Gastric cancer • D2 lymphadenectomy • Multidisciplinary • Adjuvant
• Chemotherapy

KEY POINTS

- Curative treatment for gastric cancer involves either total gastrectomy or subtotal gastrectomy with extended D2 lymph node dissection for patients who present with more localized disease.
- After resection, adjuvant chemoradiation has improved long-term survival in gastric cancer, especially for patients who did not have a complete lymph node dissection.
- Perioperative chemotherapy and radical gastrectomy improves survival and may downstage select patients from unresectable to resectable.
- Chemotherapy for advanced gastric cancer provides palliative benefits, and may provide some short-term survival advantages.

INTRODUCTION

Despite modern advances in diagnostics, surgical techniques, radiation therapy, and chemobiologic therapy, gastric cancer remains a highly fatal disease. Based on SEER data, the 5-year relative survival for gastric cancer (all stages) from 2002–2008 is 27%.[1] The presence of micrometastatic disease, even in apparent early stage disease, contributes to the poor overall survival and the need for improved chemotherapeutics. Most gastric cancers are adenocarcinoma histology (>90%). There has been a migration of gastric cancers over the past century. In the early 1900s most gastric cancers were distal and involved the gastric antrum and body. The incidence of distal gastric cancers has been declining steadily, whereas the incidence of proximal gastric cancers and esophagogastric junction (EGJ) cancers has risen. There has also been

[a] Department of Medical Oncology, Medical Oncology Hematology Consultants, Helen F. Graham Cancer Center, Christiana Care Hospital, Suite 3400, Newark, DE 19713, USA; [b] Department of Surgery, Helen F. Graham Cancer Center, Christiana Care Hospital, 4701 Ogletown-Stanton Road, Suite 4000, Newark, DE 19713, USA; [c] Department of Radiation Oncology, Helen F. Graham Cancer Center, Christiana Care Hospital, 4701 Ogletown-Stanton Road, Suite 1110, Newark, DE 19713, USA
* Corresponding author.
E-mail address: JoBennett@Christianacare.org

Surg Oncol Clin N Am 22 (2013) 247–264
http://dx.doi.org/10.1016/j.soc.2012.12.013
surgonc.theclinics.com
1055-3207/13/$ – see front matter

a corresponding increase in the number of adenocarcinomas of the distal esophagus. The rate of increase is alarmingly high and should be considered an epidemic. In regards to gastric, EGJ, and distal adenocarcinomas of the esophagus, their natural history, response to treatment, and prognosis are very similar suggesting a shared pathogenesis. Some of the possible causes include infectious pathogens (ie, *Helicobacter pylori*); Barrett esophagus; and obesity.[2] As the world continues to struggle with the obesity epidemic, there will continue to be an increase in these malignancies.

Surgical resection remains the primary therapy for gastric cancers when the goal of care is curative. More than 50% of gastric cancers have metastasized to regional lymph nodes at the time of surgery. Survival rates are correlated with the degree of lymph node involvement. Five-year survival for N0 disease is around 50%, whereas survival for N3 disease is only 10%.[3] The poor survival with advanced disease confirms the importance of developing more active systemic therapy, which can be incorporated into a multidisciplinary approach to improve outcomes. There is currently no agreed on approach (neoadjuvant vs adjuvant) for locally advanced gastric cancer. This is in part related to the numerous areas of controversy, which have not been addressed in large multicenter randomized controlled phase III trials. Some of the issues have arisen because classifications of gastric cancers and EGJ cancers have changed with time. In addition, this overlap has diluted the data pool because most of the major clinical trials have included a sizable population of distal esophageal, EGJ, and gastric cancers. In the most recent version of TNM staging system (version 7), EGJ and gastric cardia tumors (Siewert III, arise in cardia within 5 cm of EGJ and extend into esophagus or EGJ junction[4]) are classified as esophageal cancer rather than gastric cancer.[5]

THE ROLE OF SURGERY IN THE MULTIDICIPLINARY TREATMENT OF GASTRIC CANCER

Extent of Gastric Resection

Resection of the stomach has been the primary weapon in the attempt to cure gastric cancer for over a century. The advantages and potential benefits of gastrectomy allow surgery to continue to be the mainstay in the multimodality treatment of gastric adenocarcinoma. A multitude of studies have attempted to delineate the optimal extent of organ resection and lymphadenectomy in terms of potential value versus perioperative morbidity and mortality. Much debate has occurred in regards to the extent of gastric resection to reduce perioperative complications and death rates, while at the same time optimizing the patient's chance for long-term survival. Gastric body and antrum tumors are best managed by distal subtotal gastrectomy with reconstruction, and cancers arising in the fundus are routinely managed with total gastrectomy. There is some variation with regard to proximal tumors, those arising near the gastric cardia or gastroesophageal junction. In most cases, operative approach entails either transhiatal or thoracoabdominal esophagogastrectomy. Most gastroesophageal junction cancers are treated like esophageal cancers and are not the focus of this article. The debate centers around the management of tumors arising in the body and distal half of the stomach.

McNeer and colleagues[6] published their results in 1974 after performing routine total gastrectomy for all patients with cancer of the stomach, demonstrating a high morbidity and mortality associated with the procedure. This raised the question as to whether such a radical operation was indeed necessary for all patients with gastric adenocarcinoma. Subsequently, there have been several large studies comparing outcomes data between total and subtotal gastrectomy. A multicenter randomized trial was conducted by Gouzi and colleagues[7] and published in 1989. This French subtotal versus total gastrectomy trial was conducted between 1980 and 1985 and included 169 patients with distal gastric adenocarcinoma who were randomized to undergo either a distal subtotal gastrectomy or total gastrectomy. The trial showed a slightly lower perioperative mortality rate in the total gastrectomy group; however, 5-year survival outcomes data were virtually identical at 48% for both groups. The Italian Gastrointestinal Tumor Study Group conducted a similar study between 1982 and 1993, accruing patients with carcinoma confined to the gastric antrum. A total of 618 patients from 31 Italian institutions were included in the study, and were randomized to subtotal gastrectomy or total gastrectomy. D2 lymphadenectomy and omental bursectomy were recommended for both groups but not mandated by the trial design. There was median follow-up of 72 months, and the 5-year survival was found to be 65.3% for the subtotal gastrectomy group and 62.4% for the total gastrectomy group.[8] These two landmark studies solidified the theory that subtotal gastrectomy could be performed safely and effectively, with similar long-term survival to total gastrectomy. In addition, multiple publications have documented significantly better outcomes with regard to patient satisfaction and quality of life after subtotal gastrectomy compared with total gastric resection.

Extent of Lymph Node Dissection and Splenectomy

Gastric cancer has a strong predilection to spread to local and regional lymph nodes as the first site of metastatic disease. For this reason, as with many gastrointestinal cancers, lymph node harvesting is an imperative part of a proper cancer operation. Lymph node staging provides prognostic information to guide further therapy and to guide patient expectations. Lymph node dissection also has therapeutic benefits that improve locoregional control, and which may potentially improve long-term survival. The debate over the past few decades has revolved around the extent of lymph node dissection necessary for adequate staging and treatment of patients with gastric cancer, ranging from removal of only perigastric nodes (D1) to removal of the distant para-aortic nodes (D3).

The lymph node stations of the foregut in the region of the stomach are identified as D1 to D3 by the Japanese Gastic Cancer Association. The first level nodes (D1) are stations 1 to 6 and are referred to as the perigastric lymph nodes. Second level lymph nodes (D2) include stations 7 to 12 and are the regional nodes. The third level (D3) lymph nodes include stations 13 to 16, which are the para-aortic lymph nodes.[9] There is a vast body of literature comparing a more aggressive D2 lymphadenectomy with the more conservative D1 resection. A large proportion of this data comes from the Japanese, where at this time the completion of D2 lymphadenectomy is considered standard of care. Such a standard has been met with some reluctance by surgeons in the United States and Europe, and this is a topic of debate among surgical oncologists. In part, many Western surgeons believe that gastric cancer in Western patients is a different disease than what is seen in the East, making comparisons in outcome based on technique alone very difficult and potentially misleading. Tumor location, tumor histology, patient demographics, and comorbidities are all variables that potentially make gastric cancer seen in the West a biologically more aggressive disease.[10] Nonetheless, many surgical oncologists in the West are now trained to perform an extended lymphadenectomy, and based on current American Joint Committee on Cancer staging (seventh edition), a proper gastric cancer operation needs to harvest at least 15 lymph nodes, which usually requires a D2 lymphadenectomy.

The first large randomized clinical trial comparing D1 with D2 lymphadenectomy was conducted from 1986 to 1995 by Cuschieri and colleagues[11,12] (British Surgical Cooperative Group) and published in 1996 with long-term data published in 1999.

At the time of laparotomy, patients were assessed for resectability, and if resectable were then randomized to either D1 or D2 lymphadenectomy. A total of 737 cases were registered during the study period. Four hundred subjects were included for randomization after intraoperative assessment of eligibility. Median follow-up was 6.5 years. The 5-year overall survival for the D1 group was 35% compared with 33% for the D2 group. There was no difference between disease-free or recurrence-free survival. Morbidity and mortality were higher in the D2 group; however, this seemed to correlate with the much higher likelihood of concomitant pancreatectomy or splenectomy at the time of resection. Splenectomy and pancreatectomy performed during lymphadenectomy proved to be independent predictors of poor survival, perhaps negating any potential benefit that would have been seen with a D2 lymphadenectomy.

The Dutch D1 versus D2 lymphadenectomy trial took place between 1989 and 1993, with results published by Bonenkamp and colleagues[13,14] in 1995.[15,16] A total of 996 patients, after exclusions, were randomized to either D1 or D2 lymphadenectomy. Two hundred eighty-five of these patients were found to have distant metastatic disease and were excluded. The remaining 711 subjects underwent the randomly assigned operation and lymphadenectomy. Morbidity (25% D1 vs 43% D2) and in-hospital mortality (4% D1 vs 10% D2) were statistically significantly higher in the D2 group. These findings were comparable with those reported by the British trial. Rates of pancreatic and splenic resections were again much higher in the D2 group. Similar to the British trial, no statistically significant difference was found between the D1 and D2 groups in terms of survival. Five-year survival in the D1 group was 45% and 47% for the D2 group. Fifteen-year follow-up data published by Songun and colleagues[16] in 2010 has reported a benefit to completion of D2 gastrectomy in patients with more advanced stage cancer with more extensive nodal involvement.

The German Gastric Cancer Study was published in 1998 by Siewert and colleagues[17] and included 1654 patients conducted in a prospective fashion. Long-term results of D1 versus D2 lymphadenectomy were compared. D1 lymphadenectomy was defined as resection of less than or equal to 25 lymph nodes, and D2 defined as removal of 25 or more nodes. The results of this study demonstrate a statistically significant difference in long-term survival in patients with stage II (T2N1) disease for whom D2 lymphadenectomy was performed. These results were accomplished without significant increase in perioperative morbidity or mortality in the D2 group. When comparing these data with the long-term outcomes published by Songun from the Dutch trial, it seems that patients with positive nodes are the ones who benefit the most from the lymph node dissection. Because the surgeon does not know this prospectively, and considering the prevalence of lymph node metastases is high in patients with gastric cancer, in general, all such patients should undergo an extended lymphadenectomy. To address this challenge, Japanese surgeons have developed a predictive tool that gives a risk stratification to determine which patients and which nodal stations are most likely to harbor metastases based on certain tumor characteristics.

The Importance of the Maruyama Index

The Maruyama program was produced by Kampschoer and colleagues[18] and published in 1989. It was initially comprised of a database of 3843 cases of gastric cancer collected prospectively from 1969 to 1984 at the National Cancer Center, Tokyo, Japan, and has since been expanded. The program allows new cases to be matched based on seven preoperatively identifiable characteristics, including histologic type, tumor location, tumor diameter, depth of tumor invasion, age and gender of patient, and Borrmann morphologic type. It matches new cases of gastric cancer to cases within the database with similar characteristics, and based on known results gives a nodal metastasis risk for each individual lymph node station and overall survival in the form of a numerical score. The validity of the predictions made by this program has been tested using Dutch, Italian, and German populations, with published results proving it to be accurate.[18–22]

Blinded reanalysis and autopsy data from the Dutch D1-D2 trial has been reported evaluating the effect of Maruyama index in this population. The authors demonstrated that a Maruyama index of less than five results in significantly superior long-term survival, and a low index score is an independent predictor of disease-free and overall survival. Long-term (>11 years) follow-up data from autopy-based analysis of these subjects revealed that distant-only failure was no different between the Maruyama index categories (15% for MI <5 vs 13% for MI >5), but regional failure was significantly different between the groups (8% for MI <5 vs 21% for MI >5). The authors concluded that performing "low Maruyama index" surgery provides significant benefit in terms of local-regional control and survival, but does not provide long-term prevention of distant metastatic disease.[20,22] This literature suggests that planning a "low Maruyama index" surgery can be considered more crucial to overall and disease-free survival than simply the D level of lymphadenectomy completed alone. Many suggest that this piece of data should be calculated for all patients undergoing gastric resection and lymphadenectomy for adenocarcinoma of the stomach.

THE ROLE OF MINIMALLY INVASIVE TECHNIQUES IN THE TREATMENT OF GASTRIC CANCER

The use of diagnostic laparoscopy and laparoscopic ultrasound as adjuncts in the metastatic work-up of foregut cancers including gastric adenocarcinoma is now widely accepted. In patients with advanced disease, diagnostic laparoscopy is highly accurate for identification of occult metastases not visualized on preoperative computed tomography scanning. A study by Burke and colleagues[23] at Memorial Sloan Kettering Cancer Center in 1997 reported staging laparoscopy to be 94% accurate with sensitivity of 84% and specificity of 100%. A more recent study published in 2009 from Romania found strikingly similar statistics, including accuracy of 95.5%, and sensitivity and specificity of 89% and 100%, respectively.[24]

Similarly, laparoscopic gastric resection and lymphadenectomy has become a viable option in the surgical treatment of early gastric cancer. However, its use is still controversial in terms of overall oncologic quality, safety, and cost effectiveness. A large meta-analysis published by Zeng and colleagues[25] in 2012 examined results of studies comparing laparoscopic-assisted versus open distal gastrectomy for early gastric cancer. Twenty-two studies with a total of 3411 participants were included in the meta-analysis. They reported similar numbers of lymph nodes retrieved between the groups. Postoperative morbidity was significantly less after laparoscopic resection, including intraoperative blood loss, postoperative analgesic consumption, and hospital duration. Long-term survival was not statistically significant between the groups, with reported 5-year survival rates ranging between 92% and 98% for each group. The surgical techniques required for adequate laparoscopic gastric resection and lymphadenectomy, however, are operator dependant, time consuming, and have a steep learning curve as with any technically complex laparoscopic operation. This poses a challenge to cancer surgeons, because gastric cancer is not that common, limiting the number of patients available to gain experience with laparoscopic oncologic gastrectomy and lymphadenectomy.

Endoscopic mucosal resection has also emerged as an acceptable option for selected Tis and T1 lesions. Unfortunately, such early disease is rarely seen in Western patients. In Eastern countries, gastric cancer is much more prevalent, screening programs are routine, and early cancers are indeed detected frequently. Mounting evidence has shown that endoscopic mucosal resection is a safe and effective option for very early gastric cancers with favorable characteristics, because the adequacy of this modality depends on the absence of lymph node metastasis. This has proved to be a safe procedure, with evidence published by Ono and colleagues[26] in 2001. This was an 11-year case series including 445 patients. They reported no gastric cancer- or treatment-related deaths during a median follow-up period of 38 months. Endoscopic mucosal resection is, similar to laparoscopic gastrectomy, a technically challenging procedure and should be performed at only specialized centers with high volume and adequately trained operators.

THE ROLE OF CHEMOTHERAPY IN THE MULTIDISCIPLINARY TREATMENT OF GASTRIC CANCER

The role of chemotherapeutics in gastric cancer is constantly evolving. As understanding of the molecular nature of the various subtypes of gastric cancer improves, therapies will also continue to evolve and it is hoped improve outcomes and lessen the toxicity associated with therapy. There is current evidence to support the use of systemic chemotherapy in the perioperative setting and in the metastatic setting. Some of the pivotal trials, which have depicted the benefit of systemic therapies in gastric adenocarcinoma, are highlighted next. Initially discussed are perioperative treatment trials followed by adjuvant trials and finally the treatment of metastatic disease.

Treatment biases remain and treatment does vary geographically. One can refer to the surgery section for more information on the different surgical techniques and degree of lymph node resection to see how this likely affects outcome and response to chemoradiotherapy. In the United States, most patients are treated initially with surgery followed by adjuvant chemoradiotherapy based on the results of the Intergroup 0116 trial. In Northern Europe they favor a perioperative or neoadjuvant approach based on the result of the MAGIC trial and French FNLCC trial. In Japan and southern Europe they tend to favor adjuvant chemotherapy alone without radiation therapy.[27] One can argue that the patient population and the molecular characteristics of the tumor and patients also may very geographically. Clinicians need to improve the understanding of the molecular characteristics of the tumors too not only create novel targeted agents, but also to be able to appropriately test these agents and treatment strategies appropriately. Highlighted next are the major studies that have evaluated the role of the various perioperative treatment strategies.

PREOPERATIVE AND NEOADJUVANT CHEMOTHERAPY

There are several potential advantages to the neoadjuvant approach. One could downstage the patient or convert borderline resectable cases. There is perceived improved tolerance and ability to deliver the entire treatment program. For patients who are destined to develop metastatic disease one could potentially spare surgery if the patient develops metastatic disease during the chemotherapy portion of treatment. For chemotherapy-sensitive disease it allows early exposure to systemic chemotherapy and potentially improved outcomes. The major downside is delaying surgery and allowing a potentially resectable case to become unresectable.

There have been three large randomized clinical trials that have evaluated the perioperative and neoadjuvant approach to multimodality therapy in gastric adenocarcinomas. Two of the trials have shown a clear survival advantage to this approach (MAGIC and FRENCH FNLCC/FFCD) and have shaped the way gastric cancer is managed in most of Western Europe. The EORTC trial failed to show a survival advantage, although it was not powered to show a survival advantage, given poor accrual.[28–31] Two additional trials have incorporated an oral fluoropyrimidine, which also failed to show a survival advantage.[32,33]

The MAGIC trial was conducted in the United Kingdom and included 503 patients, 74% with gastric, 11% with distal esophageal, and 155 with EGJ adenocarcinomas. Patients had to have at least T2 or higher disease. The trial randomized patients to surgery alone versus surgery and perioperative chemotherapy. The chemotherapy treatment program included three preoperative and three postoperative cycles of ECF (epirubicin, 50 mg/m^2 Day 1; cisplatin, 60 mg/m^2 Day 1; 5-fluorouracil [5-FU], 200 mg/m^2 daily), each cycle lasting 21 days.

The results showed a significant improvement in 5-year survival with perioperative chemotherapy 36% versus surgery alone 23% (hazard ratio [HR], 0.75; 95% confidence interval [CI], 0.6–0.93). Progression-free survival (PFS) was also improved. The patients receiving chemotherapy also had a higher rate of potentially curative surgery (79% vs 70%). The final pathologic stage also suggested that patients were able to be downstaged with preoperative chemotherapy (T1/T2 52% vs 37%; N0/N1 84% vs 71%). Local (14% vs 21%) and systemic (24% vs 37%) failure rates were reduced with perioperative chemotherapy.

The ECF chemotherapy regimen seemed to be relatively well tolerated. The most common significant toxicity was neutropenia at a rate of 23%. Other grade 3/4 toxicities were noted in less than 12% of the patients. However, only 42% of patients were able to complete the entire treatment program including all recommended chemotherapy, surgery, then more chemotherapy.

The other large randomized trial that showed a survival advantage to perioperative chemotherapy, is the French FNLCC/FFCD trial. It randomized 224 patients with stage II or greater gastric, EGJ, and distal esophageal cancers to either surgery alone or surgery and perioperative chemotherapy. The chemotherapy program included infusional 5-FU, 800 mg/m^2 daily for 5 days, plus cisplatin, 100 mg/m^2 on Day 1 or 2 every 28 days. Two to three cycles were administered preoperatively and three to four cycles postoperatively for a total of six cycles. The results showed an increase in the number of patients achieving an R0 resection when they received preoperative chemotherapy (84% vs 73%). Five-year survival and disease-free survival were both significantly improved in the chemotherapy group (38% vs 24% and 34% vs 19%, respectively).

Some of the major criticisms of the trial mirrored those of the other perioperative treatment trials and included a large proportion of EGJ and distal esophageal cancers. In addition, only around 50% of the patients who were randomized to chemotherapy received postoperative chemotherapy.

The EORTC 40954 is the third large randomized trial that evaluated the role of perioperative chemotherapy, although this trial failed to show a survival advantage to chemotherapy in addition to surgical resection. It randomized 144 patients with stage III or IV (M0) disease and included both gastric and EGJ cancers to surgery alone versus neoadjuvant chemotherapy followed by surgery. There was no postoperative chemotherapy in this trial. Of note, a large number of patients in these trials were unable to receive postoperative chemotherapy. The chemotherapy program in this trial was two 48-day cycles of cisplatin administered on Days 1, 15, and 29, and leucovorin and 24-hour infusional FU on Days 1, 8, 15, 22, 29, and 36.

With median follow-up of 4.4 years the HR is 0.84 (CI, 0.52–1.35). There was a significant difference in the percent of patients able to achieve a complete resection favoring chemotherapy (82% vs 67%). The incidence of postoperative complications was also higher in the chemotherapy group (27% vs 16%).

The criticism of this trial is that it again included patients with EGJ cancers and the study was underpowered to show a survival advantage secondary to poor accrual (planned 360 patients). One of the problems is that in the United States most patients are treated based on the results of the Intergroup trial and are not offered perioperative chemotherapy.

ADJUVANT RADIATION THERAPY

Analyses of patterns of recurrence of gastric cancer suggest high rates of local or regional recurrences in addition to systemic spread after surgery. In other disease sites, radiation therapy has been shown to reduce local failures, and this seems to hold true in gastric cancer. Early studies of adjuvant radiotherapy demonstrated reductions in local failure when radiation therapy was used. The British Stomach Cancer Group study evaluated postoperative radiation therapy; postoperative chemotherapy (5-FU, mitomycin C, and doxorubicin); and surgery.[34] Although there was no difference in survival in this study, patients receiving radiation therapy had a lower local failure rate at 5 years compared with surgery alone (27% vs 10%). Similar results were demonstrated in a Chinese series of 370 patients randomized to preoperative radiation therapy.[35] Local control and regional nodal control were both improved with radiation therapy (61% vs 48%, and 61% vs 45%, respectively). Intraoperative series of radiation therapy have also demonstrated improved local control compared with surgery alone.[36]

The role of postoperative radiation therapy combined with chemotherapy in modern management of gastric cancer was solidified as standard of care through the results of the Intergroup 0116 study.[37] This trial randomized 556 patients with stage IB through IV gastric or gastroesophageal cancer to surgery alone or surgery followed by 5-FU–based chemoradiation (45 Gy). Most of the patients on this study had T3/T4 disease, and 85% had nodal metastases. Half of patients had a D0 dissection, with only 10% having a D2 dissection, which was the recommended surgery. Most patients unfortunately had a less than adequate surgical resection. More importantly, considering most patients did not have appropriate lymph node dissection, patients may not have been staged accurately. Stage migration is therefore a concern with this study, and it is therefore not clear if patients were randomized accurately after surgery. The data are somewhat difficult to interpret. Despite these issues with the study, this regimen gained widespread national popularity and is one of the gold standard regimens.

Patients randomized to the adjuvant treatment arm received a total of three 28-day cycles of 5-FU (425 mg/m^2/d) and leucovorin (20 mg/m^2/d) for 5 days per cycle. They received cycle 1 of chemotherapy followed 1 month later by 5 weeks of concurrent chemoradiotherapy (45 Gy; 1.8 Gy/day plus concurrent 5-FU 400 mg/m^2/d and leucovorin 20 mg/m^2/d on Days 1–4 and the last 3 days of radiation therapy). After 1 month of rest the patients completed two additional cycles of 5-FU/leucovorin.

The radiation was delivered with a four-field technique (opposed anterior-posterior portals along with opposed lateral fields). With a median follow-up of 5 years, medial overall survival was 27 months for surgery alone and 36 months for surgery followed by chemoradiation. Three-year overall survival was 41% for the surgery-alone group and 50% for surgery followed by chemoradiation group. Local failures were reduced from 29% to 19% with the addition of adjuvant chemoradiation.

The largest criticisms of this trial surround the surgery performed and toxicity of treatment. Although a D2 lymphadenectomy was recommended, only 10% of patients had a D2 dissection and more than half of patients had a D0 dissection. This likely reflects the surgical techniques that were used in the United States at the time. In addition, 36% of patients in the chemoradiation group were unable to complete their protocol treatment because of toxicity. However, this trial does demonstrate a significant overall survival benefit even in the settings of these criticisms. In fact, the survival advantage seen in the Intergroup trial is similar to that seen in the MAGIC and French trials.

This led to the question of whether further intensification of the chemotherapy backbone could improve outcomes with the chemoradiation approach. CALGB 80101 addressed this issue with the addition of the ECF regimen.[38] The study included 546 patients with locally advanced gastric and EGJ malignancies. After surgical resection patients were randomized to adjuvant chemoradiotherapy based on the INT0116 regimen (Standard arm) versus postoperative ECF, and 5-FU plus radiation therapy.

Median overall survival was 37 months versus 38 months, paralleling the Intergroup 0116 data. The ECF-containing regimen was associated with less toxicity (diarrhea, mucositis, and G4 neutropenia). The ongoing RTOG 0114 trial is evaluating a cisplatin/paclitaxel/5-FU regimen. It remains to be seen if any other regimen is a better backbone than 5-FU/leucovorin.

The ARTIST trial compared adjuvant chemotherapy with chemoradiotherapy in gastric cancers after resection with a D2 lymph node dissection.[39] It randomized 458 patients. The chemotherapy-alone arm received six cycles of cisplatin and capecitabine. The chemoradiation arm received two cycles of the same chemotherapy followed by chemoradiation (radiation therapy 45 Gy, concurrent capecitabine 825 mg/m^2 twice a day) and an additional two cycles of chemotherapy. The disease-free survival in both arms was equivalent, which questions the benefit of chemoradiotherapy in patients with a complete D2 resection. Going back to the Intergroup 0116 trial, it may be that the benefits of chemoradiation made up for the inadequate lymphadenectomy. These data indirectly stress the importance of appropriate surgical resection.

ADJUVANT CHEMOTHERAPY

There are numerous randomized phase III trials evaluating the role of adjuvant chemotherapy versus surgery alone in gastric cancer. Most of the early trials failed to show a survival advantage,[40–46] perhaps because of poor surgical technique; patients failed to receive chemotherapy (surgical complications); and the studies were underpowered. Multiple meta-analyses, however, have shown a survival benefit with chemotherapy.[47–50]

The Japanese ACTS-GC trial was a large trial that included 1059 patients with either stage II or III gastric cancer.[51] A D2 lymphadenectomy was required and is the standard surgery performed in Japan. Patients were treated with surgery alone or surgery plus S1. S1 was administered at a dose of 80 to 120 mg daily for 4 out of 6 weeks for 1 year. The 5-year overall survival was 72% versus 61% favoring S1. The survival for both groups was far superior than what has been experienced in the western population (MAGIC, 36% vs 23%; Intergroup, 43% vs 28%). This brings up the question if there is something different regarding the underlying biology of the cancer, the patient population, or the treatment. The standard of care in Japan is now surgical resection with D2 lymphadenectomy followed by 1 year of adjuvant S1.

The Classic trial is the most recent large multicenter randomized trial to be published.[52] It included 1035 patients (South Korea, China, and Taiwan). Patients had to have either stage II or stage III (A or B) gastric cancer. All patients were required to have D2 resections and were randomized to surgery alone or surgery followed by adjuvant chemotherapy. The chemotherapy consisted of eight 21-day cycles of capecitabine at 1000 mg/m^2 twice a day on Days 1 to 14 and oxaliplatin at 130 mg/m^2 on

Day 1. With median follow-up of 34 months, 3-year disease-free survival was 74% versus 59% favoring chemotherapy. Overall survival was 83% versus 78% with HR of 0.72 (95% CI, 0.52–1.00) again favoring chemotherapy. A large portion of the participants required dose modifications secondary to myeloid and gastrointestinal toxicity.

TREATMENT OF METASTATIC GASTRIC CANCER

Although the incidence of distal gastric cancer is declining in the Western population, it remains one of the most deadly malignancies. There has only been minimal progress in the improvement of survival in metastatic gastric cancer during the past 50 years. To improve on the survival and quality of life of patients with metastatic gastric cancer there is a need to derive more effective and less toxic therapy and improve on the use of supportive and palliative care tools (pain management, nutrition support, and hospice).

It has been demonstrated in multiple trials and meta-analysis that palliative systemic chemotherapy is superior to supportive care alone in patients with advanced gastric cancer.[53,54] Most chemotherapeutic agents have been used in gastric cancer and most have had limited activity. Modern chemotherapeutic regimens have emerged from the merger of traditional gastric cancer regimens with regimens used to treat head and neck cancer. In the past the primary chemotherapy agents for distal gastric cancers included 5-FU and anthracycline combinations, whereas the primary chemotherapy for esophageal and head and neck cancers included 5-FU and cisplatin. Theses later merged to form the modern three-agent regimens (ie, ECF). These regimens were shown to be superior to 5-FU–anthracycline combinations. ECF has emerged as one of the standard regimens (perioperative and metastatic) and has been used to compare novel regimens. Since the inception of ECF only marginal improvements have been made on outcomes and toxicity with more modern agents (ie, oxaliplatin, taxanes, and irenotecan). The discovery of Her2/neu overexpression and the subsequent incorporation of trastuzumab have also had an incremental improvement in outcomes in patients with advanced disease.

FLUOROPYRIMIDINES

There are now multiple oral fluoropyrimidines available (uracil-ftorafur, S-1, and capecitabine) in addition to intravenous 5-FU. The oral agents have been shown to be equivalent to infusional 5-FU. They have high response rates (up to 41%)[55–60] but median survival still does not exceed 9 months. The oral agents are briefly described next.

Uracil-ftorafur is an oral drug consisting of ftorafur and uracil. Ftorafur (Tegafur) is an oral 5-FU prodrug. It is converted into 5-FU in the liver. Uracil is a inhibitor of dihydropyrimidine dehydrogenase, which degrades 5-FU, thus increasing the potential effectiveness and toxicity of 5-FU. Secondary to the polymorphisms involving CYP2A6, the maximum tolerated dose varies wildly in individuals. This agent is currently not available in the United States.

S-1 is an oral agent and a combination of three drugs. It consist of ftorafur, 5-chloro-2,4-dihydroxypyridine, and potassium oxonate in a 1:0.4:1 ratio. Ftorafur is a prodrug for 5-FU as described previously. Although the other components either enhance the cytotoxic effect or limit the toxicity of 5-FU, 5-chloro-2,4-dihydroxypyridine inhibits dihydropyrimidine dehydrogenase, thus increasing the half-life of the drug by blocking its degradation. Finally, potassium oxonate inhibits orotate phosphoribosyl transferees, which is responsible for phosphorylating 5-FU, thereby decreasing 5-FU–associated diarrhea. It is currently not available in the United States. It is available in Europe for advanced gastric cancer and in Asia.

Capecitabine is a novel oral fluoropyrimidine that is available in the United States. It requires a three-step activation process. The initial two steps occur in the liver. The final step involves thymidine phosphorylase and occurs after it reaches tumor cells.

There now have been several trials comparing the various oral fluoropyrimidines and traditional 5-FU. There have been some minor differences, but unfortunately there has not been a major impact on overall survival and toxicity is still present. Highlighted next are a few of the trials.

JCOG 9912 is a phase III trial that included 704 patients with unresectable or recurrent gastric adenocarcinomas.[58] Patients had received no previous systemic chemotherapy. It compared three regimens including S-1 (40 mg/m^2 orally twice a day on Days 1–28 of a 6-week cycle); irinotecan plus cisplatin; and 5-FU alone. This study was powered to show noninferiority of S-1 compared with 5-FU and to show superiority of irinotecan/cisplatin over 5-FU. The PFS for S1 when compared with infusional 5-FU was 4.2 versus 2.9 months. The response rate was 28% versus 9%, again favoring S1. Median overall survival was 11.4 versus 12.3 months. S-1 had more G3–4 diarrhea (8% vs <1%), despite the design of the drug.

The First-Line Advanced Gastric Cancer Study trial was a global prospective randomized phase III trial.[61] A total of 1053 patients were randomized to cisplatin/S1 or cisplatin/5-FU. The primary endpoint was median overall survival and it was not significant (8.6 vs 7.9 months). The S1 arm was less toxic, but the dose of cisplatin was also less in that arm (75 vs 100 mg/m^2).

A Korean phase II trial including 91 patients with previously untreated advanced gastric cancer compared S1 (40–60 mg twice a day on Days 1–28 every 6 weeks) with capecitabine (1250 mg/m^2 twice a day on Days 1–14 every 3 weeks).[59] The overall response rate was 29% versus 20% favoring S1. Overall survival with S1 was 8.2 months versus 9.5 months with capecitabine. The toxicity profile was similar except for hand-foot-mouth, which was more common with capecitabine (0% vs 7%).

A randomized phase III trial including 316 patients with advanced gastric cancer compared oral capecitabine with infusional 5-FU.[62] A cycle was 21 days and included cisplatin at 80 mg/m^2 on Day 1 and either capecitabine, 1000 mg/m^2 twice a day for 14 days, or infusional 5-FU, 800 mg/m^2/day on Days 1 to 5. The study was powered for noninferiority. Median PFS was 5.6 months versus 5 months and overall survival 10.5 months versus 9.3 months. The degree of G3/G4 toxicities was similar.

Currently, the use of an oral fluoropyrimidine or traditional 5-FU is acceptable in the management of advanced gastric cancer. There are several factors that may influence a clinician's decision including availability, delivery method, patient preference, and cost. In today's world, cost is a key issue. The cost of traditional 5-FU is significantly lower than the oral agents at this time.

COMBINATION CHEMOTHERAPY

It has been demonstrated in multiple phase II trials that combination chemotherapy regimens are associated with higher response rates compared with single agents, although when single agents have been compared with combination regimens in randomized trials there has been no true survival advantage.[63–65] It is unknown if the more modern regimens (ECF, EOX, irinotecan/taxane based regimens) and the inclusion of appropriate biologic agents will have an impact on survival because they have not been tested.

ECF REGIMEN

ECF was initially shown to be highly active in gastric cancer. In 128 patients with advanced gastric cancer, ECF was associated with a high response rate of 71%.[66]

This promising result led to further investigation of this regimen. In a randomized trial including 274 patients with advanced esophagogastric adenocarcinoma, patients were treated with ECF or FAMTX.[67] Response rate was 45% versus 21%, and median survival 8.9 versus 5.7 months, favoring ECF.

ECF was also compared with a mitomycin-containing regimen (mitomycin, 7 mg/m^2 every 6 weeks; cisplatin, 60 mg/m^2 every 3 weeks; and infusional 5-FU, 300 mg/m^2 daily).[68] This trial included 580 patients with advanced esophagogastric cancer. Response rates (42% vs 44%), median survival (9.4 vs 8.7 months), and toxicity were similar. ECF was determined to be the preferred regimen because it was associated with a superior quality of life. ECF then became the preferred and reference regimen in subsequent gastric cancer trials.

The role of anthracyclines remains debatable in gastric and other malignancies with the development of more modern chemobiologic agents. A meta-analysis did suggest improved survival with the addition of epirubicin to cisplatin and 5-FU (HR for death, 0.82; 95% CI, 0.73–0.92).[69] Modern methods of delivering 5-FU may improve outcomes and alleviate the need for anthracyclines. CALGB 80403 is a randomized trial that combines cetuximiab with ECF, FOLFOX, and irinotecan plus cisplatin. Preliminary results[70] indicate that outcomes are similar between FOLFOX and ECF in terms of relative risk (RR), PFS, and overall survival.

Oxaliplatin is another platinum agent that has shown activity in various gastrointestinal malignancies, including gastric adenocarcinomas. In gastric and esophageal cancers various regimens including oxaliplatin have shown promising response rates ranging from 40% to 65%. Most of the regimens included a fluoropyrimidine. Median survival ranged from 8 to 15 months. There have been two-phase III trials that have compared oxaliplatin with cisplatin regimens.[71,72]

The REAL-2 trial is a pivotal study that compared capecitabine with 5-FU, and cisplatin with oxaliplatin.[71] It is a randomized phase III study including just over 1000 patients with advanced gastric cancer. It used a 2×2 design. Patients were either randomized to 3-week cycles of epirubicin (50 mg/m^2) plus cisplatin (60 mg/m^2) and either infusional 5-FU (200 mg/m^2 daily) (ECF) or capecitabine (625 mg/m^2 twice a day) (ECX) or epirubicin plus oxaliplatin (130 mg/m^2) and either infusional 5-FU (EOF) or capecitabine (EOX). It was designed as a noninferiority study.

Objective response rates were similar (ECF 41%, EOF 42%, ECX 46%, and EOX 48%). PFS was also similar. If one combines the overall survival of the two-capecitabine regimes there was an improvement favoring capecitabine versus infusional 5-FU (HR for death, 0.86; 95% CI, 0.8–0.99). There was no significant difference in toxicity between the capecitabine and infusional 5-FU arms.

Overall survival, PFS, and response rates in the two arms containing oxaliplatin also did not differ significantly from each other or the two cisplatin-containing arms. When comparing the previous "standard" regimen of ECF versus EOX, median survival was slightly longer at 11.2 versus 9.9 months (HR, 0.80; 95% CI, 0.66–0.97) with EOX.

The toxicities associated with oxaliplatin are somewhat different from cisplatin. Oxaliplatin was associated with more neuropathy and diarrhea, whereas cisplatin was associated with more neutropenia, thromboembolism, and renal dysfunction.

TAXANES

Paclitaxel and docetaxel have been shown to be active in gastric cancer. The taxanes, like most active agents, have had response rates around 40% to 50%, although at this time there is no clear advantage in terms of efficacy for either of the taxanes. In addition multidrug regimens including taxanes, fluoropyrimidines, and platinum agents have not been directly compared with ECF in a large randomized trial.

Docetaxel in combination with cisplatin and 5-FU (DCF) was compared with cisplatin and 5-FU alone in a large randomized trial (TAX-325).[73] A total of 457 patients with advanced gastric cancer were randomized to 21-day cycles of cisplatin, 75 mg/m^2 Day 1, infusional 5-FU, 750 mg/m^2/d Days 1 to 5, and docetaxel, 75 mg/m^2 Day 1, or cisplatin, 100 mg/m^2 Day 1, and 5-FU, 1000 mg/m^2/d Days 1 to 5.

The addition of docetaxel improved response rate (37% vs 25%), time to progression (5.6 m vs 3.7 m), and 2-year survival (18% vs 9%). Diarrhea and neutropenia were also increased with docetaxel. The group who received DCF experienced an improved clinical benefit. Based on this trial docetaxel is approved in the United States and Europe for advanced gastric cancer as the DCF regimen.

DCF was compared with ECF in a randomized phase II trial, although it involved only 81 patients with advanced gastric cancer.[74] The RR was 37% versus 26% and median overall survival 10.4 versus 8.3 months favoring DCF. More neutropenic complications were also associated with DCF. This study was not powered to determine a superior regimen.

IRINOTECAN

Irinotecan has been shown to be active in advanced gastric adenocarcinoma. It has been used in regimes including fluoropyrimidines, cisplatin/oxaliplatin, and docetaxel. Irinotecan combinations have been shown to be active, but toxic.

There is only one phase III randomized trial with irinotecan in gastric cancer.[58] The JCOG 9912 trial compared cisplatin at 80 mg/m^2 on Day 1 and irinotecan at 70 mg/m^2 on Days 1 and 15 of a 28-day cycle with 5-FU alone. The combination had improved RR (38% vs 9%) and PFS (4.8 vs 2.9 months), although it was associated with more toxicity. Unfortunately, there are no randomized phase III data comparing an irinotecan-based regimen with EOX/ECF and DCF to determine if there is a superior regimen in terms of overall survival in advanced gastric cancer.

BIOLOGIC AGENTS

Multiple biologic or targeted agents have been tested in advanced gastric cancer. Both monoclonal antibodies and small molecule tyrosine kinase inhibitors have been tested. These included agents that target Her2/neu (trastuzumab, lapatinib); epidermal growth factor receptor (cetuximab, gefitinib, erlotiniib); and vascular endothelial growth factor (bevacizumab, sunitinib, sorafenib). So far the most promising data are emerging from anti-Her2 therapy. Her2/neu (type II EFGR) is overexpressed in around 25% of gastric cancers. This is similar to breast cancer. It is more common with intestinal-type than diffuse type (32% vs 6%).[75]

The ToGA trial is a randomized phase III trial that demonstrated the efficacy of the addition of anti-Her2 therapy in patients with advanced gastric and EGJ cancers, which also overexpress Her2.[76] Patients were either randomized to six cycles of infusional 5-FU/capecitabine and cisplatin versus the same regimens and trastuzumab. Response rate (47% vs 35%) was improved with trastuzumab. Median overall survival, the primary endpoint, was also improved with trastuzumab (13.8 vs 11.1 months). The addition of trastuzumab was not associated with much toxicity. Asymptomatic decrease in cardiac ejection fraction along with diarrhea was increased in the trastuzumab arm.

SECOND-LINE CHEMOTHERAPY

There is currently no standard second-line treatment program. One would advice a regimen with agents where one would not expect cross-resistance. If a clinical trial is available it should always be considered in this setting.

The role of intraperitoneal chemotherapy in gastric cancer remains controversial. It is only applicable in highly selected patients. It is not considered a standard of care. If it is considered patients should be referred to a center with experience and expertise.

SUMMARY

Gastric cancer remains a deadly and difficult to treat malignancy. Steady progress has been made over the years through advancements in multidisciplinary treatments that combine a more locoregionally complete surgery, the incorporation of modern chemotherapeutic agents and biologic agents, and more modern radiation regimens. Western surgeons have become more willing and adept to perform a D2 lymphadenectomy. Properly conducted clinical trials that incorporate good surgical techniques and frontline chemotherapy have improved patient outcomes. As understanding of the molecular nature of individual gastric cancer improves, one can also expect the incorporation of various targeted therapies in the management of this disease. Although a cure is not yet in sight, oncologists from many different disciplines continue to make small strides that have cumulative effects over many years. The evidence is clear that a cure for gastric cancer cannot be achieved using only one treatment modality. Surgeons, medical oncologists, and radiation oncologists need to continue to work together to offer patients a comprehensive treatment plan.

REFERENCES

1. SEER Cancer Statistics. Available at: http://www.seer.cancer.gov/statistics/. Accessed January 22, 2013.
2. Wijnhoven BP, Siersema PD, Hop WC, et al. Adenocarcinomas of the distal esophagus and gastric cardia are one clinical entity. Rotterdam Esophageal Tumor Group. Br J Surg 1999;86:529.
3. Klein Kranenbarg E, Hermans J, van Krieken JH, et al. Evaluation of the 5th edition of the TNM classification for gastric cancer: improved prognostic value. Br J Cancer 2001;84:64.
4. Rudiger Siewert J, Feith M, Werner M, et al. Adenocarcinoma of the esophagogastric junction: results of the surgical therapy based on anatomical/topographic classification in 1002 consecutive patients. Ann Surg 2000;232:353.
5. Edge SB, Compton CC. American Joint Committee on Cancer staging manual. 7th edition. New York: Springer; 2010.
6. McNeer G, Bowden L, Booner RJ, et al. Elective total gastrectomy for cancer of the stomach: end results. Ann Surg 1974;180(2):252–6.
7. Gouzi JL, Huguier M, Fogniez PL, et al. Total versus subtotal gastrectomy for adenocarcinoma of the antrum. A French prospective controlled study. Ann Surg 1989;209:162–6.
8. Bozzetti F, Marubini E, Bonfanti G, et al. Subtotal versus total gastrectomy for gastric cancer: five-year survival rates in a multicenter randomized Italian trial. Italian Gastrointestinal Tumor Study Group. Ann Surg 1999;230(2):170–8.
9. Japanese Gastric Cancer Association. Japanese classification of gastric carcinoma: 3rd English edition. Gastric Cancer 2011;14:101–12.

10. Bickenbach K, Strong VE. Comparisons of gastric treatments: east vs. west. J Gastric Cancer 2012;12(2):55–62.
11. Cuschieri A, Fayers P, Fielding J, et al. Postoperative morbidity and mortality after D1 and D2 resections for gastric cancer: preliminary results of the MRC randomized surgical trial. The Surgical Cooperative Group. Lancet 1996;347(9007):995–9.
12. Cuschieri A, Weeden S, Fielding J, et al. Patient survival after D1 and D2 resections for gastric cancer: long-term results of the MRC randomized surgical trial. The Surgical Cooperative Group. Br J Cancer 1999;79(9–10):1522–30.
13. Bonenkamp JJ, Songun I, Hermans J, et al. Randomized comparison of morbidity after D1 and D2 dissection for gastric cancer in 996 Dutch patients. Lancet 1995; 345(8952):745–8.
14. Bonenkamp JJ, Hermans J, Sasako M, et al, Dutch Gastric Cancer Group. Extended lymph-node dissection for gastric cancer. N Engl J Med 1999; 340(12):908–14.
15. Hartgrink HH, Van De Velde CJ, Putter H, et al. Extended Lymph node dissection for gastric cancer: who may benefit? Final results of the Randomized Dutch Gastric Cancer Group Trial. J Clin Oncol 2004;22:2069–77.
16. Songun I, Putter H, Kranenbarg EM, et al. Surgical treatment of gastric cancer: 15 year follow-up results of the randomized nationwide Dutch D1D2 trial. Lancet Oncol 2010;11(5):439–49.
17. Siewert JR, Bottcher K, Stein JH, et al. Relevant prognostic factors in gastric cancer: ten-year results of the German Gastric Cancer Study. Ann Surg 1998; 228:449–61.
18. Kampschoer GH, Maruyama K, van de Velde CJ, et al. Computer analysis in making preoperative decisions: a rational approach to lymph node dissection in gastric cancer patients. Br J Surg 1989;76(9):905–8.
19. Bollschweiler E, Boettcher K, Hoelscher AH, et al. Preoperative assessment of lymph node metastases in patients with gastric cancer: evaluation of the Maruyama computer program. Br J Surg 1992;79(2):156–60.
20. Hundahl S, Peeters K, Kranenbarg EK, et al. Improved regional control and survival with "low Maruyama index" surgery in gastric cancer: autopsy findings from the Dutch D1-D2 Trial. Gastric Cancer 2007;10:84–6.
21. Guadagni S, de Manzoni G, Catarci M, et al. Evaluation of the Maruyama computer program accuracy for preoperative estimation of lymph node metastases from gastric cancer. World J Surg 2000;24(12):1550–8.
22. Peeters K, Hundahl S, Kranenbarg EK, et al. "Low Maruyama index" surgery for gastric cancer: a blinded re-analysis of the Dutch D1-D2 Trial. World J Surg 2005; 29:1576–84.
23. Burke EC, Karpek MS, Conlon KC, et al. Laparoscopy in the management of gastric adenocarcinoma. Ann Surg 1997;225:262–7.
24. Muntean V, Mihailov A, Iancu C, et al. Staging laparoscopy in gastric cancer. Accuracy and impact on therapy. J Gastrointestin Liver Dis 2009;18(2):189–95.
25. Zeng YK, Yang ZL, Peng JS, et al. Laparoscopy-assisted versus open distal gastrectomy for early gastric cancer: evidence from randomized and non-randomized clinical trials. Ann Surg 2012;256(1):39–52.
26. Ono H, Kondo H, Gotoda T, et al. Endoscopic mucosal resection for treatment of early gastric cancer. Gut 2001;48(2):225–9.
27. Cornelis JH, van de Velde, Koen CMJ, et al. The gastric cancer treatment controversy. J Clin Oncol 2003;21:2234.
28. Cunningham D, Allum W, Stenning S, et al. Perioperative chemotherapy versus surgery alone for resectable gastroesophageal cancer. N Engl J Med 2006;355:11.

29. Boige V, Pignon J, Saint-Aubert B, et al. Final results of a randomized trial comparing preoperative 5-fluorouracil/cisplatin to surgery alone in adenocarcinoma of stomach and lower esophagus (ASLE): FNLCC ACCORD07-FFCD 9703 trial [abstract]. J Clin Oncol 2007;25:200.
30. Ychou M, Boige V, Pignon J, et al. Perioperative chemotherapy compared with surgery alone for resectable gastroesophageal adenocarcinoma: FNCLCC and FFCD multicenter phase III trial. J Clin Oncol 2011;29:1715.
31. Cascinu S, Labiance R, Barone C, et al. Adjuvant treatment of highrisk, radically resected gastric cancer patients with 5-fluorouracil, leucovorin, cisplatin, and epidoxorubicin in a randomized controlled trial. J Natl Cancer Inst 2007;99:601.
32. Schuhmacher C, Gretschel S, Lordick F, et al. Neoadjuvant chemotherapy compared with surgery alone for locally advanced cancer of the stomach and cardia: European Organisation for Research and Treatment of Cancer randomized trial 40954. J Clin Oncol 2010;28:5210.
33. Kobayashi T, Kimura T. Long-term outcome of preoperative chemotherapy with 5'-deoxy-5fluorouridine (5'-DFUR) for gastric cancer. Gan To Kagaku Ryoho 2000;27:1521.
34. Hallisey MT, Dunn JA, Ward LC, et al. The second British Stomach Cancer Group Trial of adjuvant radiotherapy or chemotherapy in resectable gastric cancer: a five year followup. Lancet 1994;343:1309.
35. Zhang ZX, Gu XZ, Yin WB, et al. Randomized clinical trial on the combination of preoperative irradiation and surgery in the treatment of adenocarcinoma of gastric cardia (AGC) report on 370 patients. Int J Radiat Oncol Biol Phys 1998;42:929.
36. Sindelar W, Kinsela T, Chen P, et al. Intraoperative radiotherapy in retroperitoneal sarcomas: final results of a prospective, randomized clinical trial. Arch Surg 1993;128:402.
37. MacDonald JS, Smalley SR, Benedetti J, et al. Chemoradiotherapy after surgery compared with surgery alone for adenocarcinoma of the stomach or gastroesophageal junction. N Engl J Med 2001;345:725.
38. Fuchs CS, Tepper JE, Niedzwiecki D, et al. Postoperative adjuvant chemoradiation for gastric or gastroesophageal junction (GEJ) adenocarcinoma using epirubicin, cisplatin, and infusional (CI) 5-FU (ECF) before and after CI 5-FU and radiotherapy (CRT) compared with bolus 5-FU/LV before and after CRT: Intergroup trial CALGB 80101. J Clin Oncol 2011;29:4003.
39. Lee J, Lim DH, Kim S, et al. Phase III trial comparing capecitabine plus cisplatin versus capecitabine plus cisplatin with concurrent capecitabine radiotherapy in completely resected gastric cancer with D2 lymph node dissection: ARTIST trial. J Clin Oncol 2012;30:268.
40. Higgins G, Amadeo J, Smith D, et al. Efficacy of prolonged intermittent therapy with combined 5-FU and methyl-CCNU following resection for gastric carcinoma, A Veterans Administration Surgical Oncology, Group Report. Cancer 1983;52:1105–12.
41. Engstrom P, Lavin P, Douglass H, et al. Postoperative adjuvant 5-fluorouracil plus methyl-CCNU therapy for gastric cancer patients, Eastern Cooperative Oncology Group Study (EST 3275). Cancer 1985;55:1868–73.
42. Bonfanti G. Adjuvant treatments following curative resection for gastric cancer. The Italian Gastrointestinal Tumor Study Group. Br J Surg 1988;75:1100–4.
43. Allum W, Hallissey M, Ward L, et al. A controlled, prospective, randomized trial of adjuvant chemotherapy or radiotherapy in resectable gastric cancer: interim report. British Stomach Cancer Group. Br J Cancer 1989;60:739–44.
44. Coombs R, Schein P, Chilvers C, et al. A randomized trial comparing adjuvant fluorouracil, doxorubicin, and mitomycin with no treatment in operable gastric

cancer. International Collaborative Cancer Group. J Clin Oncology 1990;8: 1362–9.
45. Nitti D, Wils J, Dos Santos J, et al. Randomized Phase III trial of adjuvant FAMTX or FEMTX compared with surgery alone in resected gastric cancer. A combined analysis of the EORTC GI Group and the ICCG. Ann Oncol 2006;2:2629.
46. Nashimoto A, Nakajima T, Furukawa H, et al, Gastric Cancer Surgical Study Group, Japan Clinical Oncology Group. Randomized trial of adjuvant chemotherapy with mitomycin, fluorouracil, and cytosine arabinoside followed by oral fluorouracil in serosa-negative gastric cancer: Japan Clinical Oncology Group 9206-1. J Clin Oncol 2003;21(12):2282–7.
47. Earle CC, Maroun JA. Ajuvant chemotherapy after curative resection for gastric cancer in non-Asian patients: revisiting a meta-analysis of randomized trials. Eur J Cancer 1999;35:1059.
48. Mari E, Floriani I, Tinazzi A, et al. Efficacy of adjuvant chemotherapy after curative resection for gastric cancer: a meta-analysis of published randomized trials. A study of the GISCAD. Ann Oncol 2000;11:837.
49. Sun P, Xiang J, Chen Z. Meta-analysis of adjuvant chemotherapy after radical surgery for advanced gastric cancer. Br J Surg 2009;96:26.
50. Paoletti X, Oba K, Burzykowski T, et al, GASTRIC Group. Benefit of adjuvant chemotherapy for resectable gastric cancer: a meta-analysis. JAMA 2010;303:1729.
51. Sasako M, Sakuramoto S, Katai H, et al. Five-year outcomes of a randomized phase III trial comparing adjuvant chemotherapy with S1 versus surgery alone in stage II or III gastric cancer. J Clin Oncol 2011;29:4387.
52. Bang YJ, Kim YW, Yang HK, et al. Adjuvant capecitabine and oxaliplatin for gastric cancer after D2 gastrectomy (CLASSIC): a phase 3 open-label, randomized controlled trial. Lancet 2012;379:315.
53. Glimelius B, Ekstrom K, Hoffman K, et al. Randomized comparison between chemotherapy plus best supportive care with best supportive care in advanced gastric cancer. Ann Oncol 1997;8:163.
54. Wagner AD, Grothe W, Haerting J, et al. Chemotherapy in advanced gastric cancer: a systematic review and meta-analysis based on aggregate data. J Clin Oncol 2006;24:2903.
55. Hong YS, Song SY, Lee SI, et al. A phase II trial of capecitabine in previously untreated patients with advanced and/or metastatic gastric cancer. Ann Oncol 2004;15:1344.
56. Koizumi W, Saigenji K, Ujiie S, et al. A pilot phase II study of capecitabine in advanced or recurrent gastric cancer. Oncology 2003;64:232.
57. van Groeningen CJ, Peters GJ, Schornagel JH, et al. Phase I clinical and pharmacokinetic study of oral S-1 in patients with advanced solid tumors. J Clin Oncol 2000;18:2772.
58. Boku N, Yamamoto S, Fukuda H, et al. Fluorouracil versus combination of irinotecan plus cisplatin versus S-1 in metastatic gastric cancer: a randomized phase 3 study. Lancet Oncol 2009;10:1063.
59. Lee JL, Kang YK, Kang HJ, et al. A randomized multicenter phase II trial of capecitabine vs. S-1 as first-line treatment in elderly patients with metastatic or recurrent unresectable gastric cancer. Br J Cancer 2008;99:584.
60. Jeung HC, Rha SY, Shin SJ, et al. A phase II study of S-1 monotherapy administered for 2 weeks of a 3-week cycle in advanced gastric cancer patients with poor performance status. Br J Cancer 2007;97:458.
61. Ajani JA, Rodriguez W, Bodoky G, et al. Multicenter phase III comparison of cisplatin/S-1 with cisplatin/infusional fluorouracil in advanced gastric or

gastroesophageal adenocarcinoma study: the FLAGS trial. J Clin Oncol 2010; 28:1547.
62. Kang YK, Kang WK, Shin DB, et al. Capecitabine/cisplatin versus 5-fluorouracil/ cisplatin as first-line therapy in patients with advanced gastric cancer: a randomized phase III noninferiority trial. Ann Oncol 2009;20:666.
63. Ohtsu A, Shimada Y, Shirao K, et al. Randomized phase III trial of fluorouracil alone versus fluorouracil plus cisplatin versus uracil and tegafur plus mitomycin in patients with unresectable, advanced gastric cancer: JCOG9205. J Clin Oncol 2003;21:54.
64. Koizumi W, Narahara H, Hara T, et al. S-1 plus cisplatin versus S-1 alone for first-line treatment of advanced gastric cancer (SPIRITS) trial: a phase III trial. Lancet Oncol 2008;9:215.
65. Cullinan SA, Moertel CG, Flemming TR, et al. A comparison of three chemotherapeutic regimens in the treatment of advanced pancreatic and gastric carcinoma. Fluorouracil vs. fluorouracil and doxorubicin vs. fluorouracil, doxorubicin, and mitomycin. JAMA 1985;253:2061.
66. Findlay M, Cunningham D, Norman A, et al. A phase II study in advanced gastroesophageal cancer using epirubicin and cisplatin in combination with continuous infusion 5-fluorouracil (ECF). Ann Oncol 1994;5:609.
67. Webb A, Cunningham D, Scarffe JH, et al. Randomized trial comparing epirubicin, cisplatin, and fluorouracil versus fluorouracil, doxorubicin, and methotrexate in advanced esophagogastric cancer. J Clin Oncol 1997;15:261.
68. Ross P, Nicolson M, Cunningham D, et al. Prospective randomized trial comparing mitomycin, cisplatin, and protracted venous-infusion fluorouracil with epirubicin, cisplatin and PVI 5-FU in advanced esophagogastric cancer. J Clin Oncol 2002;20:1996.
69. Wagner AD, Unverzagt S, Grothe W, et al. Chemotherapy for advanced gastric cancer. Cochrane Database Syst Rev 2010;(3):CD004064.
70. Enzinger PC, Burtness B, Hollis D, et al. CALGB 80403/ECOG 1206: a randomized phase II trial of three standard chemotherapy regimens (SCF, IC, FOLFOX) plus cetuximab in metastatic esophageal and GE junction cancer [abstract 4006]. J Clin Oncol 2010;28:302.
71. Cunningham D, Starling N, Rao S, et al. Capecitabine and oxaliplatin for advanced esophagogastric cancer. N Engl J Med 2008;358:36.
72. Al-Batran SE, Hartmann JT, Probst S, et al. Phase III trial in metastatic gastroesophageal adenocarcinoma with fluorouracil, leucovorin plus either oxaliplatin or cisplatin: a study of the Arbeitsgemeinschaft Internistische Onkologie. J Clin Oncol 2008;26:1435.
73. van Cutsem E, Moiseyenko VM, Tjulandin S, et al. Phase III study of docetaxel and cisplatin plus fluorouracil compared with cisplatin and fluorouracil as first-line therapy for advanced gastric cancer: a report of the V325 Study Group. J Clin Oncol 2006;24:4991.
74. Roth AD, Fazio N, Stupp R, et al. Docetaxel, cisplatin, and fluorouracil; docetaxel and cisplatin; and epirubicin, cisplaitn, and fluorouracil as systemic treatment for advanced gastric carcinoma: a randomized phase II trial of the Swiss Group for Clinical Cancer Research. J Clin Oncol 2007;25:3217.
75. Takehana T, Kunitomo K, Kono K, et al. Status of c-erbB-2 in gastric adenocarcinoma: a comparative study of immunohistochemistry, fluorescence in situ hybridization and enzyme-linked immunosorbent assay. Int J Cancer 2002;98:833.
76. Bang YJ, Van Cutsem E, Feyereislova A, et al. Trastuzumab in combination with chemotherapy versus chemotherapy alone for treatment of HER2-positive advanced gastric or gastro-esophageal junction cancer (ToGA): a phase 3, open-label, randomized controlled trial. Lancet 2010;376:687.

Multidisciplinary Management of Pancreatic Cancer

Rachit Kumar, MD[a], Joseph M. Herman, MD, MS[a,b,*], Christopher L. Wolfgang, MD, PhD[c,b,d], Lei Zheng, MD, PhD[b,c,**]

KEYWORDS

• Pancreatic cancer • Multidisciplinary care • Pancreatectomy • Radiation • Chemotherapy

KEY POINTS

- Multidisciplinary evaluation of patients who have pancreatic cancer may result in a change in the diagnosis and management of patients.
- A single-day multidisciplinary clinic is an effective format for approaching this aggressive disease and should involve both physicians and ancillary staff.
- Multidisciplinary care should be applied to every stage of this disease, including resectable, borderline resectable, locally advanced, and metastatic disease.
- Multidisciplinary care should be implemented in all aspects of management, including diagnosis, initial treatment planning, and follow-up, including reevaluation throughout the course of therapy.

Disclosure: No relevant conflicts of interest to be disclosed.

[a] Department of Radiation Oncology & Molecular Radiation Sciences, The Sidney Kimmel Comprehensive Cancer Center, Johns Hopkins University School of Medicine, Baltimore, MD, USA; [b] Department of Oncology, The Sol Goldman Pancreatic Cancer Center, The Skip Viragh Center for Pancreatic Cancer, The Sidney Kimmel Comprehensive Cancer Center, Johns Hopkins University School of Medicine, Baltimore, MD, USA; [c] Department of Surgery, The Sol Goldman Pancreatic Cancer Center, The Skip Viragh Center for Pancreatic Cancer, The Sidney Kimmel Comprehensive Cancer Center, Johns Hopkins University School of Medicine, Baltimore, MD, USA; [d] Department of Pathology, The Sol Goldman Pancreatic Cancer Center, The Skip Viragh Center for Pancreatic Cancer, The Sidney Kimmel Comprehensive Cancer Center, Johns Hopkins University School of Medicine, Baltimore, MD, USA

* Corresponding author. Department of Radiation Oncology & Molecular Radiation Sciences, Sidney Kimmel Comprehensive Cancer Center, Johns Hopkins Hospital, 401 North Broadway, Weinberg Suite 1440, Baltimore, MD 21231.

** Corresponding author. Department of Oncology, The Sidney Kimmel Comprehensive Cancer Center, Johns Hopkins University School of Medicine, 1650 Orleans Street, CRB1, Room 488, Baltimore, MD 21231.

E-mail addresses: jherma15@jhmi.edu (J.M. Herman); lzheng6@jhmi.edu (L. Zheng).

Surg Oncol Clin N Am 22 (2013) 265–287
http://dx.doi.org/10.1016/j.soc.2012.12.003
surgonc.theclinics.com
1055-3207/13/$ – see front matter

INTRODUCTION

Epidemiology

Pancreatic cancer is the fourth leading cause of cancer-related deaths, despite having the 10th most common incidence of all malignancies in the United States. An estimated 43,290 new cases and 37,390 deaths are expected in 2012.[1] The median age of diagnosis in the United States is 72 years, and more than 66% are diagnosed after the age of 65 years.[2] There is a slight predominance in African Americans and Whites as opposed to Hispanics and Asians.[3] Although numerous risk factors have been researched, few have been identified. Cigarette smoking remains the clear modifiable risk factor, whereas chronic pancreatitis and genetic predisposition account for the remaining clear risk factors.[4] Obesity and a Western diet have been implicated as conferring risk, but this is less well understood.[4] The median survival for early-stage disease is 20 to 24 months, with a 5-year survival of only 15% to 20%.[5,6] Patients with locally advanced disease have a median survival of 9 to 15 months, whereas patients with metastatic disease have a median survival of 4 to 6 months.[5,6]

Staging

The American Joint Committee on Cancer (AJCC) has been the historical standard for staging of pancreatic cancer. The seventh edition of the TNM (tumor-node-metastasis) staging from the AJCC is shown in **Table 1**.[7]

In the routine practice of multidisciplinary care for pancreatic cancer, a pretreatment staging system to distinguish localized, resectable disease from unresectable disease at the time of initial diagnosis is critical. Surgically resectable tumors have a significantly improved survival compared with unresectable tumors.[1] Several institutional panels including the M.D. Anderson Cancer Center (MDACC) and National Comprehensive Cancer Network (NCCN) have proposed a staging system to separate patients based on whether they are surgically resectable, borderline resectable, unresectable, or metastatic (**Table 2**).[8] More recently, a consensus guideline modified from the MDACC staging criteria was recommended by a joint committee of the American Hepato-Pancreato-Biliary Association (AHPBA), the Society of Surgical Oncology (SSO), and the Society for the Surgery of the Alimentary Tract (SSAT).[9] This AHPBA/SSO/SSAT staging system is routinely used in the Johns Hopkins Pancreatic Multi-Disciplinary Clinic (PMDC).

The resectability of a pancreatic tumor depends on the degree of involvement of major vessels. The assessment of vascular involvement is made separately for the arterial axes and the portovenous system. With regards to the latter, any degree of involvement of the portal vein or superior mesenteric vein is considered resectable if the vessel can technically be reconstructed after en bloc resection. In contrast, involvement of the major arteries is most often made based on the degree of encasement identified on the axial plane of cross-sectional imaging. The arteries of importance include the superior mesenteric, celiac, and hepatic arteries.[5,8,10–12] Greater than 180° encasement of any of these vessels is considered locally advanced and unresectable.[8] Rarely, exceptions are made in which short-segment encasement of the hepatic artery is resected en bloc and reconstructed. Less than 180° of involvement is considered borderline resectable and is associated with an increased likelihood of a margin positive resection, higher local recurrence, and decreased survival.[8] These patients are most often offered preoperative chemoradiotherapy before resection.

The discussion of treatment options in this article uses the AHPBA/SSO/SSAT staging system as opposed to the AJCC TNM system.

Table 1
The TNM staging system of pancreatic adenocarcinoma

Stage 0	Tis	N0	M0
Stage IA	T1	N0	M0
Stage IB	T2	N0	M0
Stage IIA	T3	N0	M0
Stage IIB	T1	N1	M0
	T2	N1	M0
	T3	N1	M0
Stage III	T4	Any N	M0
Stage IV	Any T	Any N	M1

Primary Tumor (T)	**Regional Lymph Nodes (N)**	**Distant Metastasis (M)**
Tx: primary tumor cannot be assessed	Nx: regional lymph nodes cannot be assessed	M0: no distant metastasis
T0: no evidence of primary tumour	N0: no regional lymph node metastasis	M1: distant metastasis
Tis: carcinoma in situ (including PanIN)	N1: regional lymph node metastasis	
T1: tumor limited to the pancreas, ≤2 cm in greatest dimension		
T2: tumor limited to the pancreas, >2 cm in greatest dimension		
T3: tumor extends beyond the pancreas but without involvement of the celiac axis or the superior mesenteric artery		
T4: tumor involves the celiac axis or the superior mesenteric artery		

Presentation

Most patients with pancreatic adenocarcinoma present late in the course of disease, because early pancreatic cancer is often silent.[13] Typically, most patients are diagnosed incidentally via an unrelated abdominal computed tomography (CT) scan and have few or no symptoms. Most commonly, patients present with signs and symptoms of biliary obstruction, including jaundice, pruritis, light or clay-colored stools, dark urine, and scleral icterus. Occasionally, pancreatitis and cholangitis may precipitate the diagnosis of this malignancy.[4] These signs and symptoms are common for cancer of the head of the pancreas, and pancreatic body/tail lesions are often more advanced at presentation. Involvement of the celiac nerve plexus may result in epigastric abdominal pain, classically presenting as a dull pain that may radiate to the midback. Early bowel or stomach obstruction may result in early satiety, nausea, vomiting, or dyspepsia.

Some patients with pancreatic cancer may present with diabetes mellitus within 2 years of the discovery of pancreatic cancer. Migratory thrombophlebitis is an uncommon but well-recognized presenting sign in this malignancy.[14]

Table 2
The AHPBA/SSO/SSAT pretreatment staging system of pancreatic adenocarcinoma

Resectability Status	Criteria	Median Survival (mo)
Resectable	No distant metastases No radiographic evidence of SMV and portal vein abutment, distortion, tumor thrombus, or encasement Clear fat planes around the celiac axis, hepatic artery, and SMA	20–24
Borderline resectable	No distant metastases Venous involvement of the SMV/portal vein showing tumor abutment with or without impingement and narrowing of the lumen, encasement of the SMV/portal vein but without encasement of the nearby arteries, or short-segment venous occlusion resulting from either tumor thrombus or encasement but with suitable vessel proximal and distal to the area of vessel involvement, allowing for safe resection and reconstruction GDA encasement up to the hepatic artery with either short-segment encasement or direct abutment of the hepatic artery without extension to the celiac axis Tumor abutment of the SMA not to exceed >180° of the circumference of the vessel wall	Resected: ~20 Unresected: ~11
Locally advanced	Head: no distant metastases; SMA encasement exceeding >180° or any celiac axis abutment; unreconstructable SMA/portal vein occlusion/encasement; extensive hepatic artery involvement; aortic invasion or encasement Body: no distant metastases; SMA or celiac axis encasement >180°; unreconstructable SMV/portal occlusion; aortic invasion Tail: no distant metastases; SMA or celiac axis encasement >180° All: metastases to lymph node beyond the field of resection	9–15
Metastatic	Any presence of distant metastases	4–6

Abbreviations: GDA, gastroduodenal artery; SMA, superior mesenteric artery; SMV, superior mesenteric vein.

The distinction of pancreatic adenocarcinoma from the other most common solid tumors of the pancreas, which include pancreatic neuroendocrine tumor, pancreoblastoma, and solid pseudopapillary neoplasms, is often definitive based on cross-sectional imaging characteristics. In general, pancreatic adenocarcinomas tend to be hypoattenuating on venous phase CT, whereas the next most common pancreatic neoplasm, neuroendocrine, tends to enhance on arterial phase. However, variations of the common features also exist, and benign conditions such as sclerosing mesenteritis, autoimmune pancreatitis, and chronic pancreatitis may mimic pancreatic adenocarcinoma. Pancreatic adenocarcinoma can arise in association with cystic neoplasms such as intraductal papillary mucinous neoplasm and mucinous cystic neoplasm. Although a full discussion of these alternatives is beyond the scope of this article, many of these lesions can present in a similar fashion to classic pancreatic adenocarcinoma. Pancreatic neuroendocrine tumor may have systemic symptoms based on whether or not the tumor is hormone producing, as in the case of a pancreatic carcinoid tumor.[15] The discussion of appropriate treatment options in the multidisciplinary setting of a newly diagnosed pancreatic mass should recognize these alternative diagnoses.

Natural History

Analysis of the patterns of failure after the treatment of pancreatic cancer suggests that control of both local and distant disease is necessary, even in patients considered to have early-stage, surgically resectable disease. Because of their retroperitoneal location (the proximity of the pancreatic tumor to the stomach, small bowel [particularly the adjacent duodenum], spleen, and abdominal vasculature), the mass invades this tissue and may result in pain, bleeding, nausea, vomiting, and gastrointestinal obstruction.[16] Regional lymph node metastases are also common, most commonly within the pancreaticoduodenal, porta hepatis, celiac axis, superior mesenteric, and para-aortic nodes. At diagnosis, more than 80% of patients have disease that extends into adjacent organs, regional lymph nodes, or other soft tissue.[16]

The most common recognized site of metastatic disease is within the liver, followed by the lung, peritoneal cavity, and other distant sites.[4] Approximately 50% of patients have metastatic disease at the time of diagnosis.[5,6] Given that survival data after surgery alone are approximately 11.5 months with a 5-year survival of less than 17%, disease recurs in patients both locally and at distant sites.[17] The subsequent discussion introduces the modalities of treatment and their implementation at different stages of the disease.

Diagnosis and Workup

A patient with suspected pancreatic adenocarcinoma should undergo an abdominal pancreas protocol CT scan with intravenous (IV) and oral contrast along with pelvic and chest CT.[8] Abdominal pancreas protocol magnetic resonance imaging (MRI) is indicated if patients are unable to take IV contrast. Pancreas protocol CT is a multiphase contrast-enhanced set of images including a noncontrast CT scan along with arterial, pancreatic parenchymal, and portal venous phase contrast enhancement. The contrast enhancement between the pancreatic parenchyma and the tumor is greatest during the late arterial phase. Because surgical decisions regarding resectability are a direct result of the tumor-vasculature relationship identified on imaging, high-quality CT scans are preferred. MRI may be particularly helpful in identifying extrapancreatic disease, particularly in helping to identify small hepatic or peritoneal metastases.[8] The use of positron emission tomography (PET) scans is an area of ongoing research, but retrospective data show increased sensitivity of identifying metastatic disease compared with CT alone.[18] Further, recent data support the use of PET to help better characterize the extent of soft tissue extension of a pancreatic tumor before planning radiation treatment.[19]

Although a biopsy is not required before surgical resection, pathologic confirmation of malignancy is necessary before the initiation of neoadjuvant or definitive chemotherapy or radiation therapy.[8] Options for biopsy include both noninvasive (fine-needle aspiration [FNA]) and invasive approaches (open/laparoscopic), although the invasive approach should be performed only in the setting of 2 or more negative or indeterminate biopsies with a strong clinical or radiological suspicion of malignancy. FNA can be performed under CT guidance or with endoscopic ultrasonography

(EUS). Although tissue is accurately obtained from both methods, EUS is the preferred method because of a lower risk of bleeding, infection, and peritoneal seeding, as well as allowing for staging information, including an assessment of venous invasion, although it is less accurate in determining involvement of the superior mesenteric artery (SMA).[8] In addition to its diagnostic capabilities, therapeutic interventions, including celiac plexus blocks and aspiration of ascites, may be performed with EUS.

If a patient has biliary obstruction for which surgery is either delayed or not favored, biliary decompression may be performed during endoscopic retrograde cholangiopancreatography (ERCP).[8] This procedure combines endoscopic and fluoroscopic imaging and allows for palliation with stent placement. Along with ERCP, patients are recommended to undergo EUS as well.[8] The choice of metal versus plastic stents also remains a controversial issue. Although many investigators and institutions prefer metal stents because of their more durable patency, the risk of stent migration is more significant with metal stents than with plastic stents. Many NCCN member institutions prefer plastic stents in the purely palliative setting (ie, patients with a life span <3 months), whereas metal stents are preferred if patients are receiving neoadjuvant or definitive chemoradiation.[8] An ongoing prospective clinical trial seeks to better compare the choice of stent in the setting of preoperative pancreatic cancer (ClinicalTrials.gov NCT01191814).

Although many tumor-associated antigens have been studied for their diagnostic value in pancreatic cancer, none has shown as strong a connection with this disease as carbohydrate antigen 19-9 (CA 19-9).[8] This is a sialylated Lewis A blood group antigen commonly associated with pancreatic and hepatobiliary disease and with certain tumors. However, it is not pancreatic cancer specific. Because CA 19-9 may be falsely positive in cases of biliary obstruction (either benign or malignant), preoperative levels of this antigen should be measured after biliary decompression and bilirubin normalization.[8] Although CA 19-9 has not been shown to be a concrete predictor of tumor response to chemotherapy, levels of this antigen after surgical resection correlate with survival. Data from a prospective clinical trial, RTOG 9704, indicated that a CA 19-9 level greater than 180 U/mL postoperatively is associated with a significantly worse survival than levels less than this value (hazard ratio = 3.53, $P<.0001$).[20] The NCCN panel recommends the use of CA 19-9 in the preoperative setting with a normalized bilirubin, the postoperative setting to address patient prognosis, and during follow-up for surveillance monitoring.[8]

The College of American Pathologists recommends an extensive analysis of the pancreatic tumor specimen.[8] This analysis includes the histologic grade, primary tumor size (in centimeters), regional nodal involvement, and metastatic disease. Further, the extent of tumor extension into nearby vasculature, the margin status along vascular structures, the pancreatic margin, lymphovascular invasion within the tumor, and perineural invasion within the tumor, should all be identified. Pancreatic intraepithelial neoplasia (a precursor lesion to invasive pancreatic cancer) and chronic pancreatitis should be noted if present.

MULTIDISCIPLINARY MANAGEMENT BASED ON CONSENSUS STAGING

A multidisciplinary evaluation is the preferred method to properly stage a patient before initiation of therapy.[8] This evaluation ensures an objective patient assessment and improves communication between disciplines. In up to 30% of cases, a single-day multidisciplinary clinic involving multiple treatment providers and ancillary staff at a high-volume institution can result in a change in diagnosis or management.[21] Ideally, patients with nonmetastatic pancreatic cancer should undergo a multidisciplinary assessment with radiation, medical, and surgical oncology specialists. Given the huge burden that this diagnosis presents to the entire family, social work can be helpful. When indicated, nutrition should also be discussed.

Resectable Pancreatic Cancer

Surgery is the mainstay of treatment of resectable pancreatic cancer. At the Johns Hopkins PMDC, upfront surgery is routinely recommended to all resectable patients unless the patients are interested in participating in neoadjuvant therapy clinical trials or are not medically fit for surgery. The role of the multidisciplinary team (MDT) approach in the management of resectable pancreatic cancer is particularly important. Improvement in the radiographic diagnosis is one strategy to identify patients who have locally advanced or micrometastatic disease, because these patients do not benefit from aggressive upfront surgery. Resectable disease with a very high CA 19-9 level without biliary obstruction can be suggestive of systemic micrometastases, and, thus, these patients may benefit from upfront systemic therapy before local therapy (radiation or surgery).

It is still controversial whether initially resectable patients benefit from neoadjuvant (preoperative) therapy. Theoretic advantages of neoadjuvant therapies include reduction in toxicity, increase in efficacy, addressing systemic disease recurrence risk initially, and optimal patient selection for pancreatectomy through exclusion of patients with rapidly progressive metastatic disease. However, because current chemotherapy and radiation therapy have a low response rate, the concern with neoadjuvant therapy is the potential for disease progression, thus allowing initially resectable patients to become unresectable. Prospective and retrospective studies suggest that both upfront surgery and neoadjuvant therapy are associated with similar overall survival (**Table 3**). Nonetheless, patients who underwent curative surgery after neoadjuvant therapy had a longer survival (if they did not progress before surgery) compared with those who had upfront surgical resection. However, it is not known if this subpopulation of patients benefits from neoadjuvant therapy or if neoadjuvant chemotherapy merely selects those patients with a more favorable tumor biology. A randomized study comparing immediate surgery versus neoadjuvant therapy is needed to validate the role of neoadjuvant therapy in patients with resectable tumors. Neoadjuvant therapy for resectable patients should be administrated in the setting of clinical trials. An ongoing multicenter phase 3 study comparing resectable pancreatic cancer randomized to adjuvant gemcitabine or neoadjuvant gemcitabine/oxaliplatin followed by adjuvant gemcitabine (NEOPAC) may for the first time help determine the efficacy of neoadjuvant chemotherapy in pancreatic cancer.

Postoperative (adjuvant) therapy is considered to be the standard of care for resected pancreatic cancer. The role and timing of radiation, as well as the ideal chemotherapy regimen, continue to be topics of debate in the literature.[27,28] At the Johns Hopkins PMDC, both chemotherapy and radiation are favored in the adjuvant setting. However, the sequence of chemotherapy and radiation therapy is individualized. Patients with a close or positive resection margin (R1 resection) are treated with chemoradiation first, followed by further adjuvant chemotherapy. Patients with node-positive resections (regional lymph node metastasis) are treated with 4 to 6 months of systemic chemotherapy first, followed by chemoradiation if there is no evidence of disease at the completion of chemotherapy. Individuals with T1/T2 tumors and N0 resections are usually given 6 months of chemotherapy alone, although some patients also elect to receive adjuvant radiation therapy. At Johns Hopkins, these patients are

Table 3
Selected, recently published, prospective studies of neoadjuvant therapy for resectable pancreatic cancer

Study	Treatment	Patients	Median Survival (mo)	Median Survival (mo) (Number of Patients Resected)	Median Survival (mo) (Number of Patients Unresected)
Desai et al,[22] 2007	Gem/Ox + XRT → Gem/Ox	12 (44)[a]	12.5 (44 patients)	NR	NR
Varadhachary et al,[23] 2008	Gem + Cis → Gem + XRT	79	17.4	31 (52)	10.5 (27)
Evans et al,[24] 2008	Gem + XRT	86	23	34 (64)	7.1 (22)
Heinrich et al,[25] 2008	Gem + Cis	28	26.5	19.1 (25)	NR (3)
Le Scodan et al,[26] 2008	5FU/Cis + XRT	41	9.4	9.5 (26)	5.6 (15)

Abbreviations: Cis, cisplatin; Gem, gemcitabine; NR, not reported Ox, oxaliplatin; RT, radiation; XRT, X-ray radiation therapy.
[a] Twelve of a total of 44 patients were enrolled as resectable.

often treated with 2 cycles of gemcitabine-based chemotherapy, followed by chemoradiation, and concluded by another 2 cycles of gemcitabine-based chemotherapy. If patients choose not to have radiation therapy, 6 months of systemic chemotherapy is recommended. Although many data exist regarding adjuvant therapy, a consensus has not yet been reached regarding exact recommendations. A multidisciplinary assessment with radiation and medical oncologists after surgery allows patients and families to discuss the benefits and drawbacks of radiation therapy in this context.

Borderline Resectable

Patients with borderline resectable pancreatic cancer should receive neoadjuvant chemotherapy with chemoradiation. Without neoadjuvant therapy, the risk of having a positive resection margin is high for borderline tumors, because of the tumor involvement of adjacent vascular structures. With neoadjuvant therapy, most of the retrospective analyses showed that the resectability rate is approximately 30% to 40% and that the rate of margin-negative resections is approximately 80%, with survival comparable to patients with initially resectable tumors.[29] Thus, patients with locally nonresectable tumors should be included in neoadjuvant protocols and subsequently reevaluated for resection.

The role of chemotherapy or chemoradiation as a component of neoadjuvant therapy for borderline resectable tumors is not formally established. In general, both treatment modalities are considered to be part of neoadjuvant therapy. The optimal sequence of chemotherapy and chemoradiation is also not clearly defined. Induction chemotherapy followed by chemoradiation is a preferred sequence of treatment, as supported by recent studies. However, vascular involvement varies between borderline resectable tumors. Therefore, it is unlikely to define a consensus treatment strategy for all borderline resectable cases. Each individual case of borderline resectable disease should be presented in a multidisciplinary clinic or tumor board. After each treatment modality, the case should be reevaluated by the MDT. Often, radiographic changes on CT scans do not reflect tumor response after neoadjuvant therapy.[30] Other markers of tumor response, including changes in fluorodeoxyglucose (FDG) PET (maximum standardized uptake value, PERCIST [Positron Emission Tomography Response Criteria in Solid Tumors]) and CA 19-9, may assist the team in a decision regarding surgical management.[19]

Locally Advanced

There are fewer studies for locally advanced pancreatic cancer than for resectable and metastatic disease. The largest randomized study was published almost 30 years ago and showed that radiation concurrently with 5-fluorouracil (5-FU) prolonged the median overall survival from 5.7 months (with radiation alone) to 10.1 months.[31] Since this time, 5-FU combined with radiation therapy has been the standard treatment option for this population.

Subsequently, most research efforts have been made in testing the role of systemic chemotherapy in addition to chemoradiation (**Table 4**). Essentially, all randomized studies support the sequential combination of systemic chemotherapy followed by chemoradiation for locally advanced pancreatic cancer. However, these studies are limited by a small sample size and mainly tested single-agent gemcitabine after chemoradiation.

The role of systemic chemotherapy in locally advanced pancreatic cancer is emphasized by the high risk of microscopic systemic disease at the time of diagnosis or the rapid development of metastases during the course of radiation. In the last decade, induction chemotherapy with a gemcitabine-based combination was tested in

Table 4
Selected studies of locally advanced pancreatic cancer

Study	Enrollment	Treatments	Median Survival (mo)	*P* Value
GITSG Moertel et al,[31] 1981	194	60 Gy vs 60 Gy + 5-FU (bolus) or 40 Gy + 5-FU (B)	5.7 vs 10.1 or 10.6	<.01
GITSG,[32] 1988	43	Streptozocin, MMC, 5-FU vs 54 Gy + 5-FU (bolus) → streptozocin, MMC, 5-FU	8 vs 10.5	<.02
ECOG Klaassen et al,[33] 1985	91	5-FU (bolus) vs 40 Gy + 5-FU (bolus) →5-FU	8.2 vs 8.3	ns
FFCD/SFRO Chauffert et al,[34] 2008	119	Gem vs 60 Gy + 5-FU (c.i.) + Cis → Gem	13 vs 8.6	.03
ECOG Loehrer et al,[35] 2008	74	Gem vs 50.4 Gy + Gem → Gem	9.2 vs 11	.04
GERCOR Huguet et al,[36] 2007[a]	181	Gem-based chemo vs Gem-based chemo → chemorad	11.7 vs 15	.0009
MDACC Krishnan et al,[37] 2007[a]	323	Chemorad vs Gem-based chemo → chemorad	8.5 vs 11.9	<.001

Abbreviations: chemo, chemotherapy; chemorad, radiation in concurrence with 5FU, Gem, or capecitabine; Cis, cisplatin; Gem, gemcitabine; MMC, mitomycin C; c.i, continuous infusion; ns, not significant.
[a] Retrospective studies.

multiple single-arm clinical trials.[38–41] Two retrospective analyses support induction chemotherapy before chemoradiation, which is superior to upfront chemoradiation in prolonging overall survival (see **Table 4**). Therefore, locally advanced pancreatic cancer should be approached multidisciplinarily to determine the sequence of chemotherapy and radiation. Infrequently, locally advanced diseases can be downstaged with definitive chemotherapy and chemoradiation. Such patients should be evaluated for surgery by an MDT.

When it is unlikely that a patient will ever undergo surgical resection (complete encasement of the hepatic artery, celiac artery, or SMA), standard chemoradiation may be of some benefit. In these patients, innovative local therapies such as stereotactic body radiotherapy (SBRT) and irreversible electroporation are being evaluated.[42,43] With improved chemotherapy options, new modalities of local therapy may offer more durable local control.

Local Recurrence

Local recurrences are a common challenge in treating pancreatic cancer and present an area for careful coordination within the MDT. Of particular importance is the presence of an experienced radiation oncologist, medical oncologist, and radiologist.

Approximately 25% of recurrences after successful resection initially present with local recurrence (another 50% present with simultaneous local and distant recurrence). Treating this stage of disease is challenging. In general, these patients are not considered candidates for re-resection unless the recurrence is within pancreatic parenchyma. For those who recur within 6 months after the completion of adjuvant therapy, systemic recurrence is often suspected despite radiographic evidence to the contrary. Systemic chemotherapy before local radiation should be the management strategy in this population, unless they have not been treated with radiation as part of their initial adjuvant therapy. The treatment strategy follows that of locally advanced pancreatic cancer. Patients who have local recurrence more than 6 months after adjuvant therapy have a good chance of having local disease only. Therefore, it is reasonable to retreat the disease with local therapy. If the patients have received standard radiation as part of adjuvant therapy, they are often treated with SBRT at the Johns Hopkins PMDC on a clinical trial. If radiation therapy was not implemented in the adjuvant setting, standard dose radiation should be offered first.

Careful discrimination for metastatic disease is important for treating local recurrence before initiating radiation therapy. A PET scan may be valuable in this setting. A key challenge in diagnosing local recurrence is distinguishing a local recurrence from postoperative or postradiation changes. Increasing soft tissue infiltration is often the sign of local recurrence rather than posttreatment inflammatory changes, which are anticipated to attenuate over time. A PET scan may help distinguish between posttreatment fibrotic changes and local recurrence; however, posttreatment changes may be PET-avid immediately after surgery or radiation. A high-quality three-dimensional CT scan may be helpful to discern the relationship between suspected local recurrence and blood vessels. If blood vessel invasion is identified, a local recurrence is almost always present. After salvage radiation treatment, a repeat PET scan (>6 weeks after treatment) may be valuable to determine tumor response and identify metastatic disease. Treatment-responsive or stable disease may be watched without systemic chemotherapy, which can be reserved for disease progression. There are few data to guide the treatment of local recurrence. Clinical trials are required for this stage of disease.

Metastatic Disease

Newly diagnosed metastatic disease and metastatic recurrence are not curable conditions. In general, patients with metastatic disease do not benefit from surgery with a curative attempt. The multidisciplinary care for metastatic disease should be focused on supportive care and palliation, including biliary stent placement, bypass surgery, and celiac block for pain management. After adequate supportive care is provided, patients with good performance status may consider aggressive systemic chemotherapy with multiple agents. The primary goals of chemotherapy are palliation and improved survival. Although some effect on survival may be achieved, these benefits are usually limited to patients with good performance status. If patients have a poor performance status, the NCCN guidelines recommend single-agent gemcitabine or supportive care. Palliative short-course radiation (3 Gy x 10) may also be indicated if patients have local obstruction or pain.

Palliative Care

Supportive care is important for all stages of pancreatic cancer. Most patients are symptomatic at diagnosis. Pancreatectomy is associated with a high incidence of complications. Many studies have reported various prognostic factors as determinants of survival in advanced pancreatic cancer and have determined that performance status is the most relevant prognostic factor. All these studies have highlighted the importance of supportive care and palliative care in pancreatic cancer management. The multidisciplinary approach to supportive and palliative care should include nutrition counseling, pain management, biliary intervention, antiemetic treatment, psychiatric evaluation for depression, and a discussion of social and familial support systems. If patients have biliary or pancreatic obstruction and clay-colored stools, it may be important to add pancreatic enzymes to their diet. The exact dose and frequency are patient-specific and based on their caloric intake.

Accumulated data have suggested that only patients with a high performance status benefit from gemcitabine-based combinations.[44] FOLFIRINOX (infusional 5-FU/folinic acid plus irinotecan and oxaliplatin) is generally considered to be contraindicated in patients with a poor performance status because of its toxicity.[45] As a principle, patients suitable for any chemotherapy or for certain combinational chemotherapy regimens, should be carefully selected from their performance status. A deterioration of performance status occurs rapidly when pancreatic cancer progresses after the failure of first-line treatment. For patients who have a poor performance status, palliative care should be the sole focus.

MANAGEMENT OPTIONS BASED ON TREATMENT DISCIPLINE

Surgical Principles

Approximately 20% of patients with pancreas cancer are candidates for a potentially curative resection. Most resectable tumors are located in the head, neck, and uncinate process of the pancreas and are resected by a pancreaticoduodenectomy (Whipple operation). Resectable tumors in the body or tail of the pancreas undergo distal pancreatectomy and splenectomy.[46]

The goal of a potentially curative operation is to achieve a margin free of cancer (R0) in the least physiologically disruptive manner, allowing for the institution of adjuvant therapy. A margin-negative resection is achieved in 60% to 80% of operations.[16,47–49] However, although these patients are considered cleared of all known disease, their long-term survival remains poor. Even in the setting of margin-negative resections, the 5-year survival rate is 25%, and the 10-year survival rate is less than 10%.[48] Studies correlating lymph node status with survival reveal that survival is improved for lymph node-negative patients.[50–52] Wagner and colleagues[49] report a median survival time of 26 months in lymph node-negative patients compared with 16 months in lymph node-positive patients.

Postoperative Complications

Although the mortality after pancreaticoduodenectomy at specialized pancreatic surgery centers is low (2%–3%), the rate of postoperative complications remains high. In one series of 650 consecutive patients,[53] the mortality was 1.4%, but the complication rate was 41%. The most common of these complications were delayed gastric emptying (19%), pancreatic fistula (14%), and infection (10%). Similarly, in a series of more than 700 patients with a distal pancreatectomy, the morbidity was 33%, including fistula (12%), abscess (5%), small bowel obstruction (5%), and new-onset diabetes (7%).[54]

Radiation Principles

Radiation may be implemented in multiple settings of pancreatic cancer, including in neoadjuvant cases, surgically unresectable disease, as adjuvant therapy after curative resection, or as palliation for local or distant symptoms.[55] Given the rarity and severity of this diagnosis, a consultation with an experienced radiation oncologist is advised in the multidisciplinary setting. At the Johns Hopkins PMDC, a radiation oncologist meets most patients at the time of initial consultation (even some patients with metastatic disease) to discuss the role that radiation may play in the care of the patient.[21]

Standard fractionation radiation therapy is recommended at 45 to 54 Gy for up to 6 weeks at 1.8 to 2.0 Gy/day, most often with a radiosensitizer.[8] No consensus exists on specific radiosensitizers, and gemcitabine, continuous infusion of 5-FU, and capecitabine may all be considered.[8] Based on RTOG 9704 (Radiation Therapy Oncology Group), radiation is delivered in the adjuvant setting to 45 Gy to the tumor bed, surgical anastomosis, and regional lymph nodes.[56] An additional boost of 5 to 15 Gy can be directed at the tumor bed to target microscopic or macroscopic extension. The radiation volume is determined by preoperative CT scans (with oral and IV contrast) and surgical clips. Additional imaging, including an MRI and PET scan, may often help determine soft tissue extension to further assist with localization in radiation planning.[19] Although adjuvant radiotherapy has historically been avoided in patients in whom neoadjuvant chemoradiation has been delivered, recent data regarding SBRT suggests that retreatment with an acceptable risk of long-term toxicity may be a consideration.[8] This approach is recommended at high-volume, experienced radiation treatment facilities.

In the neoadjuvant, borderline, and locally advanced settings, radiation field targets the visible tumor and an adjoining margin with or without adjacent lymph nodes.[8] The radiation volume includes the gross tumor volume, an area of microscopic tumor extension (clinical target volume), and a margin for error in tumor movement or patient set-up (planning target volume [PTV]). The PTV may be reduced with optimum tumor imaging techniques, including abdominal compression and patient breath-hold to minimize internal tumor movement. Further, daily tumor imaging during radiation may also help reduce tumor movement. The reason to implement these technologies is to reduce the potential for both short-term and long-term radiation side effects.[55] The most common radiation side effects are caused by damage to the duodenum, which, along with the stomach, is one of the most radiosensitive organs in the abdomen. Short-term and long-term side effects include nausea, vomiting, abdominal pain, gastric/duodenal perforation, and malabsorption.[55]

A recent area of interest has been the use of SBRT in the treatment of pancreatic adenocarcinoma. SBRT is a radiation technology that allows the use of high doses of radiation delivered with extreme precision to a well-localized target. A pioneering study by Koong and colleagues[57] showed the safety and efficacy of this modality. Published trials evaluating this technology are outlined in **Table 5**. A recently completed, prospective, multi-institutional protocol will help determine the role of this technology in the locally advanced setting, in which significant downstaging leading to surgical resectability may be a possibility.

The use of radiation in the palliative setting has been well described. A short course of 5 to 10 fractions of radiation may be used to reduce pain associated with tumor metastases to the bones/viscera, bleeding associated with tumor infiltration into the vasculature, and obstruction as a result of tumor infiltration into the intestinal tract.[8]

Chemotherapy Principles

Pancreatic cancer is highly resistant to chemotherapy. Although systemic chemotherapy is considered to be less effective in pancreatic cancer than other gastrointestinal malignancies, its role in all stages of pancreatic cancer is well established. Fluorouracil-based chemotherapy (5-FU) was a main stay of treatment and has largely been replaced by gemcitabine. However, recent studies suggest that gemcitabine may not be superior to 5-FU.[63] Different drugs and combinations have emerged and have been incorporated with an attempt to improve treatment outcomes.

Therapy by stage

The first randomized controlled trial of adjuvant therapy in pancreatic cancer[64] concluded that treatment with bolus 5-FU plus radiation followed by 2 years of weekly 5-FU maintenance provided better outcome than surgery alone. Subsequently, 5-FU

Table 5
Selected studies of SBRT for pancreatic cancer

Study	Treatment	Pt	Toxicity	1-y FFLP (%)	Median Survival
Koong et al,[57] 2004	Phase 1 dose escalation, 3 patients: 15 Gy x 1, 5 patients: 20 Gy x 1, 7 patients: 25 Gy x 1	15	No grade 3 or 4		8.5 mo
Koong et al,[58] 2005	45 Gy IMRT + 25 Gy x 1 stereotactic boost	19	2 patients with grade 3 toxicity		33 wk
Schellenberg et al,[42] 2008	Gemcitabine + 25 Gy x 1 stereotactic	16	4 patients with grade 3 or 4	91	11.4 mo
Chang et al,[59] 2009	25 Gy x 1, 21% had received previous standard RT	77	7 patients with grade 3 or 4	84	11.9 mo
Mahadevan et al,[60] 2010	24–36 Gy in 3 fractions	36	5 patients with grade 3	78	14.3 mo
Polistina et al,[61] 2010	30 Gy in 3 fractions	23	No grade 2 or higher	NR	10.6 mo
Herman et al,[62] 2012	33 Gy in 5 fractions	32	3 patients late grade 3–4	87	14.9 mo

Abbreviations: FFLP, freedom from local progression; NR, not reported; RT, radiotherapy.

became the only standard adjuvant chemotherapy for many years. The benefit of adjuvant chemotherapy was further supported by the ESPAC-1 (European Study Group for Pancreatic Cancer 1) trial.[65] After gemcitabine was found to be superior to 5-FU for metastatic pancreatic cancer, it replaced 5-FU as first-line chemotherapy. The use of gemcitabine as an adjuvant chemotherapy is supported by the RTOG 9704 trial, which reported that the combination of gemcitabine and chemoradiation is superior to the combination of 5-FU and chemoradiation.[57] The role of gemcitabine was not established until the CONKO-001 (Charité Onkologie Clinical Studies in GI Cancer) study reported significant improvements in disease-free survival and overall survival with 6 months of adjuvant gemcitabine, versus observation, in resected pancreatic adenocarcinomas, thus determining the necessity of chemotherapy when radiation is not delivered.[66] However, the ESPAC-3 study found no significant difference in overall survival between 5-FU/leucovorin versus gemcitabine as the adjuvant therapy after surgery (**Table 6**).

The current standard of adjuvant chemotherapy is either gemcitabine or 5-FU/leucovorin alone, before or after chemoradiation, with gemcitabine more commonly used than 5-FU. The high incidence of recurrence after adjuvant chemotherapy with single-agent gemcitabine or 5-FU has led to tremendous effort in testing the combinatorial chemotherapy and innovative biologic or immune-based therapies.[70,71] However, new chemotherapy strategies have been tested only in phase 1/2 studies with a limited number of patients. Although many of these studies reported promising safety and efficacy data regarding combinatorial chemotherapy, none provided sufficiently strong evidence to support the application of any combinatorial chemotherapy in routine adjuvant therapy. Combinatorial chemotherapy should be offered through clinical trials unless metastatic disease is suspected after the pancreatectomy. Phase 3 studies to support combinatorial chemotherapy are lacking.

Among potential combinatorial chemotherapy regimens to be tested, a regimen combining gemcitabine and 5-FU is a reasonable choice. The result of the ESPAC-3 study suggested that both agents may be effective in the adjuvant setting, and therefore, the combination of both agents may offer a broad spectrum of coverage. FOLFIRINOX was shown to be superior to gemcitabine for the treatment of metastatic pancreatic cancer and may have effectiveness in the adjuvant setting. However, the high toxicity of FOLFIRINOX is a concern. The gastrointestinal toxicity may be more difficult to tolerate for postoperative patients, virtually all of whom have clinical or subclinical gastrointestinal motility issues.

Particularly intriguing are experimental therapies testing new modalities or molecular targets. Among these therapies, therapeutic vaccines and immunotherapy have emerged for this chemoresistant malignancy. Chemotherapy followed by vaccine therapy is a well-accepted sequence.[70] Sequencing chemotherapy and radiation therapy with a vaccine are still challenging because both chemotherapy and radiation therapy are associated with lymphopenia, an immunosuppressive condition.

Neoadjuvant chemotherapy

The optimal regimen for neoadjuvant chemotherapy has not been determined. The role of chemotherapy or chemoradiation as a component of neoadjuvant therapy for either borderline resectable or resectable cancers is not formally established. Gemcitabine-based combinatorial regimens have been used for neoadjuvant chemotherapy. A small, randomized phase 2 study suggested that gemcitabine-based combination chemotherapy is associated with a high resection rate (70% vs 38%) and an encouraging survival rate (62% vs 42%, 12-month survival) when compared with neoadjuvant single-agent gemcitabine.[72] Although FOLFIRINOX seems to have

Table 6
Selected randomized phase 3 studies of adjuvant chemotherapy or chemoradiation

Study	Treatment	Patients	1 y (%)	2 y (%)	5 y (%)	Median Survival (mo) (*P*)
GITSG,[64] (1985)	Obs vs chemorad	43	49 vs 63	15 vs 42	NR	11 vs 20 (.01)
Bakkevold and Kambestad,[67] (1993)	Obs vs chemo	61	45 vs 70	32 vs 43	8 vs 4	11 vs 23 (.02)
EORTC,[68] (1999)	Obs vs chemorad	114	40 vs 65	23 vs 37	10 vs 20	12.6 vs 17.1 (.099)
ESPAC-1[a,65] (2004)	2-by-2 design (no chemo vs chemo)	289	NR	30 vs 40	8 vs 21	15.5 vs 20.1 (.009)
RTOG-9704,[57] (2004)	Gem–5-FU/XRT vs 5-FU–5-FU/XRT	538	NR	NR	NR	16.9 vs 20.6 (.03)
CONKO-001,[66] (2007)	Obs vs chemo	354	72 vs 72	42 vs 47	11 vs 22	20.5 vs 22.1 (.06)
ESPAC-3,[69] (2010)	5-FU vs Gem	1088	78 vs 80	48 vs 49	NR	23.0 vs 23.6 (.39)

Abbreviations: chemo, chemotherapy; chemorad, chemoradiation; Gem, gemcitabine; NR, not reported; Obs, observation; XRT, X-ray radiation therapy.

[a] In this study with a 2-by-2 design, 147 patients were assigned to receive both chemoradiotherapy and chemotherapy or chemotherapy alone, and 142 were to receive chemoradiotherapy alone or were observed; the comparison of these 2 groups is shown here.

a higher response rate than the currently used gemcitabine-based regimen, its role in the neoadjuvant setting is still debated because of its toxicity.

Unresectable disease

The role of chemotherapy in locally advanced unresectable pancreatic cancer has been evolving. The optimal chemotherapy regimen for locally advanced pancreatic cancer has not yet been defined. However, it is reasonable to follow the same paradigm as treatment of metastatic pancreatic cancer. For both borderline resectable and locally advanced pancreatic cancer, the optimal length of induction of chemotherapy is unknown. A retrospective analysis of patients with locally advanced pancreatic cancer treated at our institution suggests that patients receiving longer than 3 cycles of induction chemotherapy have a better overall survival than those who received fewer than 3 cycles of induction chemotherapy (Faisal, Wolfgang, Herman, et al, unpublished data, 2007). These data need to be validated in a prospective clinical trial.

Metastatic disease

Systemic chemotherapy with gemcitabine has been a standard of care for advanced pancreatic cancer in the United States for decades, although the response rate remains low. Gemcitabine-based combinations with fluoropyrimidines and platin analogues have failed to provide a significant prolongation of survival, although they did demonstrate some benefits in patients with good performance status.[44,73–75] The only gemcitabine-based combination that was shown in a phase 3 clinical trial to prolong overall survival statistically compared with gemcitabine alone is the combination of gemcitabine and erlotinib; however, the magnitude of the survival improvement was not of appreciable clinical value.[76] Recently, the partenarait de recherche en oncologie digestive 4/actions concertees dans les cancer colorectaux et digestifs 11 (PRODIGE 4/ACCORD 11) trial reported that FOLFIRINOX was markedly superior to gemcitabine when tested in select good-performance patients. The median overall survival was 11.1 months in the FOLFIRINOX group compared with 6.8 months in the gemcitabine group.[45] The objective response rate was 31.6% in the FOLFIRINOX group versus 9.4% in the gemcitabine group, showing the attractiveness of FOLFIRINOX for neoadjuvant chemotherapy for borderline resectable pancreatic cancer or locally advanced pancreatic cancer. More adverse events were noted in the FOLFIRINOX group, although the patients in the FOLFIRINOX group maintained a better quality of life than those in the gemcitabine group.

New gemcitabine-based combinations are also under active investigation. The phase 1/2 studies of gemcitabine plus albumin-bound paclitaxel (nab-paclitaxel) suggest that this combination is active in patients with advanced pancreatic cancer. At the maximal tolerant dose of this combination, the response rate was 48%, with a median overall survival of 12.2 months and a 1-year survival of 48%.[77] These studies also suggest that the expression of secreted protein acidic and rich in cysteine (SPARC) in the stroma, but not in the tumor, was correlated with improved survival. A phase 3 study of nab-paclitaxel plus gemcitabine versus gemcitabine in metastatic adenocarcinoma of the pancreas has recently completed accrual with a total of 842 patients; results are forthcoming.

Another 3-drug regimen is the combination of gemcitabine, docetaxel, and capecitabine/Xeloda (GTX). The synergy of sequential treatments with these 3 drugs was supported by preclinical data. Optimized by Fine and colleagues,[78] a phase 2 study reported response rates of 21.9% and a median overall survival of 14.5 months (n = 43) in advanced pancreatic adenocarcinoma. Given the accessibility of GTX, many oncologists are now using this regimen on a routine basis. A multicenter retrospective analysis of first-line GTX showed that patients with metastatic and locally advanced disease achieved a median survival of 11.3 and 25.0 months, respectively.[79]

NOVEL BIOMARKERS/PATIENT SELECTION/FUTURE DIRECTIONS

One of the most important future aspects of multidisciplinary care for pancreatic cancer is implementing personalized medicine. Significant progress has been achieved in the last 10 years in analyzing genetic and epigenetic alterations as well as conducting a genome-wide search for biomarkers. Accumulated studies have used biomarkers to help the diagnosis, predict the prognosis, and guide the treatment. Von Hoff and colleagues[77] have tested a wide array of analytical techniques, including immunohistochemistry, fluorescence in situ hybridization, and DNA sequencing to identify biomarkers from patient specimens to help choose chemotherapy and targeted agents in clinical trials. Hidalgo and colleagues[80] have tested xenograft models in nude mice to predict sensitivity and resistance to various chemotherapy and targeted agents in patients who have pancreatic cancer. Overall, there was a remarkable correlation between drug activity in the tumor xenograft model and clinical outcome, both in terms of resistance and sensitivity. These data support the use of the personalized xenograft model as a powerful investigational platform for therapeutic decision making and to efficiently guide cancer treatment in the clinic. Many patients visiting the Johns Hopkins PMDC enquire regarding the clinical use of these tests. No guidelines exist to guide clinicians on selecting chemosensitivity prediction tests and subsequent modulation of treatment plans. Therefore, the Johns Hopkins PMDC encourages patients to use these chemosensitivity prediction tests in the setting of clinical trials, with the expectation that they may become a component of routine practice in the PMDC.

FOLLOW-UP

Given the risk of recurrence with pancreatic cancer of any stage, the NCCN consensus guidelines recommend a history and physical examination every 3 to 6 months for the first 2 years after initial therapy. The use of CA 19-9 and CT scans on a schedule of every 3 to 6 months, along with the history and physical examination, is recommended by the panel, but without data to suggest that the use of these follow-up tools improves patient outcomes. At our institution, CT scans of the abdomen and pelvis along with a CA 19-9 every 3 to 6 months, or as indicated clinically, are part of routine follow-up for this malignancy.

REFERENCES

1. Siegel R, Desantis C, Virgo K, et al. Cancer treatment and survivorship statistics, 2012. CA Cancer J Clin 2012;62:220.
2. Hayat MJ, Howlader N, Reichman ME, et al. Cancer statistics, trends, and multiple primary cancer analyses from the Surveillance, Epidemiology, and End Results (SEER) Program. Oncologist 2007;12:20.
3. Ferlay J, Shin HR, Bray F, et al. Estimates of worldwide burden of cancer in 2008: GLOBOCAN 2008. Int J Cancer 2010;127:2893.
4. Abeloff MD. Abeloff's clinical oncology. 4th edition. Philadelphia: Churchill Livingstone/Elsevier; 2008.
5. Vincent A, Herman J, Schulick R, et al. Pancreatic cancer. Lancet 2011;378:607.
6. Hidalgo M. Pancreatic cancer. N Engl J Med 2010;362:1605.
7. Edge SB. American Joint Committee on Cancer: AJCC cancer staging manual. 7th edition. New York: Springer; 2010.

8. Tempero MA, Arnoletti JP, Behrman SW, et al. Pancreatic adenocarcinoma, version 2.2012: featured updates to the NCCN guidelines. J Natl Compr Canc Netw 2012;10:703.
9. Callery MP, Chang KJ, Fishman EK, et al. Pretreatment assessment of resectable and borderline resectable pancreatic cancer: expert consensus statement. Ann Surg Oncol 2009;16:1727.
10. Buchs NC, Chilcott M, Poletti PA, et al. Vascular invasion in pancreatic cancer: imaging modalities, preoperative diagnosis and surgical management. World J Gastroenterol 2010;16:818.
11. Tseng JF, Raut CP, Lee JE, et al. Pancreaticoduodenectomy with vascular resection: margin status and survival duration. J Gastrointest Surg 2004;8:935.
12. Leach SD, Lee JE, Charnsangavej C, et al. Survival following pancreaticoduodenectomy with resection of the superior mesenteric-portal vein confluence for adenocarcinoma of the pancreatic head. Br J Surg 1998;85:611.
13. Pelaez-Luna M, Takahashi N, Fletcher JG, et al. Resectability of presymptomatic pancreatic cancer and its relationship to onset of diabetes: a retrospective review of CT scans and fasting glucose values prior to diagnosis. Am J Gastroenterol 2007;102:2157.
14. Robbins SL, Kumar V, Cotran RS. Robbins and Cotran pathologic basis of disease. 8th edition. Philadelphia: Saunders/Elsevier; 2010.
15. Crippa S, Partelli S, Boninsegna L, et al. Implications of the new histological classification (WHO 2010) for pancreatic neuroendocrine neoplasms. Ann Oncol 2012;23:1928.
16. Winter JM, Cameron JL, Campbell KA, et al. 1423 pancreaticoduodenectomies for pancreatic cancer: a single-institution experience. J Gastrointest Surg 2006; 10:1199.
17. Griffin JF, Smalley SR, Jewell W, et al. Patterns of failure after curative resection of pancreatic carcinoma. Cancer 1990;66:56.
18. Farma JM, Santillan AA, Melis M, et al. PET/CT fusion scan enhances CT staging in patients with pancreatic neoplasms. Ann Surg Oncol 2008;15:2465.
19. Wahl RL, Herman JM, Ford E. The promise and pitfalls of positron emission tomography and single-photon emission computed tomography molecular imaging-guided radiation therapy. Semin Radiat Oncol 2011;21:88.
20. Berger AC, Garcia M Jr, Hoffman JP, et al. Postresection CA 19-9 predicts overall survival in patients with pancreatic cancer treated with adjuvant chemoradiation: a prospective validation by RTOG 9704. J Clin Oncol 2008;26:5918.
21. Pawlik TM, Laheru D, Hruban RH, et al. Evaluating the impact of a single-day multidisciplinary clinic on the management of pancreatic cancer. Ann Surg Oncol 2008;15:2081.
22. Desai SP, Ben-Josef E, Normolle DP, et al. Phase I study of oxaliplatin, full-dose gemcitabine, and concurrent radiation therapy in pancreatic cancer. J Clin Oncol 2007;25:4587.
23. Varadhachary GR, Wolff RA, Crane CH, et al. Preoperative gemcitabine and cisplatin followed by gemcitabine-based chemoradiation for resectable adenocarcinoma of the pancreatic head. J Clin Oncol 2008;26:3487.
24. Evans DB, Varadhachary GR, Crane CH, et al. Preoperative gemcitabine-based chemoradiation for patients with resectable adenocarcinoma of the pancreatic head. J Clin Oncol 2008;26:3496.
25. Heinrich S, Pestalozzi BC, Schafer M, et al. Prospective phase II trial of neoadjuvant chemotherapy with gemcitabine and cisplatin for resectable adenocarcinoma of the pancreatic head. J Clin Oncol 2008;26:2526.

26. Le Scodan R, Mornex F, Partensky C, et al. Histopathological response to preoperative chemoradiation for resectable pancreatic adenocarcinoma: the French Phase II FFCD 9704-SFRO Trial. Am J Clin Oncol 2008;31:545.
27. Twombly R. Adjuvant chemoradiation for pancreatic cancer: few good data, much debate. J Natl Cancer Inst 2008;100:1670.
28. O'Reilly EM. Refinement of adjuvant therapy for pancreatic cancer. JAMA 2010; 304:1124.
29. Gillen S, Schuster T, Meyer Zum Buschenfelde C, et al. Preoperative/neoadjuvant therapy in pancreatic cancer: a systematic review and meta-analysis of response and resection percentages. PLoS Med 2010;7:e1000267.
30. Katz MH, Wang H, Balachandran A, et al. Effect of neoadjuvant chemoradiation and surgical technique on recurrence of localized pancreatic cancer. J Gastrointest Surg 2012;16:68.
31. Moertel CG, Frytak S, Hahn RG, et al. Therapy of locally unresectable pancreatic carcinoma: a randomized comparison of high dose (6000 rads) radiation alone, moderate dose radiation (4000 rads + 5-fluorouracil), and high dose radiation + 5-fluorouracil: the Gastrointestinal Tumor Study Group. Cancer 1981;48:1705.
32. Treatment of locally unresectable carcinoma of the pancreas: comparison of combined-modality therapy (chemotherapy plus radiotherapy) to chemotherapy alone. Gastrointestinal Tumor Study Group. J Natl Cancer Inst 1988;80:751.
33. Klaassen DJ, MacIntyre JM, Catton GE, et al. Treatment of locally unresectable cancer of the stomach and pancreas: a randomized comparison of 5-fluorouracil alone with radiation plus concurrent and maintenance 5-fluorouracil–an Eastern Cooperative Oncology Group study. J Clin Oncol 1985;3:373.
34. Chauffert B, Mornex F, Bonnetain F, et al. Phase III trial comparing intensive induction chemoradiotherapy (60 Gy, infusional 5-FU and intermittent cisplatin) followed by maintenance gemcitabine with gemcitabine alone for locally advanced unresectable pancreatic cancer. Definitive results of the 2000-01 FFCD/SFRO study. Ann Oncol 2008;19:1592.
35. Loehrer M, Langenbach C, Goellner K, et al. Characterization of nonhost resistance of *Arabidopsis* to the Asian soybean rust. Mol Plant Microbe Interact 2008;21:1421.
36. Huguet F, Andre T, Hammel P, et al. Impact of chemoradiotherapy after disease control with chemotherapy in locally advanced pancreatic adenocarcinoma in GERCOR phase II and III studies. J Clin Oncol 2007;25:326.
37. Krishnan S, Rana V, Janjan NA, et al. Induction chemotherapy selects patients with locally advanced, unresectable pancreatic cancer for optimal benefit from consolidative chemoradiation therapy. Cancer 2007;110:47.
38. Schneider BJ, Ben-Josef E, McGinn CJ, et al. Capecitabine and radiation therapy preceded and followed by combination chemotherapy in advanced pancreatic cancer. Int J Radiat Oncol Biol Phys 2005;63:1325.
39. Mishra G, Butler J, Ho C, et al. Phase II trial of induction gemcitabine/CPT-11 followed by a twice-weekly infusion of gemcitabine and concurrent external beam radiation for the treatment of locally advanced pancreatic cancer. Am J Clin Oncol 2005;28:345.
40. Ko AH, Quivey JM, Venook AP, et al. A phase II study of fixed-dose rate gemcitabine plus low-dose cisplatin followed by consolidative chemoradiation for locally advanced pancreatic cancer. Int J Radiat Oncol Biol Phys 2007;68: 809.
41. Moureau-Zabotto L, Phelip JM, Afchain P, et al. Concomitant administration of weekly oxaliplatin, fluorouracil continuous infusion, and radiotherapy after 2 months

of gemcitabine and oxaliplatin induction in patients with locally advanced pancreatic cancer: a Groupe Coordinateur Multidisciplinaire en Oncologie phase II study. J Clin Oncol 2008;26:1080.
42. Schellenberg D, Goodman KA, Lee F, et al. Gemcitabine chemotherapy and single-fraction stereotactic body radiotherapy for locally advanced pancreatic cancer. Int J Radiat Oncol Biol Phys 2008;72:678.
43. Martin RC 2nd, McFarland K, Ellis S, et al. Irreversible electroporation therapy in the management of locally advanced pancreatic adenocarcinoma. J Am Coll Surg 2012;215(3):361–9.
44. Cunningham D, Chau I, Stocken DD, et al. Phase III randomized comparison of gemcitabine versus gemcitabine plus capecitabine in patients with advanced pancreatic cancer. J Clin Oncol 2009;27:5513.
45. Conroy T, Desseigne F, Ychou M, et al. FOLFIRINOX versus gemcitabine for metastatic pancreatic cancer. N Engl J Med 2011;364:1817.
46. Wolfgang CL, Corl F, Johnson PT, et al. Pancreatic surgery for the radiologist, 2011: an illustrated review of classic and newer surgical techniques for pancreatic tumor resection. AJR Am J Roentgenol 2011;197:1343.
47. Neoptolemos JP, Stocken DD, Dunn JA, et al. Influence of resection margins on survival for patients with pancreatic cancer treated by adjuvant chemoradiation and/or chemotherapy in the ESPAC-1 randomized controlled trial. Ann Surg 2001;234:758.
48. Richter A, Niedergethmann M, Sturm JW, et al. Long-term results of partial pancreaticoduodenectomy for ductal adenocarcinoma of the pancreatic head: 25-year experience. World J Surg 2003;27:324.
49. Wagner M, Redaelli C, Lietz M, et al. Curative resection is the single most important factor determining outcome in patients with pancreatic adenocarcinoma. Br J Surg 2004;91:586.
50. Tomlinson JS, Jain S, Bentrem DJ, et al. Accuracy of staging node-negative pancreas cancer: a potential quality measure. Arch Surg 2007;142:767.
51. Asiyanbola B, Gleisner A, Herman JM, et al. Determining pattern of recurrence following pancreaticoduodenectomy and adjuvant 5-flurouracil-based chemoradiation therapy: effect of number of metastatic lymph nodes and lymph node ratio. J Gastrointest Surg 2009;13:752.
52. Berger AC, Watson JC, Ross EA, et al. The metastatic/examined lymph node ratio is an important prognostic factor after pancreaticoduodenectomy for pancreatic adenocarcinoma. Am Surg 2004;70:235.
53. Yeo CJ, Cameron JL, Sohn TA, et al. Six hundred fifty consecutive pancreaticoduodenectomies in the 1990s: pathology, complications, and outcomes. Ann Surg 1997;226:248.
54. Nathan H, Cameron JL, Goodwin CR, et al. Risk factors for pancreatic leak after distal pancreatectomy. Ann Surg 2009;250:277.
55. Gunderson LL, Tepper JE, Bogart JA. Clinical radiation oncology. 3rd edition. Philadelphia: Elsevier Saunders; 2012.
56. Regine WF, Winter KA, Abrams RA, et al. Fluorouracil vs gemcitabine chemotherapy before and after fluorouracil-based chemoradiation following resection of pancreatic adenocarcinoma: a randomized controlled trial. JAMA 2008;299:1019.
57. Koong AC, Le QT, Ho A, et al. Phase I study of stereotactic radiosurgery in patients with locally advanced pancreatic cancer. Int J Radiat Oncol Biol Phys 2004;58:1017.
58. Koong AC, Christofferson E, Le QT, et al. Phase II study to assess the efficacy of conventionally fractionated radiotherapy followed by a stereotactic radiosurgery

boost in patients with locally advanced pancreatic cancer. Int J Radiat Oncol Biol Phys 2005;63:320.
59. Chang DT, Schellenberg D, Shen J, et al. Stereotactic radiotherapy for unresectable adenocarcinoma of the pancreas. Cancer 2009;115:665.
60. Mahadevan A, Jain S, Goldstein M, et al. Stereotactic body radiotherapy and gemcitabine for locally advanced pancreatic cancer. Int J Radiat Oncol Biol Phys 2010;78:735.
61. Polistina F, Costantin G, Casamassima F, et al. Unresectable locally advanced pancreatic cancer: a multimodal treatment using neoadjuvant chemoradiotherapy (gemcitabine plus stereotactic radiosurgery) and subsequent surgical exploration. Ann Surg Oncol 2010;17:2092.
62. Herman JM, Chang DT, Goodman KM, et al. A phase II multi-institutional study to evaluate gemcitabine and fractionated stereotactic body radiotherapy for unresectable, locally advanced pancreatic adenocarcinoma. Poster presentation at the 2012 ASCO Annual Meeting. Chicago, June 1–5, 2012.
63. Neoptolemos JP, Moore MJ, Cox TF, et al. Effect of adjuvant chemotherapy with fluorouracil plus folinic acid or gemcitabine vs observation on survival in patients with resected periampullary adenocarcinoma: the ESPAC-3 periampullary cancer randomized trial. JAMA 2012;308:147.
64. Kalser MH, Ellenberg SS. Pancreatic cancer. Adjuvant combined radiation and chemotherapy following curative resection. Arch Surg 1985;120:899.
65. Neoptolemos JP, Stocken DD, Friess H, et al. A randomized trial of chemoradiotherapy and chemotherapy after resection of pancreatic cancer. N Engl J Med 2004;350:1200.
66. Oettle H, Post S, Neuhaus P, et al. Adjuvant chemotherapy with gemcitabine vs observation in patients undergoing curative-intent resection of pancreatic cancer: a randomized controlled trial. JAMA 2007;297:267.
67. Bakkevold KE, Kambestad B. Long-term survival following radical and palliative treatment of patients with carcinoma of the pancreas and papilla of Vater–the prognostic factors influencing the long-term results. A prospective multicentre study. Eur J Surg Oncol 1993;19:147.
68. Klinkenbijl JH, Jeekel J, Sahmoud T, et al. Adjuvant radiotherapy and 5-fluorouracil after curative resection of cancer of the pancreas and periampullary region: phase III trial of the EORTC gastrointestinal tract cancer cooperative group. Ann Surg 1999;230:776.
69. Neoptolemos JP, Stocken DD, Bassi C, et al. Adjuvant chemotherapy with fluorouracil plus folinic acid vs gemcitabine following pancreatic cancer resection: a randomized controlled trial. JAMA 2010;304:1073.
70. Lutz E, Yeo CJ, Lillemoe KD, et al. A lethally irradiated allogeneic granulocyte-macrophage colony stimulating factor-secreting tumor vaccine for pancreatic adenocarcinoma. A Phase II trial of safety, efficacy, and immune activation. Ann Surg 2011;253:328.
71. Picozzi VJ, Abrams RA, Decker PA, et al. Multicenter phase II trial of adjuvant therapy for resected pancreatic cancer using cisplatin, 5-fluorouracil, and interferon-alfa-2b-based chemoradiation: ACOSOG Trial Z05031. Ann Oncol 2011;22:348.
72. Palmer DH, Stocken DD, Hewitt H, et al. A randomized phase 2 trial of neoadjuvant chemotherapy in resectable pancreatic cancer: gemcitabine alone versus gemcitabine combined with cisplatin. Ann Surg Oncol 2007;14:2088.
73. Louvet C, Labianca R, Hammel P, et al. Gemcitabine in combination with oxaliplatin compared with gemcitabine alone in locally advanced or metastatic

pancreatic cancer: results of a GERCOR and GISCAD phase III trial. J Clin Oncol 2005;23:3509.
74. Heinemann V, Quietzsch D, Gieseler F, et al. Randomized phase III trial of gemcitabine plus cisplatin compared with gemcitabine alone in advanced pancreatic cancer. J Clin Oncol 2006;24:3946.
75. Poplin E, Feng Y, Berlin J, et al. Phase III, randomized study of gemcitabine and oxaliplatin versus gemcitabine (fixed-dose rate infusion) compared with gemcitabine (30-minute infusion) in patients with pancreatic carcinoma E6201: a trial of the Eastern Cooperative Oncology Group. J Clin Oncol 2009;27:3778.
76. Moore MJ, Goldstein D, Hamm J, et al. Erlotinib plus gemcitabine compared with gemcitabine alone in patients with advanced pancreatic cancer: a phase III trial of the National Cancer Institute of Canada Clinical Trials Group. J Clin Oncol 2007;25:1960.
77. Von Hoff DD, Ramanathan RK, Borad MJ, et al. Gemcitabine plus nab-paclitaxel is an active regimen in patients with advanced pancreatic cancer: a phase I/II trial. J Clin Oncol 2011;29:4548.
78. Fine RL, Fogelman DR, Schreibman SM, et al. The gemcitabine, docetaxel, and capecitabine (GTX) regimen for metastatic pancreatic cancer: a retrospective analysis. Cancer Chemother Pharmacol 2008;61:167.
79. De Jesus-Acosta A, Oliver GR, Blackford A, et al. A multicenter analysis of GTX chemotherapy in patients with locally advanced and metastatic pancreatic adenocarcinoma. Cancer Chemother Pharmacol 2012;69:415.
80. Hidalgo M, Bruckheimer E, Rajeshkumar NV, et al. A pilot clinical study of treatment guided by personalized tumorgrafts in patients with advanced cancer. Mol Cancer Ther 2011;10:1311.

Colorectal Cancer Metastases

A Surgical Perspective

Paul H. Sugarbaker, MD, FRCS

KEYWORDS

- Lymph node metastases • Liver metastases • Peritoneal metastases
- Peritoneal carcinomatosis • Lung metastases
- Hyperthermic intraperitoneal chemotherapy
- Early postoperative intraperitoneal chemotherapy

KEY POINTS

- The survival of patients with peritoneal metastases is reduced when compared with other sites of metastatic disease such as the liver or lymph nodes.
- Isolated sites of metastatic disease can be resected by surgery with curative intent. These sites include the lungs, liver, and lymph nodes.
- If they are of limited extent, peritoneal metastases are treated with combined cytoreductive surgery and perioperative chemotherapy.
- The management strategies for synchronous metastases at numerous anatomic sites are different from metachronous metastases at numerous sites. Careful evaluation of individualized treatments by the multidisciplinary team is necessary.

INTRODUCTION

The management of colorectal cancer has continued to evolve over approximately 1 century. The most effective strategy to combat this disease is prevention. Prevention involves the identification of high-risk groups, dietary changes, and possible dietary supplements.[1] The next most effective management strategy is screening for disease to confirm a diagnosis in its early stages. The use of the hemoccult test on a regular basis has been proved effective.[2] Better yet for screening is complete colonoscopy.[3] In symptomatic patients, the management strategies have been well defined for both colon cancer and rectal cancer. The surgery must provide a complete clearance of the primary cancer and its lymph node groups at risk for metastatic disease. The resection must be accomplished with perfect containment of the process.[4,5] A patient may enter the operating room with a contained process and leave with disseminated disease. This situation results from trauma to the surgical specimen so that cancer cells are lost from the specimen into the resection site or free peritoneal cavity.[6] This loss can occur with open colorectal surgery or with laparoscopic resection.

Washington Cancer Institute, Washington Hospital Center, 106 Irving Street, Northwest, Suite 3900, Washington, DC 20010, USA
E-mail address: paul.sugarbaker@medstar.net

Surg Oncol Clin N Am 22 (2013) 289–298
http://dx.doi.org/10.1016/j.soc.2012.12.007 surgonc.theclinics.com
1055-3207/13/$ – see front matter

This article is not a commentary on the 70% of patients who have an uncomplicated colorectal cancer resection and a favorable prognosis. It concerns the approximately 30% of patients who have advanced disease at the time of presentation and the 50% of patients who months or years after resection fail treatment of primary disease. The focus is on local recurrence and metastases from colon and rectal cancer.

LYMPH NODAL METASTASES FROM COLORECTAL CANCER

In the past, extensive lymphadenectomy as part of a colorectal cancer resection was believed to be unnecessary. The rationale was that patients with metastases to the intermediate or para-aortic nodes could not survive, even if these nodes were resected as part of the primary colorectal surgical intervention. Recent data suggest that this retreat to a conservative resection is not indicated; rather, a wide resection should be performed of lymph nodes to the superior mesenteric vessels on the right and left to the origin of the inferior mesenteric artery on the left. Swanson and colleagues[7] reported on the survival of 35,787 prospectively collected cases of T3N0 colon cancers that were surgically treated and pathologically reported from 1985 to 1991. T3 cancers are expected to be at a higher risk for lymph nodal metastases compared with T1 or T2 lesions and, therefore, adequate lymphadenectomy is of greater benefit in this subgroup of patients. The 5-year survival of patients with T3N0M0 colon cancer varied from 64% if 1 or 2 lymph nodes were examined to 86% if more than 25 lymph nodes were examined. Three strata of lymph nodes (1–7, 8–12, and >13) distinguished significantly different observed 5-year survival rates. These investigators concluded that the prognosis of patients with T3N0 colon cancer is dependent on the number of lymph nodes examined and suggest a minimum of 13 lymph nodes to be resected.

Le Voyer and colleagues[8] reported on survival from an intergroup trial, INT-0089. In 3411 assessable patients, 648 had no evidence of lymph node metastases. Multivariate analyses were performed on both the node-positive and node-negative groups separately to ascertain the effect of extent of lymph node resection on survival. Survival decreased with increasing number of lymph nodes involved (P = .0001), as might be expected. After controlling for the number of nodes involved, survival increased as more nodes were analyzed (P = .0001). Even when no nodes were involved, overall survival and cause-specific survival improved as more nodes were analyzed (P = .0005 and P = .007, respectively). These investigators concluded that the number of lymph nodes resected and available for analysis for staging colon cancer is a prognostic variable on outcome.

West and colleagues[4] looked at the plane of surgical resection of colonic cancer. The complete mesocolic excision with central vascular ligation produced a survival of greater than 89%. There was a greater yield of lymph nodes in 49 specimens from Erlangen, Germany compared with 40 standard specimens from Leeds, United Kingdom; a lymph node yield of 30 in Erlangen was compared with 18 in Leeds (P<.0001). These investigators concluded that the plane of colon cancer resection and the extent of lymphadenectomy are important in optimal surgical technique. A mesocolic resection contained along with the associated greater lymph node yield was suggested as the explanation for increased survival rates reported in Erlangen.

HEPATIC METASTASES FROM COLORECTAL CANCER

As a result of the pioneering efforts of Wilson and Adson,[9] Foster and Berman,[10] and Hughes and colleagues,[11] the benefits that occur with the resection of liver metastases from metastatic colorectal cancer have been established as a standard of practice. Nevertheless, there has been no verification of the evidence in terms of a phase 3 randomized controlled study.[12] Overall, the 5-year survival after hepatic resection is 30% to 50%. There may be some improvement in this statistic as a result of repeat hepatic resections that have been shown to be successful.[13] In some patients with liver metastases that are unresectable because of a large extent of disease, systemic chemotherapy can downsize the liver metastases so that an R-0 resection is possible. The survival of this group of patients receiving neoadjuvant chemotherapy is nearly identical to patients having surgery as an initial treatment.[14]

Patient-related factors associated with poor outcome include increase in serum carcinoembryonic antigen (CEA), positive lymph node status of the primary tumor, lymph nodes present in the regional periportal lymph nodes, and disease-free interval of less than 1 year. Factors in respect to liver metastases that carry a poor prognosis are increasing number of lesions, increasing size of the largest lesion, bilobar distribution, and percentage of hepatic replacement by cancer. Also, technical factors such as a positive or close margins of resection carry a reduced prognosis.[11,15]

The technology used to destroy the liver metastases may vary greatly from institution to institution. Also, the anatomic location, size, and number of metastases may favor 1 method of ablation over another. With multiple metastases limited to either the right or left lobe, a right or left hepatectomy is indicated. Also, a lesion greater than 5 cm usually requires hemihepatectomy. However, segmental resection with clear margins may be indicated if an R-0 resection is possible. Radiofrequency ablation is an option if metastases are less than 5 cm and are not immediately adjacent to a major bile duct or major vascular structure.[16] Indications for a cryogenic ablation are similar to those for radiofrequency ablation.[17] A frequent indication for an ablative procedure in combination with resection is 1 or 2 metastases deep in the residual liver after a hemihepatectomy.

Recently, percutaneous ablation procedures have been reported.[18] Results in properly selected patients seem to be acceptable. Also, laparoscopic liver resection has been reported and associated with a reduced hospital stay.[19]

MULTIPLE SITES OF COLORECTAL METASTASES

Synchronous Metastases

Frequently, patients with simultaneous liver metastases and lung metastases or liver metastases and peritoneal metastases must be considered for treatment. In general, the Elias rule of 5s can be applied in this situation. If the patient can be made clinically disease-free and there are 5 or fewer sites of metastases, then the attempt at resection should occur. The clinician needs to realize that the morbidity and mortality from combined metastasectomy in liver, lung, or peritoneal space is increased. Also, 30% of patients are brought to the operating room for an exploratory laparotomy through a long abdominal incision and complete resection is found to be impossible.[20]

Metachronous Metastases

Patients who present with metachronous metastases present less of problem. The benefits seem to be worth the risk if an R-0 resection of all sites of metastatic disease is possible. Resection of liver metastases after previous lung metastases has been reported,[21] as well as resection of pulmonary metastases after liver metastases sequentially with R-0 resections.[22] Also the use of cytoreductive surgery and hyperthermic perioperative chemotherapy to treat peritoneal metastases before or after resection of liver metastases is common. However, the occurrence of more than 1 anatomic site of metastatic disease is associated with a reduced prognosis.[23] Palliative as well as curative benefits may occur.

MANAGEMENT OF PERITONEAL METASTASES

Survival benefits for peritoneal metastases from colon and rectal cancer using cytoreductive surgery and perioperative chemotherapy began to appear in publications in the 1990s. In 1995, Sugarbaker and Jablonski[24] showed a 3-year survival of 35% in patients with peritoneal metastases from colon cancer treated with cytoreductive surgery plus intraperitoneal mitomycin C and fluorouracil. In 2003, Verwaal and colleagues[25] from Amsterdam published a 3-year projected survival of 38% in 54 patients treated by cytoreductive surgery and hyperthermic intraperitoneal mitomycin C with adjuvant systemic 5-fluorouracil. Shen and colleagues[26] accumulated patients between 1991 and 2002. Seventy-seven patients with nonappendiceal colorectal cancer underwent the combined treatment. These investigators concluded that one-third of patients with complete resection have long-term survival and that systemic chemotherapy did not contribute to the control of peritoneal metastases. These studies performed in the absence of modern colorectal cancer chemotherapy (oxaliplatin and irinotecan) document the efficacy of cytoreductive surgery and perioperative chemotherapy to rescue approximately one-third of patients with peritoneal metastases.

Since that time, multiple publications confirming the efficacy of the combination of cytoreductive surgery and perioperative chemotherapy to benefit patients with colorectal metastases have been published. Glehen and colleagues, in a multi-institutional retrospective study of 506 patients from 28 institutions,[27] reported an overall median survival of 19.2 months in patients with peritoneal metastases from colorectal cancer treated with the combined approach. Patients in whom the cytoreductive surgery was complete had a median survival of 32.4 months compared with 8.4 months in patients in whom cytoreduction was not completed ($P<.001$). The morbidity was 22.9% and mortality 4%. These investigators concluded that the therapeutic approach of combining cytoreductive surgery with perioperative intraperitoneal chemotherapy achieved long-term survival in a selected group of patients with peritoneal metastases of colorectal origin with acceptable morbidity and mortality. The complete cytoreduction was the most important prognostic indicator.

Elias and colleagues[28] reported on colorectal peritoneal metastases in a retrospective analysis of 523 patients from 23 French-speaking centers. The overall median survival was 30.1 months and the 5-year overall survival was 27%. Eighty-four percent of the patients had a complete cytoreduction, with a median survival of 33 months. These investigators concluded that cytoreductive surgery and perioperative chemotherapy is now considered the gold standard in the French guidelines for management of peritoneal metastases. Similarly, Verwaal[29] reported a long-term Dutch multicenter data analysis. The survival of 562 patients at 10 years was 37%.

At the top of the list regarding evidence-based medicine for this treatment strategy is the phase 3 study reported by Verwaal and colleagues[30] in 2003. This landmark study compared 105 patients with colorectal peritoneal metastases who were randomly assigned to receive either standard treatment with systemic 5-fluorouracil and leucovorin compared with an aggressive cytoreductive surgery with perioperative chemotherapy using hyperthermic mitomycin C. The patients in the experimental therapy arm also had systemic 5-fluorouracil chemotherapy. After a median follow-up of 21.6 months, the median survival was 12.6 months with systemic chemotherapy and 22.3 months with cytoreduction and perioperative chemotherapy ($P = .032$). These investigators reported that a complete cytoreduction and a limited extent of disease were important determinants of benefit. The durability of the benefit of cytoreductive surgery and perioperative chemotherapy was confirmed in a follow-up article in 2008.[31]

Recently, these benefits have been called into question by Ryan.[32] He has questioned the relevance of cytoreductive surgery and perioperative chemotherapy now that oxaliplatin, irinotecan, and molecular agents are available. He contends that the benefits of systemic chemotherapy alone are so great that cytoreduction plus perioperative chemotherapy is no longer indicated. However, current data confirm that for a limited extent of peritoneal metastases, a multidisciplinary approach using the best surgical and best chemotherapy treatments is preferable. Franko and colleagues[33] presented data to show that these 2 options work best when used together. They showed that the median survival was longer in patients treated by modern systemic chemotherapy when cytoreductive surgery and hyperthermic intraperitoneal chemotherapy were added to the clinical pathway. Currently, standard of care, until more data become available, indicates that patients with peritoneal metastases from colorectal cancer have the right to be informed of a possible curative treatment option. It is the oncologist's obligation to provide the relevant information in a timely fashion.[34]

LUNG METASTASES FROM COLORECTAL CANCER

Thoracotomy to remove metastatic colorectal cancer has been advocated since the early 1980s. Lung metastases, in the absence of metastases at other sites, occur in a few patients with colorectal cancer . In 1 series of 1578 patients who underwent a potentially curative resection of colorectal cancer, 137 (8.7%) developed lung metastases and only 16 (1%) were candidates for thoracotomy.[35] The incidence of lung metastases from colon cancer and lung metastases from rectal cancer are different. Eleven and a half percent were resected from rectal cancer and only 3.6% from patients with colon cancer.[35] Currently, favorable factors for resection include solitary metastases, CEA less than 5 ng/mL, and a disease-free interval of greater than 3 years.[36]

Technology of Pulmonary Metastases Resection or Ablation

Originally, lung metastases were resected through a lateral thoracostomy incision. In selected patients with bilateral pulmonary metastases a bilateral thoracotomy may facilitate the resection by eradication of disease from both lungs with a single intervention.[37]

Also, thoracoscopic intervention may identify and then resect the pulmonary metastases in the absence of a thoracotomy. The lesion should be 3 cm or less in size, well identified on computed tomography and away from major vessels or bronchi.[38]

Recently, percutaneous ablation of lung nodules has been reported.[39] This technology in properly selected patients is reported to be well tolerated and effective in long-term follow-up. If the expertise is available, percutaneous ablation may be the treatment of choice in selected patients.

METASTASES FROM METASTASES

Frequently, surgical judgments regarding the timing of surgical resection of metastatic disease are not obvious to the clinician. The surgeon does not want to proceed with a resection that carries moderate to high morbidity and mortality if in the near future, metastatic disease at several other anatomic sites becomes evident. However, the watch-and-wait management strategy carries with it the danger of a larger extent of disease and the possibility for further dissemination of the malignant process. The concept of metastases from metastases is a phenomenon that has been reported in patients with colorectal cancer. August and colleagues[40] reviewed their records of

81 patients who had liver resection for colorectal metastases. In 7 patients (9%), at the time of surgery, lymph node metastases within the lymphatic drainage of the liver were documented. All 7 of these patients had their extrahepatic lymphatic disease limited to nodes draining the liver, implicating lymphatic dissemination of the hepatic metastases as the mechanism of cancer spread. In this situation, the likelihood of long-term benefit from a liver resection is reduced.[41] August and colleagues[40] suggested that a need for frequent and thorough follow-up of patients after resection of primary colorectal cancer is indicated and that an urgency in the definitive management (surgical resection) of liver metastases should occur if possible.

Evers and colleagues[42] studied the pattern of relapse in women with colorectal peritoneal carcinomatosis that showed ovarian metastases. One hundred and five women underwent cytoreductive surgery combined with hyperthermic intraoperative chemotherapy. Sixty-two of the 105 (60%) had ovarian metastases. The median overall survival of the women with or without ovarian metastases was not statistically significant at 36 and 40 months, respectively. However, the pattern of relapse was different in the 2 groups. There were 19 patients who had retroperitoneal lymph nodal relapse, and 18 of these 19 patients had ovarian metastases. The only predictive factor for retroperitoneal relapse was a history of ovarian metastases (P = .0012). The investigators concluded that retroperitoneal lymph node recurrence was linked to ovarian metastases originating from the colorectal malignancy. Early intervention or an intervention combined with systematic lymphadenectomy was suggested as a treatment option for this group of patients. Evers and Verwaal showed that the disease-free survival after a cytoreductive surgery plus HIPEC (heated intraperitoneal chemotherapy) procedure for colorectal or appendiceal peritoneal metastases was significantly lower in women with ovarian metastases. These data may also suggest that retroperitoneal metastases are a sequela of peritoneal metastases being present within the ovaries.

In patients with resectable lung metastases from primary colorectal cancer, Okumura and colleagues[43] reported that approximately one-third had mediastinal lymph node involvement documented at the time of thoracotomy. Yedibela and colleagues[44] documented mediastinal involvement in 5% of patients. Documentation of hilar metastases from lung metastases indicates a reduced prognosis with resection of pulmonary metastases. Inoue and colleague[45] reported a 5-year survival of 50% in patients with negative mediastinal or hilar lymph nodes compared with 14% with positive lymph nodes.

LOCALLY RECURRENT RECTAL CANCER

Rectal cancer may progress to an advanced stage with few or no symptoms. The large caliber of the midrectum and lower rectum can result in an absence of obstructive symptoms. Blood per rectum may be attributed to hemorrhoids and fail to cause the patient to seek medical assistance. Even with preoperative chemoradiation therapy, T3 and T4 rectal cancer may result in locally recurrent disease.[46,47]

The anatomic location of the recurrence is an important determinant of treatment options.[47,48] Lateral extension after previous total mesorectal excision is seldom resectable with an adequate margin of resection. Intraoperative radiation therapy may be added to the surgery in selected patients.[49] If the recurrence is anterior in the female patient, a vaginectomy is usually required. With posterior extension, partial sacrectomy may result in negative margins. In nearly all patients with a previous low anterior resection, an abdominoperineal resection of the residual rectum is necessary. Long-term survival is observed in approximately 10% of these patients.[47]

BRAIN METASTASES

Metastases to the brain are important because they may represent the final site of metastases, with successful control of metastatic disease at several other anatomic sites. For example, patients with successfully treated liver metastases and lung metastases may succumb to disease spread to the brain. Brain metastases are important because they show the significance of the anatomic location of the dissemination in terms of prognosis. Patients with brain metastases rarely live more than several months after diagnosis. Metastases to this site rapidly cause demise of the patient; in contrast, a larger metastasis to the liver is usually not symptomatic, may be successfully removed surgically, and has a different prognosis. The difference in prognosis of metastases located within the liver versus metastases located within the peritoneal space has already been shown.[50]

SUMMARY

All Metastases are not the Same

In this review, the differences in management of colorectal metastases at different anatomic sites have been emphasized. One of the major goals of this article is to convince the oncologist that the management of metastatic disease from colorectal cancer must be an individualized plan. The concept that systemic chemotherapy is the adequate solution to all sites of colorectal metastatic disease is not a reasonable management strategy. The treatments must be more sophisticated and individualized.

Knowledgeable Management During Follow-Up

Patients who must undergo treatment of colon and rectal cancer require a knowledgeable assessment of their disease process not only to determine prognosis but also to predict likely sites for disease progression. Some patients (eg, those in whom peritoneal seeding was documented at the time of the primary colorectal cancer resection) are recommended for second-look surgery combined with hyperthermic perioperative chemotherapy. All patients with stage II, III, or IV disease require meticulous follow-up to identify progression of disease and then evaluation for additional surgical procedures, which may result in an R-0 intervention. Lymph nodal metastases, liver metastases, peritoneal metastases, lung metastases, and locally recurrent disease have treatment options for palliation and in selected patients for cure. The treatments with long-term benefit frequently combine an R-0 resection with local-regional and systemic chemotherapy.

REFERENCES

1. Willet WC, Stampfer MJ, Colditz GA, et al. Relation of meat, fat, and fiber intake to the risk of colon cancer in a progressive study among women. N Engl J Med 1990;323:1664–72.
2. Mandel JS, Bond JH, Church TR, et al. Reducing mortality from colorectal cancer by screening for fecal occult blood. N Engl J Med 1993;328:1365–71.
3. Lieberman DA, Weiss DG, Bond JH, et al. Use of colonoscopy to screen asymptomatic adults for colorectal cancer. N Engl J Med 2000;343:162–8.
4. West NP, Hohenberger W, Weber K, et al. Complete mesocolic excision with central vascular ligation produces an oncologically superior specimen compared with standard surgery for carcinoma of the colon. J Clin Oncol 2010;28(2):272–8.

5. Quirke P, Durdey P, Dixon M, et al. Local recurrence of rectal adenocarcinoma due to inadequate surgical resection: histopathological study of lateral tumour spread and surgical excision. Lancet 1986;2:996–9.
6. Sugarbaker PH. Successful management of microscopic residual disease in large bowel cancer. Cancer Chemother Pharmacol 1999;43(Suppl):S15–25.
7. Swanson RS, Compton CC, Stewart AK, et al. The prognosis of T3N0 colon cancer is dependent on the number of lymph nodes examined. Ann Surg Oncol 2003;10(1):65–71.
8. Le Voyer TE, Sigurdson ER, Hanlon AL, et al. Colon cancer survival is associated with increasing number of lymph nodes analyzed: a secondary survey of intergroup trial INT-0089. J Clin Oncol 2003;21(15):2912–9.
9. Wilson SM, Adson MA. Surgical treatment of hepatic metastases from colorectal cancers. Arch Surg 1976;111:330–4.
10. Foster JH, Berman MM. Solid liver tumors. Philadelphia: WB Saunders; 1977.
11. Hughes KS, Simon RM, Songhorabodi S, et al. Resection of the liver for colorectal carcinoma metastases: a multi-institutional study of indications for resection. Registry of Hepatic Metastases. Surgery 1987;103:278–88.
12. Kaido T. Verification of evidence in surgical treatment for colorectal liver metastases. Hepatogastroenterology 2008;55:378–80.
13. Fernandez-Trigo V, Shamsa F, Sugarbaker PH. Repeat liver resections from colorectal metastasis. Repeat Hepatic Metastases Registry. Surgery 1995;117:296–304.
14. Adam R, Delvart V, Pascal G, et al. Rescue surgery for unresectable colorectal liver metastases downstaged by chemotherapy: a model to predict long-term survival. Ann Surg 2004;240:644–57.
15. Sugarbaker PH. Surgical management of primary and metastatic cancer of the liver. In: Shiff E, editor. Diseases of the liver. Philadelphia: JB Lippincott; 1993. p. 1297–319.
16. Abdalla EK, Vauthey JN, Ellis LM, et al. Recurrence and outcomes following hepatic resection, radiofrequency ablation, and combined resection/ablation for colorectal liver metastases. Ann Surg 2004;239(6):818–25.
17. Joosten J, Jager G, Oyen W, et al. Cryosurgery and radiofrequency ablation for unresectable colorectal liver metastases. Eur J Surg Oncol 2005;31(10):1152–9.
18. Solbiati L, Livraghi T, Goldberg SN, et al. Percutaneous radio-frequency ablation of hepatic metastases from colorectal cancer: long-term results in 117 patients. Radiology 2001;221(1):159–66.
19. Buell JF, Cherqui D, Geller DA, et al. The international position on laparoscopic liver surgery: the Louisville Statement, 2008. Ann Surg 2009;250:825–30.
20. Elias D, Liberale G, Vernerey D, et al. Hepatic and extrahepatic colorectal metastases: when resectable, their localization does not matter, but their total number has a prognostic effect. Ann Surg Oncol 2005;12(11):900–9.
21. Headrick JR, Miller DL, Nagorney DM, et al. Surgical treatment of hepatic and pulmonary metastases from colon cancer. Ann Thorac Surg 2001;71(3):975–9.
22. Robinson BJ, Rice TW, Strong SA, et al. Is resection of pulmonary and hepatic metastases warranted in patients with colorectal cancer? J Thorac Cardiovasc Surg 1999;117(1):66–75.
23. Elias D, Sideris L, Pocard M, et al. Results of R0 resection for colorectal liver metastases associated with extrahepatic disease. Ann Surg Oncol 2004;11(3):274–80.
24. Sugarbaker PH, Jablonski KA. Prognostic features of 51 colorectal and 130 appendiceal cancer patients with peritoneal carcinomatosis treated by cytoreductive surgery and intraperitoneal chemotherapy. Ann Surg 1995;221(2):124–32.

25. Verwaal VJ, van Ruth S, Witkamp A, et al. Long-term survival of peritoneal carcinomatosis of colorectal origin. Ann Surg Oncol 2005;12(1):65–71.
26. Shen P, Hawksworth J, Lovato J, et al. Cytoreductive surgery and intraperitoneal hyperthermic chemotherapy with mitomycin C for peritoneal carcinomatosis from nonappendiceal colorectal carcinoma. Ann Surg Oncol 2004;11(2):178–86.
27. Glehen O, Kwiatkowski F, Sugarbaker PH, et al. Cytoreductive surgery combined with perioperative intraperitoneal chemotherapy for the management of peritoneal carcinomatosis from colorectal cancer: a multi-institutional study. J Clin Oncol 2004;22(16):3284–92.
28. Elias D, Gilly F, Boutitie F, et al. Peritoneal colorectal carcinomatosis treated with surgery and perioperative intraperitoneal chemotherapy: retrospective analysis of 523 patients from a multicentric French study. J Clin Oncol 2010;28(1):63–8.
29. Verwaal VJ. Long-term results of cytoreduction and HIPEC followed by systemic chemotherapy. Cancer J 2009;15:212–5.
30. Verwaal VJ, van Ruth S, de Bree E, et al. Randomized trial of cytoreduction and hyperthermic intraperitoneal chemotherapy versus systemic chemotherapy and palliative surgery in patients with peritoneal carcinomatosis of colorectal cancer. J Clin Oncol 2003;21:3737–43.
31. Verwaal VJ, Bruin S, Boot H, et al. 8-year follow up of a randomized trial: cytoreduction and hyperthermic intraperitoneal chemotherapy versus systemic chemotherapy in patients with peritoneal carcinomatosis of colorectal cancer. Ann Surg Oncol 2008;15:2426–32.
32. Ryan DP. Cytoreductive surgery and hyperthermic intraperitoneal chemotherapy: history repeating itself or a new standard? American Society of Clinical Oncology 2011. p. 127–8.
33. Franko J, Ibrahim Z, Gusani NJ, et al. Cytoreductive surgery and hyperthermic intraperitoneal chemotherapy versus systemic chemotherapy alone for colorectal peritoneal carcinomatosis. Cancer 2010;116(16):3756–62.
34. Sugarbaker PH. Achieving long-term survival with cytoreductive surgery and perioperative chemotherapy to peritoneal surfaces for metastatic colon cancer. American Society of Clinical Oncology 2011. p. 122–6.
35. Pihl E, Hughes ES, McDermott FT, et al. Lung recurrence after curative surgery for colorectal cancer. Dis Colon Rectum 1987;30(6):417–9.
36. Jarabo JR, Fernandez E, Calatayud J, et al. More than one pulmonary resections or combined lung-liver resection in 79 patients with metastatic colorectal carcinoma. J Surg Oncol 2011;104:781–6.
37. Welter S, Jacobs J, Krbek T, et al. Long-term survival after repeated resection of pulmonary metastases from colorectal cancer. Ann Thorac Surg 2007;84(1):203–10.
38. De Giacomo T, Rendina EA, Venuta F, et al. Thoracoscopic resection of solitary lung metastases from colorectal cancer is a viable therapeutic option. Chest 1999;115:1441–3.
39. King J, Glenn D, Clark W, et al. Percutaneous radiofrequency ablation of pulmonary metastases in patients with colorectal cancer. Br J Surg 2004;91(2):217–23.
40. August DA, Sugarbaker PH, Schneider PD. Lymphatic dissemination of hepatic metastases. Cancer 1985;55:1490–4.
41. Iwatsuki S, Dvorchik I, Madariaga JR, et al. Hepatic resection for metastatic colorectal adenocarcinoma: a proposal of a prognostic scoring system. J Am Coll Surg 1999;189:291–9.
42. Evers DJ, Verwaal VJ. Indication for oophorectomy during cytoreduction for intraperitoneal metastatic spread of colorectal or appendiceal origin. Br J Surg 2011;98:287–92.

43. Okumura S, Kondo H, Tsuboi M, et al. Pulmonary resection for metastatic colorectal cancer: experiences with 159 patients. J Thorac Cardiovasc Surg 1996; 112(4):867–74.
44. Yedibela S, Klein P, Feuchter K, et al. Surgical management of pulmonary metastases from colorectal cancer in 153 patients. Ann Surg Oncol 2006;13(11): 1538–44.
45. Inoue M, Kotake Y, Nakagawa K, et al. Surgery for pulmonary metastases from colorectal carcinoma. Ann Thorac Surg 2000;70(2):380–3.
46. Sauer R, Becker H, Hohenberger W, et al. Preoperative versus postoperative chemoradiotherapy for rectal cancer. N Engl J Med 2004;351:1731–40.
47. Verrees JF, Fernandez-Trigo V, Sugarbaker PH. Rectal cancer recurrence after prior resection and radiation therapy: palliation following additional surgery. Int J Colorectal Dis 1996;11(5):211–6.
48. Mukherjee A. Total pelvic exenteration for advanced rectal cancer. S D J Med 1999;52:153–6.
49. Haddock MG, Nelson H, Donohue JH, et al. Intraoperative electron radiotherapy as a component of salvage therapy for patients with colorectal cancer and advanced nodal metastases. Int J Radiat Oncol Biol Phys 2003;56:966–73.
50. Chua TC, Moran BJ, Sugarbaker PH, et al. Early and long-term outcome data on 2298 patients with pseudomyxoma peritonei of appendiceal origin by a strategy of cytoreductive surgery and hyperthermic intraperitoneal chemotherapy. J Clin Oncol 2012;30(20):2449–56.

Multidisciplinary Care of Patients with Early-Stage Breast Cancer

Gary H. Lyman, MD, MPH, FRCP(Edin)[a,*], Jay Baker, MD[b],
Joseph Geradts, MD, MA[c], Janet Horton, MD[d],
Gretchen Kimmick, MD[e], Jeffrey Peppercorn, MD[e],
Scott Pruitt, MD[f], Randall P. Scheri, MD[f],
E. Shelley Hwang, MD, MPH[f]

KEYWORDS

• Breast cancer • Multidisciplinary • Mammography • Chemotherapy • Survivorship

KEY POINTS

- The management of early-stage breast cancer represents one of the most complete examples of the value of multidisciplinary cancer care, and includes a wide range of disciplines beginning with, but not limited to, radiology, pathology, surgery, radiation therapy, and medical oncology.
- Optimal evaluation, diagnosis, staging, treatment, and surveillance of patients with breast cancer require integration of a broad range of specialized expertise.
- The considerable progress made in clinical outcomes for patients with breast cancer may likely relate in large part to the success of multidisciplinary and integrated delivery of health care to these patients.

INTRODUCTION

The management of early-stage breast cancer (ESBC) represents arguably the earliest and most complete example of the value of multidisciplinary cancer care. It goes far beyond the disciplines of diagnostics and interventional radiology, pathology, surgery, radiation oncology, and medical oncology discussed in the paragraphs to come. It

[a] Comparative Effectiveness and Outcomes Research Program, Department of Medicine, Duke Cancer Institute, Duke University School of Medicine, 2424 Erwin Road, Durham, NC 27705, USA; [b] Department of Radiology, Duke Cancer Institute, Duke University School of Medicine, 2424 Erwin Road, Durham, NC 27705, USA; [c] Department of Pathology, Duke Cancer Institute, Duke University School of Medicine, 2424 Erwin Road, Durham, NC 27705, USA; [d] Department of Radiation Oncology, Duke Cancer Institute, Duke University School of Medicine, 2424 Erwin Road, Durham, NC 27705, USA; [e] Department of Medicine, Duke Cancer Institute, Duke University School of Medicine, 2424 Erwin Road, Durham, NC 27705, USA; [f] Department of Surgery, Duke Cancer Institute, Duke University School of Medicine, 2424 Erwin Road, Durham, NC 27705, USA
* Corresponding author.
E-mail address: gary.lyman@duke.edu

Surg Oncol Clin N Am 22 (2013) 299–317
http://dx.doi.org/10.1016/j.soc.2012.12.005
surgonc.theclinics.com
1055-3207/13/$ – see front matter

also includes other primary care specialties such as family medicine, internal medicine, obstetrics and gynecology, as well as the important participation of nursing, social work, and physical and occupational therapy, among many others. The optimal evaluation, diagnosis, staging, primary treatment, adjunctive therapy, supportive care, and long-term monitoring or surveillance require access to a broad wealth of specialized expertise and the integrated involvement of nearly all participants of modern health care delivery. In fact, it is in no small part the success of multidisciplinary and integrated care of patients with ESBC to which we can attribute the outstanding progress in clinical outcomes for patients with this disease, far outpacing successes in many other adult solid tumors. Within the limitations of this summary, this article focuses attention on the role of the radiologist, pathologist, surgeon, radiation oncologist, and medical oncologist in the management of patients during the initial presentation of breast cancer.

BREAST IMAGING

Breast imaging plays a central role in the multidisciplinary care of patients with breast cancer. With advances in conventional imaging, the advent of new imaging modalities, and the introduction of percutaneous needle biopsy techniques, the breast imager must be fully integrated into the care team to optimize planning for surgical, medical, and radiation therapy for patients with a new diagnosis of breast cancer. Detection of breast cancer, particularly in its earliest stages, is especially dependent on high-quality imaging. One of the fundamental advances in breast imaging is the development of full-field digital mammography, providing substantially better contrast than conventional analog imaging and providing an excellent platform for additional image evaluation such as computer-aided detection.[1] State-of-the-art ultrasound systems now offer high-resolution imaging with high-frequency transducers and digital processing techniques such as spatial compounding and harmonic imaging.[2] More recent imaging advances include dynamic contrast-enhanced breast magnetic resonance imaging (MRI) with dedicated breast-imaging coils and, most recently, molecular imaging techniques that provide contemporary versions of earlier nuclear medicine techniques.

The Breast Imaging Reporting and Data System, or BI-RADS, includes a lexicon of terms for describing the morphology of breast lesions, including 7 standardized final-assessment categories from 0 to 6, along with a final conclusion of the level of suspicion and any recommendation for additional imaging or biopsy-reducing ambiguity in breast-imaging reports.[3] New image-guided tissue sampling techniques allow histologic evaluation of almost any breast lesion, and large-core needle biopsies are now routinely performed.[4] Close communication between radiologists and pathologists is essential to confirm concordance between imaging and histology and avoid false-negative results.[5]

Optimal surgical planning requires the breast imager to accurately determine the size of the primary lesion, the presence of multifocal or multicentric lesions, and the presence of contralateral disease. Mammography and ultrasound imaging are very useful but MRI may provide more accurate assessment of preoperative staging, although the high rate of false-positive findings remains a concern.[6] In addition to diagnostic confirmation and accurate imaging measurements of cancer size, evaluation of needle biopsy samples provides hormone receptor and HER2 status of cancerous lesions, all of which are essential for the medical oncologist when considering hormonal therapy and whether to administer neoadjuvant rather than adjuvant therapy.[7]

Preoperative MRI is clearly more accurate in the determination of the size of the primary lesion, the presence of multifocal and multicentric disease, the presence of contralateral disease, and the presence of axillary adenopathy.[8] However, MRI has not been shown to reduce rates of reoperation or in-breast recurrence, and no survival benefit has been demonstrated.[9,10] Conversely, studies have demonstrated that patients undergoing preoperative MRI have higher mastectomy rates than those not undergoing MRI.[11–13] It is important that the multidisciplinary care team decide whether preoperative MRI is warranted in patients with a new diagnosis of breast cancer.

PATHOLOGY

The pathologist, though arguably the least visible member of the multidisciplinary breast team, plays a crucial role in patient management. Pathologic diagnosis represents the critical first step for subsequent evaluation and treatment of patients with breast cancer. However, the role of the pathologist extends far beyond providing accurate and complete information on the biology of a given breast carcinoma (grade, biomarkers) and the extent of disease (tumor size, regional lymph node involvement). Without appropriate clinical and radiologic information, a proper pathologic workup is often not possible and may be inaccurate. The pathologist acts as a consultant to the clinicians, as illustrated by the importance of multidisciplinary patient-care conferences where the pathologist clarifies and elaborates on diagnostic reports. The pathologist also directs and oversees quality assurance of biomarker testing and the selection of optimal tissue blocks for special studies and clinical research protocols that have a correlative science component involving human tissues. At referral institutions, pathologic material from other hospitals is reviewed, providing a second opinion and leading to a change in treatment recommendations in a significant percentage of cases.[14–18] **Fig. 1** illustrates 2 examples of significant diagnostic discrepancies. **Fig. 1**A shows a needle-core biopsy that had been diagnosed elsewhere as high-grade ductal carcinoma in situ (DCIS) but revealing a patchy infiltrate of small discohesive atypical cells that had not been appreciated. A cytokeratin immunostain (see **Fig. 1**B) demonstrated the epithelial origin of the infiltrate, and a diagnosis of invasive lobular carcinoma was made. Another needle-core biopsy came with a diagnosis of invasive ductal carcinoma (see **Fig. 1**C). However, at higher power the small nests of atypical cells clearly were enveloped by myoepithelial cells (see **Fig. 1**D) that were further highlighted on immunohistochemical (IHC) stains, and a diagnosis of papillary carcinoma in situ was rendered with entrapment of atypical epithelium within the sclerosing stroma.

The most important distinction a pathologist has to make and, fortunately, the area of highest interobserver concordance (95.5%–98%) is between invasive mammary carcinoma and noninvasive disease.[14,17–19] However, the distinction between invasive carcinoma and noninvasive disease is sometimes difficult even with the help of IHC stains, especially when there is a paucity of diagnostic material.[20,21] Perhaps the lowest degree of concordance is in the area of atypical intraductal proliferations such as the distinction between DCIS and atypical ductal hyperplasia (ADH).[19,22–25] Likewise, precise determination of tumor size may be surprisingly difficult, especially for DCIS lesions, tumors with a multinodular architecture, and carcinomas treated with neoadjuvant chemotherapy.[20,21] While the importance of wide surgical margins remains in dispute, a change in margin status on pathology review is uncommon (2%–6.5%).[14] Significant interobserver variability has been reported when assessing lymphovascular invasion.[14,24] The College of American Pathologists and the American

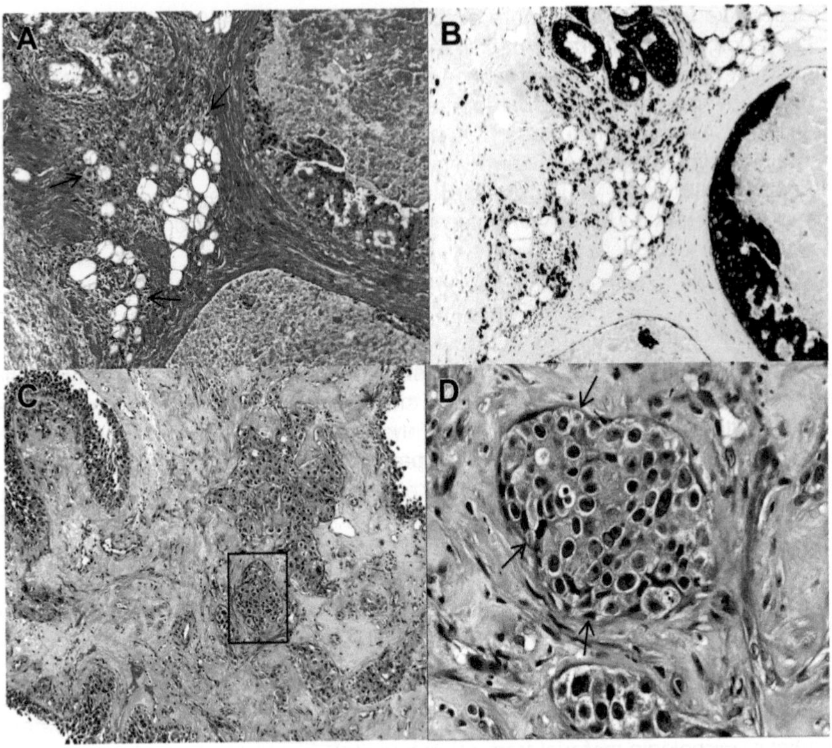

Fig. 1. Two examples of significant diagnostic discrepancies. (*A, B*) Original diagnosis: high-grade ductal carcinoma in situ (DCIS). There is a patchy infiltrate of small atypical cells (*arrows*) between the ducts involved by DCIS. On a cytokeratin stain (*B*), these cells are found to represent invasive lobular carcinoma. (*C, D*) Original diagnosis: invasive ductal carcinoma. A low-power view (*C*) shows the papillary architecture of the lesion with irregular epithelial nests within the stroma. A high-power view (*D*) demonstrates the presence of myoepithelial cells at the periphery of the atypical nests (*arrows*). Diagnosis: papillary carcinoma in situ with entrapment of atypical epithelium.

Society of Clinical Oncology (ASCO) issued guidelines for HER2 and ER/PR testing in 2007 and 2010 in an effort to reduce the well-documented interlaboratory variability in ER/PR/HER2 testing.[26–31] Although breast tumor grade is a powerful prognostic factor, its clinical utility is diminished by the well-described interobserver variability.[24,32,33] Although centrally performed multigene tests such as the Oncotype DX have good technical reproducibility, they may be subject to significant intratumor variability.[34] Moreover, much of the information provided by commercial multigene assays may be redundant and may overlap with routine data elements in pathology reports.[35] The complexity and often subjective nature of the reported results makes review of the pathologic material by an expert breast pathologist an essential part of multidisciplinary management of breast cancer.[14–18]

SURGERY

The mainstay of treatment for ESBC including invasive disease and DCIS continues to be surgery, in the form of either breast-conserving therapy (BCT, lumpectomy) or mastectomy following or before adjuvant therapy. Clearly the trajectory of the surgical management of ESBC has been toward less aggressive and debilitating surgical procedures. Current guidelines from the National Comprehensive Cancer Network (NCCN) offer 2 options for the surgical treatment of the breast for ESBC: (1) BCT with or without adjuvant radiation or (2) mastectomy. Important determinants of breast treatment are patient preference, the size and/or multifocality of tumor, competing comorbidities, and patient age.

The area of greatest controversy in breast surgery is the management of the axillary nodes. One of the most important prognostic factors with respect to survival from ESBC is the presence of axillary lymph node involvement. Therefore, determining the status of the axillary lymph nodes is critically important and is used to guide further therapy. Until the 1970s, essentially all breast cancers were treated with a radical mastectomy, including excision of level-I, -II, and -III nodes as well as the pectoralis major muscle and overlying skin. With respect to metastases to axillary nodes, this technique was both diagnostic and therapeutic but was associated with significant morbidity. Once studies demonstrated that modified radical mastectomy was equally effective in prolonging survival, this procedure replaced radical mastectomy with axillary dissection largely limited to excision of level I and level II lymph nodes.[36] Similarly, once the combination of lumpectomy and axillary dissection with postlumpectomy radiation therapy was found to be equivalent to modified radical mastectomy with respect to survival from breast cancer, all patients continued to undergo standard axillary dissection of level-I and -II nodes.[37] Subsequent large retrospective studies suggested a small survival advantage for patients with breast cancer undergoing axillary node dissection, whereas other studies failed to demonstrate any such advantage.[38,39]

At the same time, lymphatic mapping with sentinel node biopsy (SNB) was developed and was quickly adopted by surgeons throughout the Unites States. Although the combined use of radiolabeled sulfur-colloid and isosulfan blue dye increases the success of identifying the sentinel nodes, the routine use of SNB has been associated with a false-negative rate of approximately 2% to 10%, which should be discussed with the patient.[40,41] In situations where the surgeon is unable to identify the sentinel nodes, axillary node dissection is generally recommended. SNB is now the standard of care for most patients with clinically node-negative ESBC. For those patients with negative sentinel nodes, no further lymph node dissection is necessary. In patients with a positive SNB node undergoing completion lymph node dissection (CLND), additional nodal involvement has been found in approximately 20% to 50% of patients.[42] Although a CLND continues to represent the standard of care in patients with a positive SNB, it may not confer benefit in all patients based on the results of ACOSOG Z0011, which showed equivalent disease-free survival and overall survival in patients with clinical T1-T2 disease with 1 to 2 positive sentinel nodes randomized to CLND and radiation or to radiation alone.[43] For those patients with positive sentinel nodes who do not undergo CLND, many radiation oncologists include the axillary nodes in the radiation field, which may reduce axillary recurrence.[44] At present, it is recommended that women undergoing mastectomy with a positive SNB undergo excision of level-I and -II axillary nodes.

The pathologic evaluation of the nodes has also undergone notable changes in recent years. Based on several studies, and as defined in the most recent American Joint Cancer Committee staging manual, a SNB with micrometastases (<0.2 mm diameter) is now considered negative. Likewise, breast-cancer cells detected only by IHC staining, but not visualized by hematoxylin and eosin staining, are also now considered negative, with many institutions no longer performing IHC analysis of sentinel nodes. Additional clinical trials should help clearly determine which patients with breast cancer and with positive SNB can avoid further axillary dissection. SNB is generally not recommended for DCIS and is of uncertain benefit even in patients with microinvasive breast cancer.[45] On the other hand, in patients with clinically involved axillary nodes, metastatic involvement should be confirmed by fine-needle aspiration (FNA) or core-needle biopsy, and a standard axillary dissection should be performed with no role for SNB.

Locally advanced disease includes breast cancers that present with large primary tumors (>5 cm), skin or chest-wall involvement, or advanced lymph node disease. The initial approach to locally advanced breast cancer is similar to ESBC, with special attention to physical examination and imaging to evaluate the extent of local involvement including skin involvement, fixation to the chest wall, and fixed or matted nodes that will dictate locoregional management. Additional imaging to rule out distant metastases is important, as these patients are at increased risk for metastatic disease. A multidisciplinary team approach is particularly important for these complex patients who require multimodality therapy. Neoadjuvant chemotherapy has become the standard approach for patients with nonoperable breast cancer to convert them to operative candidates and facilitate local control. For patients with operable breast cancer, neoadjuvant chemotherapy has been shown to improve rates of resectability if undergoing BCT, with disease-free and overall survival similar to that of adjuvant chemotherapy.[46] Recently, neoadjuvant endocrine therapy with aromatase inhibitors has been shown to provide comparable response rates and breast-conservation rates in selected patients.[47] Following chemotherapy, either mastectomy or BCT is performed based on tumor response and patient choice. Contraindications to breast conservation include multicentric tumors, extensive calcifications, extensive skin involvement, and inability to obtain negative margins. Radiation therapy is standard after BCT, whereas postmastectomy radiation is based on disease stage at presentation. Inflammatory breast cancer (IBC) must be distinguished from both locally advanced breast cancer, which arises more slowly with infrequent or focal skin involvement, and mastitis, which may delay treatment. Although the diagnosis of IBC is based on clinical findings, dermal lymphatic involvement caused by tumor emboli within the dermal lymphatics is specific for inflammatory breast cancer but is seen in only 75% of cases.[48] Clinically suspicious lymph nodes should be biopsied to confirm nodal involvement and accurately stage the patient. SNB is not indicated for IBC because of a high false-negative rate likely attributable to involvement and consequent occlusion of the dermal lymphatics by tumor emboli.[49] Additional imaging to evaluate involvement of distant sites should be performed, as more than 30% of patients may have metastatic disease.[50] Neoadjuvant chemotherapy followed by modified radical mastectomy then by postmastectomy chest-wall radiation should be performed for patients who respond to chemotherapy and in whom complete resection can be performed. Patients with inoperable tumors despite chemotherapy should be treated with preoperative radiation followed by mastectomy if feasible.

Although surgery remains an important mainstay of treatment for locally advanced breast cancer, the more widespread use of effective and targeted systemic therapy before surgery has allowed for more successful treatment of advanced disease as well as improved understanding of tumor biology in vivo. It is hoped that systemic therapy will continue to improve disease-specific mortality in these high-risk patients, allowing for further reduction of surgical extent without compromise of patient outcomes.

RADIATION ONCOLOGY

Radiation therapy has been used, in conjunction with surgery, as a critical component of BCT since the 1970s.[44,51,52] The initial goal of radiation in this setting was to minimize the risk of local recurrence and, therefore, the need for either immediate or delayed mastectomy. Over time, as data have matured and long-term follow-up has accumulated, it has become clear that a significant reduction in the risk of local recurrence also improves survival.[53] As a result, postlumpectomy radiotherapy is indicated for almost all patient subgroups to reduce the risk of local regional recurrence by approximately two-thirds and improve overall survival over lumpectomy alone.

Historically, postlumpectomy radiotherapy has been delivered over 4.5 to 5 weeks to the whole breast followed by a 1 to 1.5-week "boost" focused on the lumpectomy cavity.[44,52,54–58] However, recent international clinical trials have demonstrated that an accelerated whole-breast treatment delivering larger doses per treatment over a shorter period of time and to an overall lower total dose is comparable with standard treatment in both efficacy and toxicity.[54,59] Although the overall total dose is lower, the treatment is believed to be "biologically equivalent," owing to the more profound impact of larger daily treatments. In the Canadian study that recently reported outcomes at 10 years, recurrence rates in both the standard and accelerated arms were just over 6%, with approximately 70% of women in both arms experiencing good or excellent cosmetic results.[55] This regimen has become a widely accepted alternative to standard therapy in the appropriate patient.

Another evolving technique designed to limit normal tissue toxicity and patient inconvenience is partial breast irradiation (PBI). PBI focuses treatment only on the resected tumor cavity and a surrounding small margin of normal breast tissue. Multiple PBI delivery techniques have evolved, spanning from 1 day to 1 week of twice-daily treatments, based on the rationale that the majority of recurrences occur in close proximity to the original site of disease.[60–63] Two randomized trials, as well as a multitude of institutional and registry trials, have published early outcomes data, and multiple randomized trials are ongoing.[64,65] Early data suggest that in the properly selected patient, efficacy and toxicity outcomes are similar to those of standard treatment. To guide clinicians in choosing the most appropriate patients, the American Society for Radiation Oncology issued a consensus statement defining patients who were "suitable," "cautionary," and "unsuitable" for PBI.[65]

In the most significant deescalation of therapy, omission of radiotherapy has been evaluated in certain subgroups. Historically it has been difficult to define a subgroup of patients in which the addition of radiotherapy did not result in a significant reduction in in-breast tumor recurrence. However, recently the Cancer and Leukemia Group B reported their data evaluating treatment of women older than 70 years with lumpectomy followed by tamoxifen alone versus lumpectomy, radiotherapy, and tamoxifen. Although a statistically significant decrease in local recurrence was noted, the overall rate of breast tumor recurrence was quite low and the major cause of mortality was unrelated to breast cancer.[66]

Although postmastectomy radiotherapy has historically been reserved for patients with more advanced primary disease, several series suggest that patients with aggressive tumor biology (HER2+ or triple negative) have higher risks of locoregional recurrence.[67,68] Investigators from China recently reported a significant increase in overall survival (90.4% vs 78.7%) in patients with triple-negative breast cancer receiving adjuvant chemotherapy and radiotherapy versus those receiving only chemotherapy after mastectomy.[69] These data require confirmation in prospective cohorts with strict eligibility criteria and modern chemotherapy.

MEDICAL ONCOLOGY

ESBC is a heterogeneous group of related disorders to which systemic therapy is tailored based, in part, on the biological or biomarker differences between subtypes, for example, estrogen and/or progesterone receptor positive or negative and HER2 overexpressed/amplified or not. Broadly speaking, systemic therapies can be grouped together as hormonal therapies, chemotherapy, or targeted therapies such as monoclonal antibodies or tyrosine kinase inhibitors. In very general terms, the hormone receptor–positive subtype is treated with endocrine treatment, although chemotherapy is also effective in most cases. Chemotherapy, but not endocrine therapy, is used in treating hormone receptor–negative breast cancers. Anti-HER2 therapies are used in tumors that overexpress HER2, typically in combination with chemotherapy and/or endocrine therapy, depending on the tumor's hormone receptor status.

Tamoxifen, a selective estrogen receptor modulator, has the longest use as a hormonal therapy and, therefore, has the most well understood toxicity profile including thromboembolic phenomenon and endometrial cancer.[70,71] The aromatase inhibitors (AIs) include the nonsteroidal AIs such as anastrozole and letrozole and the steroidal AI, exemestane. Though reserved for postmenopausal settings, these agents are thought by many to be slightly more effective than tamoxifen in treating postmenopausal hormone receptor–positive breast cancer.[72–74] While demonstrating no increased risk of endometrial cancer or thrombotic phenomenon, the AIs decrease the level of systemic estrogen, resulting in exacerbation of menopausal symptoms, loss of bone density, and an adverse effect on the cholesterol profile.[75–79] No convincing data support that one aromatase inhibitor is more effective than another. Other endocrine therapies including fulvestrant, megesterol, estrogen, androgens, and corticosteroids are generally reserved for patients with advanced hormonally sensitive disease. Gonadotropin-releasing hormone agonists, which induce medical menopause, can also be effective in premenopausal women. Adherence to endocrine therapy is a major challenge in the long-term management of breast cancer. Indeed, studies have suggested that up to 50% of patients discontinue endocrine therapy before completing 5 years.[80]

The most effective chemotherapeutic agents for breast cancer are the anthracyclines, including doxorubicin and epirubicin, and the taxanes, including paclitaxel and docetaxel, although many other agents are approved for the treatment of breast cancer. Short-term toxicities of therapy include alopecia, myelosuppression (which increases the risk of potentially life-threatening infection), nausea and vomiting, neurotoxicity, and fatigue, among others, depending on the agent. Possible long-term side effects include left ventricular dysfunction, primarily from anthracyclines, amenorrhea, and infertility, cognitive dysfunction and other cancers, including myelodysplastic syndrome; and leukemia.

For tumors in which there is amplification of HER2, anti-HER2 therapies improve long-term outcome. Approved anti-HER2 therapies now include the recombinant humanized monoclonal antibodies trastuzumab and pertuzumab and the small-molecule tyrosine kinase inhibitor, lapatinib.[81,82] An antibody chemotherapy conjugate, trastuzumab-emtansine (T-DM1), has demonstrated encouraging results in patients with advanced disease. Only trastuzumab is approved at this time in patients with ESBC. The monoclonal antibody bevacizumab inhibits angiogenesis and has been shown to have some efficacy in the treatment of metastatic breast cancer.[83] Its toxicity profile, which includes hypertension, thromboembolism, and bleeding, among others, limits its potential in the adjuvant setting.[84]

The purpose of adjuvant systemic therapy is to prevent recurrent disease, prolong disease-free survival, and increase survival rates. All patients with ESBC should meet with a medical oncologist to review the available diagnostic and prognostic information and discuss the need for adjuvant systemic therapy, as well as the appropriate choice of therapy if indicated. Any recommendation should be based on a discussion of the estimated risk of disease recurrence based on tumor type and stage and the potential benefit and harms associated with available systemic therapies. Endocrine therapy, with tamoxifen or an AI, decreases the risk of recurrence of breast cancer and death in women whose breast cancer is hormone receptor positive.[85] Guidelines from ASCO recommend that adjuvant endocrine therapy for postmenopausal women with ESBC include an AI at some point during adjuvant therapy, either as up-front therapy or as sequential treatment after tamoxifen.[86] Although chemotherapy may further reduce the risk of recurrence or death in ESBC, the proportional reduction is generally less in women with hormone receptor–positive disease than that seen with hormonal therapies.[87] As not all patients in this setting appear to benefit from the addition of systemic chemotherapy, predictive measures of chemotherapy benefit are being explored, including gene expression profiling such as the 21-gene assay Oncotype DX,[88–90] the Amsterdam 70-gene profile Mammaprint,[91–93] and the Rotterdam 76-gene signature.[94,95] The most widely used of these is Oncotype DX, which reports a recurrence score (RS) associated with an estimate of distant recurrence-free survival. Available data suggest that tamoxifen-treated patients derive little or no benefit if their tumor is associated with a low RS (Oncotype DX RS <18), whereas they are likely to derive considerable benefit from adjuvant chemotherapy in addition to tamoxifen if a high RS is found (>31). The relative benefit of chemotherapy in patients whose tumor has an intermediate-risk Oncotype DX RS is unclear and is the subject of a randomized controlled trial of hormonal therapy with or without chemotherapy (TAILORx). Although preliminary results suggest that Oncotype DX is prognostic and may be predictive of chemotherapy benefit in patients with positive lymph nodes, the level of risk in this group of patients is sufficiently high to warrant consideration of chemotherapy at present.[96]

Although the choices of chemotherapy regimens for patients with hormone receptor–negative tumors are similar to those for patients with hormone receptor-positive disease, the incremental benefit of adjuvant chemotherapy is generally greater, while hormonal therapy has no role to play in the management of hormone receptor–negative disease.[87] The decision as to whether to treat ESBC patients with chemotherapy is based on the estimated risk of cancer recurrence balanced by the estimated risk of toxicity from treatment. In patients with a low risk of recurrence and for those with a relative contraindication to anthracyclines, a combination of docetaxel and cyclophosphamide (TC) is often used, based on data from a single controlled clinical trial.[97] In patients at greater risk of disease recurrence who have no contraindication, an anthracycline is often combined with a taxane along with cyclophosphamide.[98–101] In elderly patients and those with serious medical comorbidities, a more nuanced discussion of available chemotherapy regimens and the associated benefit and harms is warranted. However, available evidence supports the use of standard chemotherapy regimens in healthy older women with few competing comorbidities.[102,103]

Adjuvant trastuzumab added to adjuvant systemic chemotherapy has demonstrated significant improvements in progression-free and overall survival in patients with HER2-positive ESBC.[104,105] Although trastuzumab is relatively safe, significant declines in cardiac function occur in approximately 20% of patients, and regularly scheduled monitoring of cardiac function is necessary.[106]

Neoadjuvant or primary systemic therapy can be used in cases where decreasing the tumor size would allow for a better cosmetic result or more successful surgery.[107] Although neoadjuvant chemotherapy is advantageous in patients with large tumors and provides an early assessment of chemotherapy responsiveness, no impact of such chemotherapy on patient survival has been demonstrated. Chemotherapy regimens used are similar to those used in the adjuvant setting, with response rates to modern chemotherapy reaching 60% to 70% and pathologic complete response rates ranging from 10% to 30%.[108,109] Response to chemotherapy, especially response in the lymph nodes, is associated with a better prognosis.[110] In patients with hormone receptor–positive tumors, neoadjuvant endocrine therapy, most notably with an aromatase inhibitor, can be effective and may also be used to answer research questions about tumor biology.[111,112] Treatment is continued for a minimum of 3 months in the absence of tumor progression, although a maximum response may not be seen for 6 to 12 months.[107,113]

SURVEILLANCE OF BREAST CANCER AND SURVIVORSHIP

Through a combination of early detection and more effective therapy, survival rates for patients with breast cancer have continued to improve over time. The vast majority of women diagnosed with ESBC are expected to survive for years or decades following the initial diagnosis and treatment. With nearly 1.4 million new cases of breast cancer reported annually worldwide, the number of breast cancer survivors is projected to grow by close to 1 million per year.[114] At present there are more than 2.7 million patients with a history of breast cancer in the United States alone.[115] Important issues to consider include surveillance for cancer recurrence, management of ongoing and late-onset toxicity from initial therapy with surgery, radiation and/or systemic therapy, management of psychosocial issues, and assistance with returning the patient to a focus on healthy living. Overlying these issues is the question of how to optimally organize delivery of health care to patients with diverse issues following treatment among multiple health care providers.

It is important to note that breast cancer that recurs locally is potentially curable and that patients with a history of breast cancer are at higher risk for a second breast cancer primary in comparison with the general population. Beyond a careful history and physical examination and annual mammography, there is no proven benefit from additional imaging or laboratory evaluation in asymptomatic patients. Rosselli Del Turco and colleagues[116] randomly assigned 1243 women to a standard follow-up strategy of routine physical examination and mammography versus a more intensive strategy of examination and mammography plus chest radiograph and bone scan every 6 months. Although thoracic and bone metastasis were identified earlier in the intensive screening arm, there was no difference in 5-year survival. Similarly, the GIVIO trial randomized 1320 women to standard follow-up care versus standard care plus screening routine blood work, chest radiograph, bone scan, and hepatic ultrasonography. Although screening asymptomatic patients led to earlier diagnosis in some patients, the majority of distant recurrences presented with symptoms, and there was no difference in survival or quality of life among patients in the intensive screening arm.[117]

Another goal of long-term follow-up is the management of ongoing and late-onset toxicity from initial therapy including that from surgery and/or radiation, such as lymphedema and multiple side effects from systemic therapy. Among patients surveyed 5 years or more after initial management for breast cancer, the most common reported side effects included depression, fatigue, and sexual dysfunction.[118] These side effects are often initially assessed by a member of the multidisciplinary breast-cancer team but may require referral to subspecialists for assistance. Fatigue is arguably the most common posttreatment symptom reported. Anthracyclines and trastuzumab may result in reduced cardiac ejection fraction or actual congestive heart failure presenting with fatigue, dyspnea, tachycardia, and elevated brain natriuretic peptide. Anthracyclines and cyclophosphamide carry a rare risk of leukemia or myelodysplasia and are associated with anemia, whereas radiation therapy may cause hypothyroidism. Menopausal symptoms such as hot flashes may contribute to insomnia which, in turn, may present as fatigue. Depression has been reported in more than 15% of patients with breast cancer and may be more common among younger women.[119] Moreover, tamoxifen metabolism and efficacy may be limited by CYP2D6 inhibitors used as antidepressants, including most selective serotonin-release inhibitors.

Menopausal symptoms can arise because of indirect ovarian suppression as a result of chemotherapy or direct effects of endocrine therapy. Hot flashes, with or without sleep disturbance, are among the most frequent complaints. In randomized trials, venlafaxine has proved superior to placebo, clonidine, and gabapentin with up to 66% reduction in hot flashes.[120] The use of topical vaginal estrogen creams to reduce symptoms of dyspareunia or vaginal dryness is somewhat controversial.[121] There is evidence of systemic absorption, making the safety among patients with breast cancer unclear, particularly for women with endocrine receptor–positive disease.[122] If a topical estrogen cream is used, patients should apply the minimal amount to achieve improvement in symptoms.

The impact of lifestyle changes on the risk of recurrence of breast cancer has also been investigated in recent studies. The Nurses Health Study found that women who walked for 3 to 5 hours per week after diagnosis experienced a lower risk of death from breast cancer in comparison with women with very low levels of physical activity.[123] The American College of Sports Medicine recommends 150 minutes of moderate exercise or 75 minutes of vigorous exercise per week among cancer survivors.[124] There is limited evidence that a specific diet can reduce the risk of recurrence of breast cancer. In the WINS trial, investigators attempted to study the impact of a low-fat diet without change in overall caloric intake among women with a history of breast cancer. With careful attention to diet, women reduced their dietary fat intake and lost weight, and experienced a modest reduction in recurrence risk, seen most prominently among women with endocrine receptor–negative breast cancer.[125] Other studies have shown that lower dietary fat intake is associated with improved prognosis.[126] Alcohol is associated with a modest increase in the risk of breast cancer, and patients can be advised of this association.[127]

An important debate has been conducted as to how to best deliver a plan of survivorship care that addresses these long-term issues. Whereas Canadian studies have demonstrated that patients may be safely referred to their primary care clinician without detrimental impact on complications among the few patients who will experience recurrence and require further breast-cancer care,[128] patient care preference surveys in the United States indicate that most still look to their oncology team for surveillance and management of ongoing symptoms from cancer therapy.[129] ASCO guidelines recommend performance of a history and physical examination every 3 to 6 months for 3 years following initial diagnosis, then annual or biannual follow-up for 2 years, followed by annual ongoing follow-up.[130] Transition to primary care follow-up alone after the first year following initial therapy is also considered acceptable as per ASCO guidelines. Many cancer centers are introducing specialized clinics for survivors of breast cancer. The future challenge will be to provide the necessary care to the growing numbers of survivors; more organized models of survivorship clinics will create opportunities for better research and more comprehensive and cost-effective care in this important setting.

SUMMARY

As our understanding of the biology and behavior as well as the complexity of diagnostic, prognostic, and therapeutic interventions for patients with ESBC has increased, the compelling need for close coordination and integration of multiple specialty fields has become increasingly apparent. Optimal care and clinical outcomes depend on the sequential and often simultaneous involvement and interchange of specialists in imaging, pathologic and molecular diagnostic and prognostic stratification, and the therapeutic specialties of surgery, radiation oncology, and medical oncology. While remaining central to the care of patients with ESBC, these are but a few of the various disciplines that are needed for providing modern, sophisticated management to patients, and the importance of the entire care team including nursing, social work, nutritional support, genetic counseling, and physical and occupational therapy, among others, cannot be overstated. Likewise, the continuing and expanding role of the primary care specialties in establishing early diagnosis, assisting with the coordination of care, and providing posttreatment surveillance of patients with ESBC in both survivorship specialty centers and general practice is increasingly appreciated. As we move further and deeper into the era of molecular biology and genomics with increasingly sophisticated novel targeted therapies and preventive strategies, the important role for coordinated involvement of the entire modern health care team in the optimal management of patients with ESBC will become even more apparent, leading to the best possible outcomes for patients.

REFERENCES

1. Pisano ED, Yaffe MJ, Hemminger BM, et al. Current status of full-field digital mammography. Acad Radiol 2000;7(4):266–80.
2. Athanasiou A, Tardivon A, Ollivier L, et al. How to optimize breast ultrasound. Eur J Radiol 2009;69(1):6–13.
3. D'Orsi CJ, Newell MS. BI-RADS decoded: detailed guidance on potentially confusing issues. Radiol Clin North Am 2007;45(5):751–63, v.
4. Liberman L. Centennial dissertation. Percutaneous imaging-guided core breast biopsy: state of the art at the millennium. AJR Am J Roentgenol 2000;174(5): 1191–9.
5. Idowu MO, Hardy LB, Souers RJ, et al. Pathologic diagnostic correlation with breast imaging findings: a College of American Pathologists Q-Probes study of 48 institutions. Arch Pathol Lab Med 2012;136(1):53–60.
6. Kuhl C, Kuhn W, Braun M, et al. Pre-operative staging of breast cancer with breast MRI: one step forward, two steps back? Breast 2007;16(Suppl 2):S34–44.
7. Li S, Yang X, Zhang Y, et al. Assessment accuracy of core needle biopsy for hormone receptors in breast cancer: a meta-analysis. Breast Cancer Res Treat 2012;135(2):325–34.
8. Bilimoria KY, Cambic A, Hansen NM, et al. Evaluating the impact of preoperative breast magnetic resonance imaging on the surgical management of newly diagnosed breast cancers. Arch Surg 2007;142(5):441–5 [discussion: 445–7].
9. Solin LJ. Counterview: pre-operative breast MRI (magnetic resonance imaging) is not recommended for all patients with newly diagnosed breast cancer. Breast 2010;19(1):7–9.
10. Solin LJ, Orel SG, Hwang WT, et al. Relationship of breast magnetic resonance imaging to outcome after breast-conservation treatment with radiation for women with early-stage invasive breast carcinoma or ductal carcinoma in situ. J Clin Oncol 2008;26(3):386–91.
11. Pettit K, Swatske ME, Gao F, et al. The impact of breast MRI on surgical decision-making: are patients at risk for mastectomy? J Surg Oncol 2009; 100(7):553–8.

12. Itakura K, Lessing J, Sakata T, et al. The impact of preoperative magnetic resonance imaging on surgical treatment and outcomes for ductal carcinoma in situ. Clin Breast Cancer 2011;11(1):33–8.
13. Katipamula R, Degnim AC, Hoskin T, et al. Trends in mastectomy rates at the Mayo Clinic Rochester: effect of surgical year and preoperative magnetic resonance imaging. J Clin Oncol 2009;27(25):4082–8.
14. Kennecke HF, Speers CH, Ennis CA, et al. Impact of routine pathology review on treatment for node-negative breast cancer. J Clin Oncol 2012;30(18):2227–31.
15. Newman EA, Guest AB, Helvie MA, et al. Changes in surgical management resulting from case review at a breast cancer multidisciplinary tumor board. Cancer 2006;107(10):2346–51.
16. Price JA, Grunfeld E, Barnes PJ, et al. Inter-institutional pathology consultations for breast cancer: impact on clinical oncology therapy recommendations. Curr Oncol 2010;17(1):25–32.
17. Rakovitch E, Mihai A, Pignol JP, et al. Is expert breast pathology assessment necessary for the management of ductal carcinoma in situ? Breast Cancer Res Treat 2004;87(3):265–72.
18. Staradub VL, Messenger KA, Hao N, et al. Changes in breast cancer therapy because of pathology second opinions. Ann Surg Oncol 2002;9(10):982–7.
19. Verkooijen HM, Peterse JL, Schipper ME, et al. Interobserver variability between general and expert pathologists during the histopathological assessment of large-core needle and open biopsies of non-palpable breast lesions. Eur J Cancer 2003;39(15):2187–91.
20. Behjatnia B, Sim J, Bassett LW, et al. Does size matter? Comparison study between MRI, gross, and microscopic tumor sizes in breast cancer in lumpectomy specimens. Int J Clin Exp Pathol 2010;3(3):303–9.
21. Shin SJ, Osborne MP, Moore A, et al. Determination of size in invasive breast carcinoma: pathologic considerations and clinical implications. Am J Clin Pathol 2000;113(5 Suppl 1):S19–29.
22. Jain RK, Mehta R, Dimitrov R, et al. Atypical ductal hyperplasia: interobserver and intraobserver variability. Mod Pathol 2011;24(7):917–23.
23. Putti TC, Pinder SE, Elston CW, et al. Breast pathology practice: most common problems in a consultation service. Histopathology 2005;47(5):445–57.
24. Sloane JP, Amendoeira I, Apostolikas N, et al. Consistency achieved by 23 European pathologists from 12 countries in diagnosing breast disease and reporting prognostic features of carcinomas. European Commission Working Group on Breast Screening Pathology. Virchows Arch 1999;434(1):3–10.
25. Wells WA, Carney PA, Eliassen MS, et al. Statewide study of diagnostic agreement in breast pathology. J Natl Cancer Inst 1998;90(2):142–5.
26. Hammond ME, Hayes DF, Dowsett M, et al. American Society of Clinical Oncology/College of American Pathologists guideline recommendations for immunohistochemical testing of estrogen and progesterone receptors in breast cancer (unabridged version). Arch Pathol Lab Med 2010;134(7):e48–72.
27. Press MF, Finn RS, Cameron D, et al. HER-2 gene amplification, HER-2 and epidermal growth factor receptor mRNA and protein expression, and lapatinib efficacy in women with metastatic breast cancer. Clin Cancer Res 2008; 14(23):7861–70.
28. Thomson TA, Hayes MM, Spinelli JJ, et al. HER-2/neu in breast cancer: interobserver variability and performance of immunohistochemistry with 4 antibodies compared with fluorescent in situ hybridization. Mod Pathol 2001;14(11): 1079–86.

29. Viale G, Regan MM, Maiorano E, et al. Prognostic and predictive value of centrally reviewed expression of estrogen and progesterone receptors in a randomized trial comparing letrozole and tamoxifen adjuvant therapy for postmenopausal early breast cancer: BIG 1-98. J Clin Oncol 2007;25(25):3846–52.
30. Hammond ME. ASCO-CAP guidelines for breast predictive factor testing: an update. Appl Immunohistochem Mol Morphol 2011;19(6):499–500.
31. Wolff AC, Hammond ME, Schwartz JN, et al. American Society of Clinical Oncology/College of American Pathologists guideline recommendations for human epidermal growth factor receptor 2 testing in breast cancer. J Clin Oncol 2007;25(1):118–45.
32. Meyer JS, Alvarez C, Milikowski C, et al. Breast carcinoma malignancy grading by Bloom-Richardson system vs proliferation index: reproducibility of grade and advantages of proliferation index. Mod Pathol 2005;18(8):1067–78.
33. Robbins P, Pinder S, de Klerk N, et al. Histological grading of breast carcinomas: a study of interobserver agreement. Hum Pathol 1995;26(8):873–9.
34. Barry WT, Kernagis DN, Dressman HK, et al. Intratumor heterogeneity and precision of microarray-based predictors of breast cancer biology and clinical outcome. J Clin Oncol 2010;28(13):2198–206.
35. Geradts J, Bean SM, Bentley RC, et al. The oncotype DX recurrence score is correlated with a composite index including routinely reported pathobiologic features. Cancer Invest 2010;28(9):969–77.
36. Turner L, Swindell R, Bell WG, et al. Radical versus modified radical mastectomy for breast cancer. Ann R Coll Surg Engl 1981;63(4):239–43.
37. Fisher B, Redmond C, Poisson R, et al. Eight-year results of a randomized clinical trial comparing total mastectomy and lumpectomy with or without irradiation in the treatment of breast cancer. N Engl J Med 1989;320(13):822–8.
38. Orr RK. The impact of prophylactic axillary node dissection on breast cancer survival—a Bayesian meta-analysis. Ann Surg Oncol 1999;6(1):109–16.
39. Sanghani M, Balk EM, Cady B. Impact of axillary lymph node dissection on breast cancer outcome in clinically node negative patients: a systematic review and meta-analysis. Cancer 2009;115(8):1613–20.
40. Bergkvist L, Frisell J, Liljegren G, et al. Multicentre study of detection and false-negative rates in sentinel node biopsy for breast cancer. Br J Surg 2001;88(12):1644–8.
41. Linehan DC, Hill AD, Akhurst T, et al. Intradermal radiocolloid and intraparenchymal blue dye injection optimize sentinel node identification in breast cancer patients. Ann Surg Oncol 1999;6(5):450–4.
42. Kim T, Giuliano AE, Lyman GH. Lymphatic mapping and sentinel lymph node biopsy in early-stage breast carcinoma: a metaanalysis. Cancer 2006;106(1):4–16.
43. Giuliano AE, Hunt KK, Ballman KV, et al. Axillary dissection vs no axillary dissection in women with invasive breast cancer and sentinel node metastasis: a randomized clinical trial. JAMA 2011;305(6):569–75.
44. Fisher B, Anderson S, Bryant J, et al. Twenty-year follow-up of a randomized trial comparing total mastectomy, lumpectomy, and lumpectomy plus irradiation for the treatment of invasive breast cancer. N Engl J Med 2002;347(16):1233–41.
45. Lyons JM 3rd, Stempel M, Van Zee KJ, et al. Axillary node staging for microinvasive breast cancer: is it justified? Ann Surg Oncol 2012;19(11):3416–21.
46. Wolmark N, Wang J, Mamounas E, et al. Preoperative chemotherapy in patients with operable breast cancer: nine-year results from National Surgical Adjuvant Breast and Bowel Project B-18. J Natl Cancer Inst Monogr 2001;(30):96–102.

47. Olson JA Jr, Budd GT, Carey LA, et al. Improved surgical outcomes for breast cancer patients receiving neoadjuvant aromatase inhibitor therapy: results from a multicenter phase II trial. J Am Coll Surg 2009;208(5):906–14 [discussion: 915–6].
48. Resetkova E. Pathologic aspects of inflammatory breast carcinoma: part 1. Histomorphology and differential diagnosis. Semin Oncol 2008;35(1):25–32.
49. Lyman GH, Giuliano AE, Somerfield MR, et al. American Society of Clinical Oncology guideline recommendations for sentinel lymph node biopsy in early-stage breast cancer. J Clin Oncol 2005;23(30):7703–20.
50. Yang WT, Le-Petross HT, Macapinlac H, et al. Inflammatory breast cancer: PET/CT, MRI, mammography, and sonography findings. Breast Cancer Res Treat 2008;109(3):417–26.
51. Veronesi U, Maisonneuve P, Rotmensz N, et al. Italian randomized trial among women with hysterectomy: tamoxifen and hormone-dependent breast cancer in high-risk women. J Natl Cancer Inst 2003;95(2):160–5.
52. Veronesi U, Marubini E, Mariani L, et al. Radiotherapy after breast-conserving surgery in small breast carcinoma: long-term results of a randomized trial. Ann Oncol 2001;12(7):997–1003.
53. Darby S, McGale P, Correa C, et al. Effect of radiotherapy after breast-conserving surgery on 10-year recurrence and 15-year breast cancer death: meta-analysis of individual patient data for 10,801 women in 17 randomised trials. Lancet 2011;378(9804):1707–16.
54. Bentzen SM, Agrawal RK, Aird EG, et al. The UK Standardisation of Breast Radiotherapy (START) Trial B of radiotherapy hypofractionation for treatment of early breast cancer: a randomised trial. Lancet 2008;371(9618):1098–107.
55. Clark RM, Whelan T, Levine M, et al. Randomized clinical trial of breast irradiation following lumpectomy and axillary dissection for node-negative breast cancer: an update. Ontario Clinical Oncology Group. J Natl Cancer Inst 1996;88(22):1659–64.
56. Liljegren G, Holmberg L, Bergh J, et al. 10-Year results after sector resection with or without postoperative radiotherapy for stage I breast cancer: a randomized trial. J Clin Oncol 1999;17(8):2326–33.
57. Veronesi U, Cascinelli N, Mariani L, et al. Twenty-year follow-up of a randomized study comparing breast-conserving surgery with radical mastectomy for early breast cancer. N Engl J Med 2002;347(16):1227–32.
58. Vrieling C, Collette L, Fourquet A, et al. The influence of the boost in breast-conserving therapy on cosmetic outcome in the EORTC "boost versus no boost" trial. EORTC Radiotherapy and Breast Cancer Cooperative Groups. European Organization for Research and Treatment of Cancer. Int J Radiat Oncol Biol Phys 1999;45(3):677–85.
59. Bentzen SM, Agrawal RK, Aird EG, et al. The UK Standardisation of Breast Radiotherapy (START) Trial A of radiotherapy hypofractionation for treatment of early breast cancer: a randomised trial. Lancet Oncol 2008;9(4):331–41.
60. Clark RM, McCulloch PB, Levine MN, et al. Randomized clinical trial to assess the effectiveness of breast irradiation following lumpectomy and axillary dissection for node-negative breast cancer. J Natl Cancer Inst 1992;84(9):683–9.
61. Liljegren G, Holmberg L, Adami HO, et al. Sector resection with or without post-operative radiotherapy for stage I breast cancer: five-year results of a randomized trial. Uppsala-Orebro Breast Cancer Study Group. J Natl Cancer Inst 1994;86(9):717–22.
62. Schnitt SJ, Hayman J, Gelman R, et al. A prospective study of conservative surgery alone in the treatment of selected patients with stage I breast cancer. Cancer 1996;77(6):1094–100.

63. Veronesi U, Luini A, Del Vecchio M, et al. Radiotherapy after breast-preserving surgery in women with localized cancer of the breast. N Engl J Med 1993;328(22):1587–91.
64. Polgar C, Fodor J, Major T, et al. Breast-conserving treatment with partial or whole breast irradiation for low-risk invasive breast carcinoma—5-year results of a randomized trial. Int J Radiat Oncol Biol Phys 2007;69(3):694–702.
65. Smith BD, Arthur DW, Buchholz TA, et al. Accelerated partial breast irradiation consensus statement from the American Society for Radiation Oncology (ASTRO). Int J Radiat Oncol Biol Phys 2009;74(4):987–1001.
66. Hughes KS, Schnaper LA, Berry D, et al. Lumpectomy plus tamoxifen with or without irradiation in women 70 years of age or older with early breast cancer. N Engl J Med 2004;351(10):971–7.
67. Nguyen PL, Taghian AG, Katz MS, et al. Breast cancer subtype approximated by estrogen receptor, progesterone receptor, and HER-2 is associated with local and distant recurrence after breast-conserving therapy. J Clin Oncol 2008;26(14):2373–8.
68. Voduc KD, Cheang MC, Tyldesley S, et al. Breast cancer subtypes and the risk of local and regional relapse. J Clin Oncol 2010;28(10):1684–91.
69. Wang J, Shi M, Ling R, et al. Adjuvant chemotherapy and radiotherapy in triple-negative breast carcinoma: a prospective randomized controlled multi-center trial. Radiother Oncol 2011;100(2):200–4.
70. Osborne CK. Tamoxifen in the treatment of breast cancer. N Engl J Med 1998;339(22):1609–18.
71. Riggs BL, Hartmann LC. Selective estrogen-receptor modulators—mechanisms of action and application to clinical practice. N Engl J Med 2003;348(7):618–29.
72. Dowsett M, Cuzick J, Ingle J, et al. Meta-analysis of breast cancer outcomes in adjuvant trials of aromatase inhibitors versus tamoxifen. J Clin Oncol 2010;28(3):509–18.
73. Forbes JF, Cuzick J, Buzdar A, et al. Effect of anastrozole and tamoxifen as adjuvant treatment for early-stage breast cancer: 100-month analysis of the ATAC trial. Lancet Oncol 2008;9(1):45–53.
74. Winer EP, Hudis C, Burstein HJ, et al. American Society of Clinical Oncology technology assessment on the use of aromatase inhibitors as adjuvant therapy for postmenopausal women with hormone receptor-positive breast cancer: status report 2004. J Clin Oncol 2005;23(3):619–29.
75. Amir E, Seruga B, Niraula S, et al. Toxicity of adjuvant endocrine therapy in postmenopausal breast cancer patients: a systematic review and meta-analysis. J Natl Cancer Inst 2011;103(17):1299–309.
76. Crew KD, Greenlee H, Capodice J, et al. Prevalence of joint symptoms in postmenopausal women taking aromatase inhibitors for early-stage breast cancer. J Clin Oncol 2007;25(25):3877–83.
77. Howell A, Cuzick J, Baum M, et al. Results of the ATAC (Arimidex, Tamoxifen, Alone or in Combination) trial after completion of 5 years' adjuvant treatment for breast cancer. Lancet 2005;365(9453):60–2.
78. Mao JJ, Stricker C, Bruner D, et al. Patterns and risk factors associated with aromatase inhibitor-related arthralgia among breast cancer survivors. Cancer 2009;115(16):3631–9.
79. Presant CA, Bosserman L, Young T, et al. Aromatase inhibitor-associated arthralgia and/or bone pain: frequency and characterization in non-clinical trial patients. Clin Breast Cancer 2007;7(10):775–8.

80. Partridge AH, Wang PS, Winer EP, et al. Nonadherence to adjuvant tamoxifen therapy in women with primary breast cancer. J Clin Oncol 2003;21(4):602–6.
81. Baselga J, Cortes J, Kim SB, et al. Pertuzumab plus trastuzumab plus docetaxel for metastatic breast cancer. N Engl J Med 2012;366(2):109–19.
82. Geyer CE, Forster J, Lindquist D, et al. Lapatinib plus capecitabine for HER2-positive advanced breast cancer. N Engl J Med 2006;355(26):2733–43.
83. Miller K, Wang M, Gralow J, et al. Paclitaxel plus bevacizumab versus paclitaxel alone for metastatic breast cancer. N Engl J Med 2007;357(26):2666–76.
84. Scappaticci FA, Skillings JR, Holden SN, et al. Arterial thromboembolic events in patients with metastatic carcinoma treated with chemotherapy and bevacizumab. J Natl Cancer Inst 2007;99(16):1232–9.
85. Davies C, Godwin J, Gray R, et al. Relevance of breast cancer hormone receptors and other factors to the efficacy of adjuvant tamoxifen: patient-level meta-analysis of randomised trials. Lancet 2011;378(9793):771–84.
86. Burstein HJ, Prestrud AA, Seidenfeld J, et al. American Society of Clinical Oncology clinical practice guideline: update on adjuvant endocrine therapy for women with hormone receptor-positive breast cancer. J Clin Oncol 2010; 28(23):3784–96.
87. Peto R, Davies C, Godwin J, et al. Comparisons between different polychemotherapy regimens for early breast cancer: meta-analyses of long-term outcome among 100,000 women in 123 randomised trials. Lancet 2012;379(9814):432–44.
88. Goldstein LJ, Gray R, Badve S, et al. Prognostic utility of the 21-gene assay in hormone receptor-positive operable breast cancer compared with classical clinicopathologic features. J Clin Oncol 2008;26(25):4063–71.
89. Paik S, Shak S, Tang G, et al. A multigene assay to predict recurrence of tamoxifen-treated, node-negative breast cancer. N Engl J Med 2004;351(27): 2817–26.
90. Paik S, Tang G, Shak S, et al. Gene expression and benefit of chemotherapy in women with node-negative, estrogen receptor-positive breast cancer. J Clin Oncol 2006;24(23):3726–34.
91. Buyse M, Loi S, van't Veer L, et al. Validation and clinical utility of a 70-gene prognostic signature for women with node-negative breast cancer. J Natl Cancer Inst 2006;98(17):1183–92.
92. Mook S, Schmidt MK, Weigelt B, et al. The 70-gene prognosis signature predicts early metastasis in breast cancer patients between 55 and 70 years of age. Ann Oncol 2010;21(4):717–22.
93. van de Vijver MJ, He YD, van't Veer LJ, et al. A gene-expression signature as a predictor of survival in breast cancer. N Engl J Med 2002;347(25):1999–2009.
94. Desmedt C, Piette F, Loi S, et al. Strong time dependence of the 76-gene prognostic signature for node-negative breast cancer patients in the TRANSBIG multicenter independent validation series. Clin Cancer Res 2007;13(11):3207–14.
95. Foekens JA, Atkins D, Zhang Y, et al. Multicenter validation of a gene expression-based prognostic signature in lymph node-negative primary breast cancer. J Clin Oncol 2006;24(11):1665–71.
96. Albain KS, Barlow WE, Shak S, et al. Prognostic and predictive value of the 21-gene recurrence score assay in postmenopausal women with node-positive, oestrogen-receptor-positive breast cancer on chemotherapy: a retrospective analysis of a randomised trial. Lancet Oncol 2010;11(1):55–65.
97. Jones SE, Savin MA, Holmes FA, et al. Phase III trial comparing doxorubicin plus cyclophosphamide with docetaxel plus cyclophosphamide as adjuvant therapy for operable breast cancer. J Clin Oncol 2006;24(34):5381–7.

98. Martin M, Pienkowski T, Mackey J, et al. Adjuvant docetaxel for node-positive breast cancer. N Engl J Med 2005;352(22):2302–13.
99. Martin M, Rodriguez-Lescure A, Ruiz A, et al. Randomized phase 3 trial of fluorouracil, epirubicin, and cyclophosphamide alone or followed by paclitaxel for early breast cancer. J Natl Cancer Inst 2008;100(11):805–14.
100. Roche H, Fumoleau P, Spielmann M, et al. Sequential adjuvant epirubicin-based and docetaxel chemotherapy for node-positive breast cancer patients: the FNCLCC PACS 01 Trial. J Clin Oncol 2006;24(36):5664–71.
101. Sparano JA, Wang M, Martino S, et al. Weekly paclitaxel in the adjuvant treatment of breast cancer. N Engl J Med 2008;358(16):1663–71.
102. Muss HB, Berry DA, Cirrincione C, et al. Toxicity of older and younger patients treated with adjuvant chemotherapy for node-positive breast cancer: the Cancer and Leukemia Group B Experience. J Clin Oncol 2007;25(24):3699–704.
103. Muss HB, Berry DA, Cirrincione C, et al. Adjuvant chemotherapy in older women with early-stage breast cancer. N Engl J Med 2009;360(20):2055–65.
104. Romond EH, Perez EA, Bryant J, et al. Trastuzumab plus adjuvant chemotherapy for operable HER2-positive breast cancer. N Engl J Med 2005;353(16):1673–84.
105. Yin W, Jiang Y, Shen Z, et al. Trastuzumab in the adjuvant treatment of HER2-positive early breast cancer patients: a meta-analysis of published randomized controlled trials. PLoS One 2011;6(6):e21030.
106. Perez EA, Suman VJ, Davidson NE, et al. Cardiac safety analysis of doxorubicin and cyclophosphamide followed by paclitaxel with or without trastuzumab in the North Central Cancer Treatment Group N9831 adjuvant breast cancer trial. J Clin Oncol 2008;26(8):1231–8.
107. Gralow JR, Burstein HJ, Wood W, et al. Preoperative therapy in invasive breast cancer: pathologic assessment and systemic therapy issues in operable disease. J Clin Oncol 2008;26(5):814–9.
108. Guarneri V, Frassoldati A, Giovannelli S, et al. Primary systemic therapy for operable breast cancer: a review of clinical trials and perspectives. Cancer Lett 2007;248(2):175–85.
109. Sachelarie I, Grossbard ML, Chadha M, et al. Primary systemic therapy of breast cancer. Oncologist 2006;11(6):574–89.
110. Kimmick GG, Shelton BJ, Case LD, et al. Long-term follow-up of a phase II trial studying a weekly doxorubicin-based multiple drug adjuvant therapy for stage II node-positive carcinoma of the breast. Breast Cancer Res Treat 2002;72(3):233–43.
111. Chia YH, Ellis MJ, Ma CX. Neoadjuvant endocrine therapy in primary breast cancer: indications and use as a research tool. Br J Cancer 2010;103(6):759–64.
112. Mathew J, Asgeirsson KS, Jackson LR, et al. Neoadjuvant endocrine treatment in primary breast cancer—review of literature. Breast 2009;18(6):339–44.
113. Kaufmann M, Hortobagyi GN, Goldhirsch A, et al. Recommendations from an international expert panel on the use of neoadjuvant (primary) systemic treatment of operable breast cancer: an update. J Clin Oncol 2006;24(12):1940–9.
114. Jemal A, Bray F, Center MM, et al. Global cancer statistics. CA Cancer J Clin 2011;61(2):69–90.
115. Howlader N NA, Krapcho M, Neyman N, et al. SEER cancer statistics review, 1975-2009. 2012. Available at: http://seer.cancer.gov/csr/1975_2009_pops09/. Accessed May 1, 2012.
116. Rosselli Del Turco M, Palli D, Cariddi A, et al. Intensive diagnostic follow-up after treatment of primary breast cancer. A randomized trial. National Research Council Project on Breast Cancer follow-up. JAMA 1994;271(20):1593–7.

117. Impact of follow-up testing on survival and health-related quality of life in breast cancer patients. A multicenter randomized controlled trial. The GIVIO Investigators. JAMA 1994;271(20):1587–92.
118. Ganz PA, Desmond KA, Leedham B, et al. Quality of life in long-term, disease-free survivors of breast cancer: a follow-up study. J Natl Cancer Inst 2002;94(1):39–49.
119. Howard-Anderson J, Ganz PA, Bower JE, et al. Quality of life, fertility concerns, and behavioral health outcomes in younger breast cancer survivors: a systematic review. J Natl Cancer Inst 2012;104(5):386–405.
120. Loprinzi CL, Kugler JW, Sloan JA, et al. Venlafaxine in management of hot flashes in survivors of breast cancer: a randomised controlled trial. Lancet 2000;356(9247):2059–63.
121. Moegele M, Buchholz S, Seitz S, et al. Vaginal estrogen therapy in postmenopausal breast cancer patients treated with aromatase inhibitors. Arch Gynecol Obstet 2012;285(5):1397–402.
122. Labrie F, Cusan L, Gomez JL, et al. Effect of one-week treatment with vaginal estrogen preparations on serum estrogen levels in postmenopausal women. Menopause 2009;16(1):30–6.
123. Holmes MD, Chen WY, Feskanich D, et al. Physical activity and survival after breast cancer diagnosis. JAMA 2005;293(20):2479–86.
124. Jones LW, Eves ND, Peppercorn J. Pre-exercise screening and prescription guidelines for cancer patients. Lancet Oncol 2010;11(10):914–6.
125. Chlebowski RT, Blackburn GL, Thomson CA, et al. Dietary fat reduction and breast cancer outcome: interim efficacy results from the Women's Intervention Nutrition Study. J Natl Cancer Inst 2006;98(24):1767–76.
126. Beasley JM, Newcomb PA, Trentham-Dietz A, et al. Post-diagnosis dietary factors and survival after invasive breast cancer. Breast Cancer Res Treat 2011;128(1):229–36.
127. Chen WY, Rosner B, Hankinson SE, et al. Moderate alcohol consumption during adult life, drinking patterns, and breast cancer risk. JAMA 2011;306(17):1884–90.
128. Grunfeld E, Levine MN, Julian JA, et al. Randomized trial of long-term follow-up for early-stage breast cancer: a comparison of family physician versus specialist care. J Clin Oncol 2006;24(6):848–55.
129. Mao JJ, Bowman MA, Stricker CT, et al. Delivery of survivorship care by primary care physicians: the perspective of breast cancer patients. J Clin Oncol 2009;27(6):933–8.
130. Khatcheressian JL, Wolff AC, Smith TJ, et al. American Society of Clinical Oncology 2006 update of the breast cancer follow-up and management guidelines in the adjuvant setting. J Clin Oncol 2006;24(31):5091–7.

Multimodality Approach to Management of Stage III Non–Small Cell Lung Cancer

Anthony Scarpaci, MD[a,*], Priya Mitra, MD[b], Doraid Jarrar, MD[c], Gregory A. Masters, MD[d]

KEYWORDS

• Non–small cell lung cancer • Neoadjuvant treatment • Multimodality approach

KEY POINTS

- Non–small cell lung cancer is a serious health condition requiring multidisciplinary input from surgical oncology, radiation oncology, and medical oncology.
- Appropriate staging studies are required to develop the optimal strategy for an individual patient. This strategy includes positron emission tomography/computed tomography scan and endobronchial ultrasonography or mediastinoscopy for locally advanced disease to determine resectability.
- Chemoradiation is the standard approach in stage III lung cancer, with surgery as an option in some cases. Concurrent chemoradiation has been proved to be superior to sequential therapy.
- Cisplatin doublet therapy is considered standard for chemotherapy selection.
- Pathologic review of biopsy samples now includes testing for EGFR gene mutations and EML4-ALK gene rearrangements.

INTRODUCTION

According to the American Cancer Society, there were an estimated 222,520 new cases of lung cancer in 2010. It is the second most prevalent cancer in men and women, behind prostate cancer and breast cancer, respectively. It is responsible for the most cancer-related deaths in both men and women. Lung cancer was responsible for 157,300 deaths in 2010.[1] The mortality data are impressive when compared with other cancers (**Table 1**).

[a] Medical Oncology, Albert Einstein Medical Center Philadelphia, 5501 Old York Road, Philadelphia, PA 19141, USA; [b] Radiation Oncology, Albert Einstein Medical Center Philadelphia, 5501 Old York Road, Philadelphia, PA 19141, USA; [c] Thoracic Surgery, Albert Einstein Medical Center Philadelphia, 5501 Old York Road, Philadelphia, PA 19141, USA; [d] Helen F. Graham Cancer Center, 4701 Ogletown-Stanton Road, Suite 3400, Newark, DE 19713, USA
* Corresponding author.
E-mail address: apscarpaci@gmail.com

Surg Oncol Clin N Am 22 (2013) 319–328
http://dx.doi.org/10.1016/j.soc.2012.12.014
surgonc.theclinics.com

Table 1
American Cancer Society: cancer statistics 2010

Cancer	Incidence	Mortality
Lung	222,520	157,300
Colorectal	142,570	51,370
Breast	209,060	40,230
Prostate	217,730	32,050
Pancreatic	43,140	36,800
Colorectal, breast, prostate, pancreatic combined	612,500	160,450

There are nearly as many deaths from lung cancer yearly as there are from the combined total of colorectal, breast, prostate, and pancreatic cancers. As a contributing factor to the high mortality, many patients present with advanced disease. According to the National Cancer Database report on lung cancer, 30% of patients with non–small cell lung cancer (NSCLC) present with locally advanced, stage IIIA/B disease, and 40% of patients present with metastatic disease at diagnosis.[2]

This article reviews staging and clinical evaluation of patients with lung cancer, with a focus on those with locally advanced disease. Patients should have routine staging studies, including pathology review, history, and physical examination, computed tomography (CT) of the chest and upper abdomen (including adrenals), positron emission tomography (PET) or integrated PET-CT, bronchoscopy, evaluation of the mediastinum by mediastinoscopy or endobronchial ultrasonography (EBUS)/endoscopic ultrasonography as recommended by National Comprehensive Cancer Network (NCCN) guidelines plus brain magnetic resonance imaging (MRI). In addition, for some locally advanced, but potentially resectable cancer, chest MRI may delineate the depth of invasion better (Pancoast tumor, pericardial invasion, involvement of vertebral bodies).

Most patients with stage III disease are recognized based on clinical staging, especially because the addition of integrated PET-CT to the staging armentarium has increased the accuracy of preoperative evaluation. A few patients are found on pathologic review to have unsuspected N2 or N3 disease; this usually constitutes microscopic metastasis that is too small to be fluorodeoxyglucose (FDG)-avid and, therefore, PET-negative. Once the pretreatment clinical staging has been completed, patients should be discussed at a multidisciplinary tumor board, which includes but is not limited to medical oncology, radiation oncology, and a dedicated thoracic surgeon. In addition, it improves patient care and communication if representatives from pulmonary medicine, pathology, social services, and radiology are present.

SURGICAL EVALUATION

Advanced local and regional cancer includes the following: any T stage with ipsilateral (N2; stage IIIA) or contralateral (N3; stage IIIB) or any scalene or supraclavicular node involvement (N3; stage IIIB). In addition, tumors that are more than 5 cm (T2b, T3>7.0 cm) or any tumor that directly invades resectable structures (T3 invasion) should be considered locally advanced and require a multimodality approach to increase the cure rate. Some tumors that invade the mediastinum, heart, great vessels, trachea, recurrent laryngeal nerve, esophagus, vertebral body, or carina (all T4) may be resectable. Some lobe nodules (formerly considered T4; *TNM Classification of Malignant Tumours, Sixth Edition*) are now surgical disease (T3; stage IIB if node-negative).

Special consideration should be given to separate tumor nodule(s) in a different ipsilateral lobe to that of the primary. In the *TNM Classification of Malignant Tumours, Sixth Edition*, this condition was considered incurable stage IV disease (M1); in the current edition, after reviewing more than 100,000 patients with lung cancer and stratifying them according to survival, this condition is now considered T4 disease and potentially curable by bilobectomy or pneumonectomy. Most locally advanced lung cancer constitutes stage IIIA and B disease.

Stage IIIA (positive ipsilateral N2 nodes, T3 invasion [N1 or N2], T4 extension, and N1 disease [+N2, considered stage IIIB]) is considered for multimodality treatment (ie, neoadjuvant chemoradiation followed by restaging and possible resection). Consideration of possible resection requires special attention on how to stage the mediastinum. Based on the findings that the positive predictive value of integrated PET-CT is only in the range of 60%, patients need cytologic or pathologic confirmation of N2 disease. Mediastinoscopy has been considered the gold standard for this purpose. It provides pathologic evaluation of FDG-avid lymph nodes in the paratracheal compartment (including subcarinal, ie, nodal station 7); at least 3 nodal stations should be biopsied during mediastinoscopy. Surgical mediastinoscopy is not repeatable; after neoadjuvant chemoradiation and restaging (integrated PET-CT), FDG uptake in the mediastinum may be caused by tumor necrosis and not recalcitrant disease. EBUS has enormous value. It only provides cytologic evaluation, but is repeatable before and after induction chemoradiation. Because surgical mediastinoscopy is still considered the gold standard of N2/N3 evaluation, mediastinoscopy can be reserved for the final evaluation after neoadjuvant therapy before surgical resection.

Stage IIIA disease is overall a heterogeneous group; on the one end of the spectrum, it encompasses patients with single nodal station microscopic disease, and on the other hand, patients with bulky multistation involvement (ie, subcarinal plus levels 2 and 4 on the right and levels 5, 6, and 7 and L2, L4 on the left). Surgical therapy alone has a poor outcome. The exception to this claim is nonclinical N2 disease, which means micrometastasis in a single nodal station on final pathologic review after lobectomy and thoracic lymphadenectomy, with negative CT and integrated PET-CT beforehand. The Intergroup trial INT0139[3] confirmed that surgery (lobectomy, but not pneumonectomy) has a role after induction concurrent chemoradiotherapy. Based on several studies, the 5-year survival for stage IIIA NSCLC can vary between 3% (clinical N2 disease; bulky, multiple stations) and 34% (single-station N2 involvement, microscopic disease). Anatomic resection for advanced lung cancer can be performed either with a minimally invasive approach (video-assisted thoracic surgery [VATS]) or through a traditional posterolateral thoracotomy. Because more experience has been gained with VATS, this approach can be offered even after induction chemotherapy and radiation therapy. Many trials require an open approach (ie, thoracotomy) and coverage of the bronchial stump with an intercostal muscle flap to prevent the complication of a bronchopleural fistula. It has been shown in the adjuvant setting that if the VATS approach is used, chemotherapy can be given earlier because of the expedited recovery from a minimally invasive approach. This strategy may translate into an overall survival benefit, because more patients are likely to finish adjuvant therapy.

With the contemporary staging (integrated PET-CT, EBUS), 85% of advanced lung cancers are assigned the correct stage before treatment. Only a few undergo upfront surgical resection and on pathologic examination are upstaged to a higher stage. Surgery does play a role in the treatment of advanced lung cancer as part of a multimodality approach. Stage IIIA disease, the most common stage of advanced NSCLC for which surgery could be considered, is heterogeneous and, therefore, survival rates vary widely (depending on N2 disease burden).

For patients with clinical stage IIIA disease (T1–3, N2), the standard of care is definitive concurrent chemoradiation (category I recommendation in the NCCN guidelines). For stage IIIB, the standard of care is definitive chemoradiation followed by chemotherapy.

Once the standard for chemoradiation therapy was established, several studies were performed to evaluate concurrent versus sequential treatment. One of the key studies was LAMP (Locally Advanced Multimodality Protocol), a randomized phase II study.[4] It was closed prematurely because of limited accrual but did provide some important data and median follow-up of approximately 40 months. The study enrolled 257 patients with unresectable stage III NSCLC and randomized the patients to 1 of 3 arms: sequential chemotherapy followed by radiation therapy, induction chemotherapy followed by concurrent chemoradiation, or concurrent chemoradiation followed by consolidative chemotherapy. The median survival for the 3 groups was 13, 12.7, and 16.4 months, respectively. The differences were not statistically significant different between the arms, although the data suggest an improved outcome in the third group.

Radiation therapy is a treatment modality that directs ionizing radiation toward tumors, mostly malignant, with the objective of tumor cell kill. The goal of radiation therapy is to deliver a maximally safe dose to the target volume and minimize dose to surrounding normal structures; the target volume is delineated by the radiation oncologist using diagnostic imaging. The total dose is divided into multiple treatments, or fractions, so that the same dose is delivered each day.

In NSCLC, radiation therapy is used either in the postoperative setting, as definitive treatment with or without chemotherapy, or in a palliative manner. In patients with early-stage and potentially resectable tumors who are medically inoperable, stereotactic ablative radiation therapy may be a reasonable treatment option. This technique delivers a high dose per fraction over a shorter period and fewer treatments.

In locally advanced NSCLC, the standard of care is concurrent chemoradiation therapy. These patients typically receive daily treatment, 5 days per week, with the same dose per fraction for approximately 6 weeks. Patients requiring radiation therapy for palliation of symptoms, such as obstruction of the mainstem bronchus, are commonly treated over 1 to 3 weeks.

Radiation therapy is delivered by either teletherapy or brachytherapy. Teletherapy typically uses a linear accelerator, which is situated approximately 100 cm from the patient; the large machine emits radiation and is directed toward the target. Teletherapy is the primary method of treatment delivery in patients with locally advanced lung cancer. Brachytherapy uses a radioactive source, which is juxtaposed against, or within, the tumor. An example of brachytherapy in lung cancer is endobronchial radiation, delivered with the assistance of a bronchoscope, in patients with an obstructing intraluminal mass.

Treatment planning for external beam radiation therapy with teletherapy is CT-based. A CT simulation is performed with the patient in the treatment position, thus simulating how the actual treatment is delivered. Patients are often supine with arms raised above their head, resting on the treatment table, so that the arms do not obstruct any portion of the torso. A wing board is a common device used at the time of simulation; it is placed under the patient's upper body and has a spot for a head rest as well as adjustable bars to grasp with the hands. A customized mold can also be created for the torso to help ensure that the patient is lying in the same position daily. Once the scan has been completed, the patient is marked with small but permanent tattoos as a positioning verification tool that is checked each day when setting the patient up for treatment. The images are linked to the treatment-planning software, and the physician delineates the target volumes, and surrounding normal tissue structures, on each axial CT slice. Next, a treatment plan is generated to deliver a maximally safe dose to the tumor and minimize dose to the surrounding critical structures; **Figs. 1** and **2** show an example of 2 treatment fields in a patient with locally advanced NSCLC.

Tumor motion of lung tumors can become problematic if there is significant variation with respiration, because the target volumes may be underdosed if they move out of the path of the radiation beam. Different methods have been used to minimize motion, including treating patients prone and using abdominal compression. Both techniques limit abdominal excursion and are easily reproducible; if either of these techniques is being considered, it must be used at the time of CT simulation.

Once the patient is undergoing daily radiation treatment, radiographic images are regularly taken on the linear accelerator before treatment to verify setup positioning. These images are matched to a digitally reconstructed radiograph (DRR) from the time of CT simulation; bony anatomy or carina positioning is used to match the DRR with the most recently obtained radiograph. This verification process has resulted in improved accuracy of treatment delivery. An area being explored is bronchoscopic placement of gold fiducial markers in or around the tumor so that this can be used instead of bony or carina anatomy.

The recommended dose of radiation therapy for definitive treatment of locally advanced NSCLC is 60 to 70 Gy (ie, 6000–7000 rad). The minimum dose of 60 Gy, in 2-Gy fractions, was established as the standard of care in 1980.[5] RTOG 73-01 (Radiation Therapy Oncology Group 73-01) was a randomized study of 375 patients with stage III NSCLC. Patients were randomized to 1 of 4 treatment regimens: 40-Gy split course or continuous dosing of 40, 50, and 60 Gy. The split course delivered 20 Gy in 1 week, then a 2-week break, followed by 20 Gy in 1 week. Each regimen used 5 fractions per week. Patients treated with split course radiation had the worst overall survival (10% at 2 years); the other groups' 2-year survival ranged between 14% and 18%. Local tumor regression increased with dose; patients treated with either 50 or

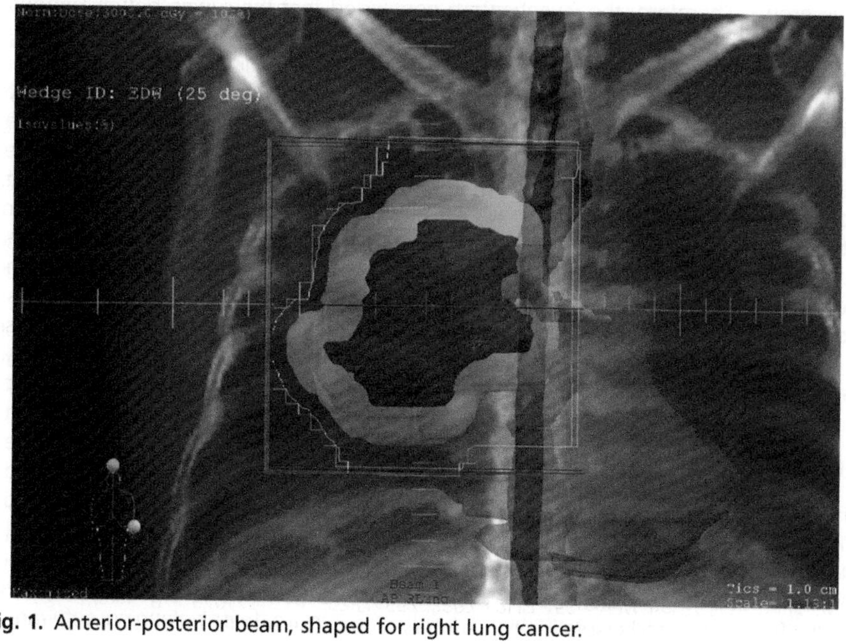

Fig. 1. Anterior-posterior beam, shaped for right lung cancer.

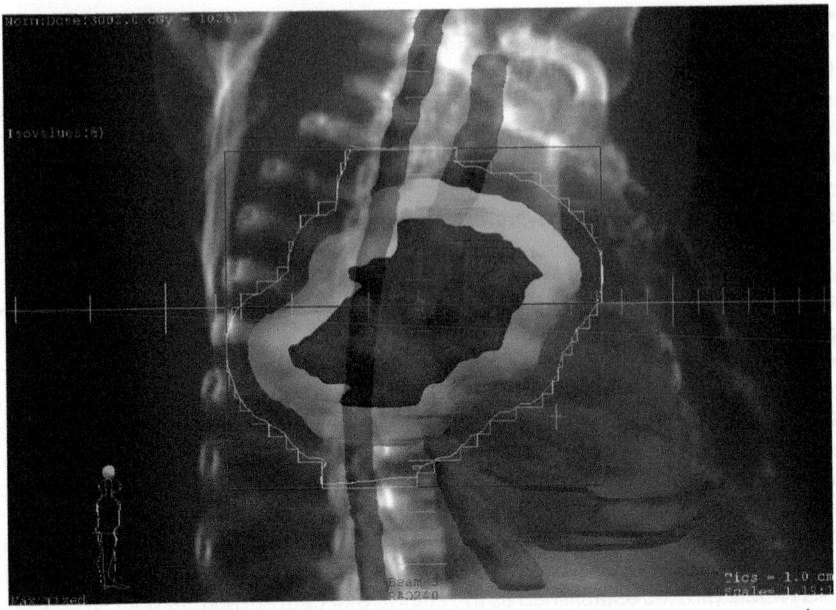

Fig. 2. Oblique beam, shaped for right lung cancer. Color key: red, gross tumor volume; turquoise, planning target volume, incorporates motion; blue, spinal cord; purple, esophagus; pink, heart; orange, carina.

60 Gy had a statistically significant increase in response rate compared with those receiving 40 Gy (69% vs 50%, respectively). The rate of intrathoracic disease recurrence also correlated with dose; the incidence was 38% in the 60-Gy group, 45% in the 50-Gy group, 51% in the 40-Gy split course group, and 64% in the 40-Gy continuous group. Therefore, the investigators concluded that there was better response and tumor control with dose escalation.

A recently closed protocol, RTOG 0617, tested the possibility of increasing the total radiation therapy dose beyond 60 Gy as well as the usefulness of adding cetuximab to the chemotherapeutic regimen. The study compared standard-dose (60-Gy) with high-dose (74-Gy) conformal radiation therapy with concurrent and consolidation chemotherapy using carboplatin and paclitaxel with or without cetuximab. Eligible patients included those with stage IIIA/IIIB NSCLC and they underwent randomization to 1 of 4 treatment arms: standard chemotherapy with 60 Gy or 74 Gy (arms A and B) and standard chemotherapy with cetuximab with 60 Gy or 74 Gy (arms C and D). The preliminary data, after a median follow-up of 9.1 months, determined that high-dose radiation therapy does not improve overall survival; this finding led to the early closure of the high-dose arms. There has been no discernible link between toxicity and decreased survival in the 74-Gy arm. Final results are still pending continued follow-up.

CHEMOTHERAPEUTIC EVALUATION

One of the major controversies in lung cancer management is the order in which therapeutic modalities are delivered. A study by Rosell and colleagues from 1994[6] and its follow-up study from 1999[7] investigated preoperative chemotherapy followed by surgery versus surgery alone. Sixty patients were randomized to preoperative mitomycin, ifosfamide, and cisplatin or to surgery alone. The results favored preoperative chemotherapy, with a significant difference in overall survival (22 months vs 10 months) after 7 years of follow-up. A study by Roth and colleagues from 1994[8] showed similar results. This trial evaluated patients with IIIA disease randomized to preoperative chemotherapy with cyclophosphamide, etoposide, and cisplatin and surgery or surgery alone. Patients receiving preoperative chemotherapy experienced median overall survival of 64 months. Patients receiving surgery alone experienced median survival of 11 months.

In 2010, Pisters and colleagues[9] published the SWOG 9900 (Southwest Oncology Group 9900) trial, which was designed to evaluate neoadjuvant chemotherapy. In this phase III trial, 354 patients were randomized to preoperative chemotherapy with carboplatin and paclitaxel followed by surgery or to surgery alone. Patients with early-stage cancers (stage IB, II, or IIIA) were evaluated for overall survival. The patients with preoperative chemotherapy were found to have improved overall survival and performance-free survival, although the results were not statistically significant. The trial was prematurely closed because of other evidence from the International Adjuvant Lung Trial and ANITA (Adjuvant Navelbine International Trialist Association) trials establishing the benefit of adjuvant chemotherapy. There was noted to be a trend toward improved overall survival in the arm with preoperative treatment.

Adjuvant chemotherapy has become the current standard of care for operable lung cancers, primarily because of the results of the ANITA and the International Adjuvant Lung Trial. Doulliard and colleagues[10] in the ANITA trial evaluated postoperative chemotherapy in the management of early-stage lung cancer. A total of 804 patients with stage IB to IIIA NSCLC were randomized to observation or adjuvant chemotherapy with vinorelbine and cisplatin. A dramatic increase in overall survival was noted in the chemotherapy arm (65.7 months vs 43.7 months). The International Adjuvant Lung Trial led by Arrigada[11] also evaluated chemotherapy versus observation. A total of 1867 patients with stage I, II, or III NSCLC were randomized to cisplatin-based chemotherapy or observation after surgery. The chemotherapy arm had superior survival compared with the observation arm (44.5% vs 40.4% at 5 years).

The SWOG 8805 trial investigated the role of trimodality therapy in the management of advanced NSCLC (stages IIIA and IIB).[12] A total of 126 patients were evaluated in this study (75 patients with stage IIIA disease and 51 patients with stage IIIB disease). Patients were treated with 2 cycles of cisplatin and etoposide and concurrent radiation followed by thoracotomy and adjuvant chemoradiation if their NSCLC was incompletely resectable or unresectable. This approach yielded a 26% 3-year survival rate.

A current Eastern Cooperative Oncology Group trial, E1505, is being conducted to evaluate the use of adjuvant chemotherapy and targeted therapy after resected early-stage NSCLC. This is a randomized phase III trial of adjuvant chemotherapy with or without bevacizumab for patients with completely resected stage IB to IIIA NSCLC. Any 1 of 4 chemotherapy regimens can be used: vinorelbine/cisplatin, docetaxel/cisplatin, gemcitabine/cisplatin, or pemetrexed/cisplatin. The patients are randomized in a 1:1 scheme with or without bevacizumab. The primary end point is overall survival. Estimated accrual is 1500 patients.

BIOMARKERS/NEW AGENTS

As more is learned about the molecular origins of lung cancer, specific genetic targets have been isolated for prognostic and predictive value. Among these biomarkers are EGFR gene mutations, ERCC1 expression, KRAS mutations, EML4-ALK gene rearrangement, and RRM1 expression. Of these genetic tests, the most significant for therapy are the EGFR mutations and EML4-ALK gene rearrangement. Current NCCN guidelines recommend that specimens from all patients with adenocarcinoma should be tested for EGFR gene mutations as well as the ALK gene mutation.

The EGFR gene mutations (exon 19 deletion and exon 21 L858R mutation) are not prognostic indicators of survival but are predictive indicators of treatment benefit from targeted therapy such as the tyrosine kinase inhibitors gefitinib and erlotinib. The EML4-ALK gene rearrangement also has predictive value for response to therapy with tyrosine kinase inhibitors such as crizotinib.

Erlotinib is indicated for patients with advanced-stage NSCLC as maintenance therapy in stable disease and for patients who have progressed through initial therapy. The tarceva results in conjuction with paclitaxel and carboplatin (TRIBUTE) trial evaluated the efficacy of erlotinib with carboplatin and paclitaxel in stage IIIB/IV NSCLC for first-line therapy.[13] TRIBUTE was a randomized phase III trial of 1059 patients with stage IIIB/IV NSCLC. Patients were randomized to a standard treatment arm of carboplatin and paclitaxel with oral placebo followed by placebo maintenance therapy or experimental treatment with carboplatin and paclitaxel and 150-mg erlotinib followed by erlotinib maintenance. There was no survival advantage seen in the experimental arm over the treatment arm (10.6 months vs 10.5 months).

Crizotinib has been approved by the US Food and Drug Administration for use in locally advanced or metastatic NSCLC. The recent cohort study by Kwak and colleagues[14] evaluated the efficacy of crizotinib in 82 patients with advanced NSCLC and the presence of the EML4-ALK mutation. Patients were treated with 250 mg twice daily. The predominant histologic subtype was adenocarcinoma (79/82 patients). There was a 57% overall response rate after median treatment duration of 6.4 months. Forty-six patients had partial response, 1 patient had a complete response, and 27 patients had stable disease.

Cetuximab has been evaluated as a potential therapeutic agent in the treatment of lung cancer. The FLEX trial evaluated the use of cetuximab when added to chemotherapy in patients with advanced NSCLC.[15] A total of 1125 patients with advanced NSCLC (stage IIIB or IV) were randomized to either chemotherapy alone (cisplatin and vinorelbine) or chemotherapy and cetuximab. There was an increase in response rate in the experimental arm (36% vs 29%) but no difference in progression-free survival. There was a slightly better overall survival rate (11.3 months vs 10.1 months); however, it was at the expense of increased episodes of grade 3 or 4 febrile neutropenia.

Vascular endothelial growth factor (VEGF) inhibitors such as bevacizumab have been evaluated in advanced lung cancer in E4599 by Sandler and colleagues.[16] A total of 878 patients with stage IIIB or IV lung adenocarcinoma were randomized to chemotherapy alone or chemotherapy with bevacizumab. The median survival of the chemotherapy alone arm was 10.3 months. The median survival of the combination therapy arm was 12.3 months with $P = .003$.

SURVEILLANCE/RECURRENCE

The management of recurrence, whether locoregional or distant, is dependent on the involved region. Locoregional recurrences can cause superior vena cava syndrome, severe hemoptysis, and endobronchial obstruction. Treatment options include endobronchial stent, photodynamic therapy, surgery, brachytherapy, external beam radiotherapy, and concurrent chemoradiation if not previously given.

Distant metastases commonly involve the brain or bone. Surgical intervention may be indicated for both brain and bone metastases; palliative external beam radiotherapy is often indicated for both situations regardless of surgery. Bisphosphonate therapy is typically recommended for patients with bone metastases.

REFERENCES

1. Jernal A, Siegel R, Xu J, et al. Cancer statistics, 2010. CA Cancer J Clin 2010;60: 277–300.
2. Fry W, Menck H, Winchester D. The National Cancer Data Base report on lung cancer. Cancer 1996;77:1947–55.
3. Albain KS, Swann RS, Rusch VR, et al. Phase III study of concurrent chemotherapy and radiotherapy (CT/RT) vs CT/RT followed by surgical resection for stage IIIA (pN2) non-small cell lung cancer (NSCLC): outcomes update of North American Intergroup 0139 (RTOG 9309). J Clin Oncol 2005;23:16S.
4. Belani CP, Choy H, Bonomi P, et al. Combined chemoradiotherapy regimens of paclitaxel and carboplatin for locally advanced non-small-cell lung cancer: a randomized phase II locally advanced multi-modality protocol. J Clin Oncol 2005;23:5883–91.
5. Perez CA, Stanley K, Rubin P, et al. A prospective randomized study of various irradiation doses and fractionation schedules in the treatment of inoperable non-oat cell carcinoma of the lung: preliminary report by Radiation Therapy Oncology Group. Cancer 1980;45:2744–53.
6. Rosell R, Gómez-Codina J, Camps C, et al. A randomized trial comparing preoperative chemotherapy plus surgery with surgery alone in patients with non-small-cell lung cancer. N Engl J Med 1994;220(3):153–8.
7. Rosell R, Gómez-Codina J, Camps C, et al. Preresectional chemotherapy in stage IIIA non-small-cell lung cancer: a 7-year assessment of a randomized controlled trial. Lung Cancer 1999;26(1):7–14.
8. Roth JA, Fossella F, Komaki R, et al. A randomized trial comparing perioperative chemotherapy and surgery with surgery alone in resectable stage IIIA non-small-cell lung cancer. J Natl Cancer Inst 1994;86(9):673–80.
9. Pisters KM, Vallières E, Crowley JJ, et al. Surgery with or without preoperative paclitaxel and carboplatin in early-stage non-small-cell lung cancer: Southwest Oncology Group Trial S9900, an intergroup, randomized, phase III trial. J Clin Oncol 2010;28(11):1843–9.
10. Douillard JY, Rossell R, De Lena M, et al. Adjuvant vinorelbine plus cisplatin versus observation in patients with completely resected stage IB-IIIA non-small cell lung cancer (Adjuvant Navelbine International Trialist Association [ANITA]): a randomized controlled trial. Lancet Oncol 2006;7:719–27.
11. Arriagada R, Bergman B, Dunant A, et al. Cisplatin-based adjuvant chemotherapy in patients with completely resected non-small-cell lung cancer. N Engl J Med 2004;350:351–60.
12. Albain KS, Rusch VW, Crowley JJ, et al. Concurrent cisplatin/etoposide plus chest radiotherapy followed by surgery for stages IIIA (N2) and IIIB non-small-cell lung cancer: mature results of Southwest Oncology Group phase II study 8805. J Clin Oncol 1995;13:1880–92.
13. Herbst RS, Prager D, Hermann R, et al. TRIBUTE: a phase III trial of erlotinib hydrochloride combined with carboplatin and paclitaxel chemotherapy in advanced non-small-cell lung cancer. J Clin Oncol 2005;23:5892–9.
14. Kwak EL, Bang YJ, Camidge DR, et al. Anaplastic lymphoma kinase inhibition in non-small-cell lung cancer. N Engl J Med 2010;363:1693–703.

15. Pirker R, Pereira JR, Szczesna A, et al. Cetuximab plus chemotherapy in patients with advanced non-small-cell lung cancer (FLEX): an open-label randomized phase III trial. Lancet 2009;373:1525–31.
16. Sandler A, Gray R, Perry MC, et al. Paclitaxel-carboplatin alone or with bevacizumab for non-small-cell lung cancer. N Engl J Med 2006;355:2542–50.

Multidisciplinary Management of Small Cell Lung Cancer

Sarah B. Goldberg, MD, MPH[a], Henning Willers, MD[b], Rebecca S. Heist, MD, MPH[c,*]

KEYWORDS

• Small cell lung cancer • Multidisciplinary management • Surgical resection
• Cranial irradiation

KEY POINTS

- Small cell lung cancer is an aggressive malignancy with a propensity for rapid growth and early metastases.
- Concurrent chemotherapy and thoracic radiation therapy are the standard treatment option for patients with limited-stage small cell lung cancer.
- Surgical resection is an option for very early disease (typically small lesions with uninvolved lymph nodes), but there are conflicting results in the literature on its usefulness.
- Extensive-stage small cell lung cancer is treated with combination chemotherapy, which improves survival and quality of life; the usual first-line treatment regimen is etoposide plus a platinum compound.
- Prophylactic cranial irradiation prolongs survival in patients with limited-stage and extensive-stage disease and should be considered in all patients who respond to initial chemotherapy.

INTRODUCTION

More than 226,000 cases of lung cancer will be diagnosed in 2012, with more than 160,000 deaths attributed to this diagnosis, making it the second most common cancer and the most common cause of cancer death in the United States.[1] The epidemiology of lung cancer has been shifting, given the decline in cigarette smoking in this

Funding Sources: None.
Conflict of Interest: None.
[a] Department of Hematology/Oncology, Yale Cancer Center, 333 Cedar Street, FMP-130, PO Box 208032, New Haven, CT 06520, USA; [b] Clark Center for Radiation Oncology, Department of Radiation Oncology, Massachusetts General Hospital Cancer Center, 100 Blossom Street, Cox 302, Boston, MA 02114, USA; [c] Department of Hematology/Oncology, Massachusetts General Hospital Cancer Center, 55 Fruit Street, Yawkey 7B, Boston, MA 02114, USA
* Corresponding author.
E-mail address: rheist@partners.org

Surg Oncol Clin N Am 22 (2013) 329–343
http://dx.doi.org/10.1016/j.soc.2012.12.002
surgonc.theclinics.com
1055-3207/13/$ – see front matter

country; although small cell lung cancer (SCLC) was previously a common histologic subtype, it now represents approximately 13% of all cases.[2] Also because of changes in smoking trends, SCLC used to be a disease found predominantly in men, but currently it is seen equally in men and women.

SCLC has a distinct natural history and treatment response pattern compared with non–small cell lung cancer (NSCLC). It tends to have a rapid doubling time and high propensity for early metastases. In contrast to NSCLC and many other solid tumors, it is commonly very chemosensitive initially, although it almost always recurs after a period of response. Given the various specialists involved in the care of patients with SCLC, it is clear that the evaluation and treatment of this disease require a multidisciplinary approach.

SCLC BACKGROUND

Pathologic Diagnosis

SCLC exists along a continuum of other neuroendocrine neoplasms of the lung, with carcinoid at one end of the spectrum, given its indolent nature, and large cell neuroendocrine carcinoma and SCLC at the other end, given their rapid growth and aggressive behavior. Histologically, SCLC typically appears as small round or oval blue monotonous cells with hyperchromatic nuclei, a salt-and-pepper chromatic pattern, and foci of necrosis. The mitotic count is frequently high, indicating the rapid growth kinetics that is seen clinically. Almost all SCLCs stain positively for keratin, thyroid transcription factor 1, and epithelial membrane antigen. Markers of neuroendocrine differentiation are also commonly seen, including chromogranin A, synaptophysin, CD56, and neuron-specific enolase.[3] A subset of NSCLC also stains positive for neuroendocrine markers, so histologic as well as immunohistochemical evaluation is important in diagnosis: tumors that appear to be NSCLC by light microscopy but stain with neuroendocrine markers may be classified as having neuroendocrine differentiation, whereas tumors with neuroendocrine histologic features as well as staining pattern are considered SCLC or large cell neuroendocrine carcinoma.[3]

Staging

SCLC can be staged based on the TNM staging system that is used for NSCLC,[4] but more commonly it is divided into just 2 stages: limited-stage SCLC (LS-SCLC) and extensive-stage SCLC (ES-SCLC) based on the Veterans Administration Lung Group's classification introduced in 1957. In this staging system, LS-SCLC is defined as disease that is confined to the ipsilateral hemithorax and is safely encompassable within a radiation field (including potentially contralateral mediastinal and ipsilateral supraclavicular nodes), whereas ES-SCLC is considered disease that is not encompassable within a radiation field, typically beyond the ipsilateral hemithorax, including malignant pleural or pericardial effusion or distant metastases. Recently, there has been an impetus toward using TNM staging for SCLC, given the prognostic information it provides as well as the usefulness when surgical resection is being considered[5]; however, most practitioners continue to use the limited or extensive staging classification, because treatment options tend to be the same within just those 2 groupings.

To fully stage patients, those with LS-SCLC should have a positron emission tomography (PET) scan to rule out occult nodal or metastatic disease, which occurs in more than 30% of patients,[6] as well as brain imaging, given the propensity of SCLC to travel to the central nervous system. More than half of patients with SCLC are diagnosed with extensive-stage disease,[2] a point at which their disease is incurable. This pattern has not changed significantly over the past few decades, but may change in the future with the new lung cancer screening guidelines. Patients with ES-SCLC may benefit from brain imaging because the incidence of asymptomatic brain metastases is common at this stage; PET scans may not be necessary once patients are already determined to have distant disease.

Signs and Symptoms

Most SCLCs present with bulky hilar and mediastinal lymphadenopathy; extrinsic bronchial compression often occurs, but the presence of an endobronchial component is rare.[3] The symptoms at presentation can often be attributed to this pattern of disease and commonly include dyspnea, cough, chest pain, and pulmonary infections. Because patients commonly present with metastatic disease, presenting symptoms are often attributable to involved sites: bone pain, neurologic symptoms, and systemic symptoms such as anorexia, weight loss, and fatigue.

Paraneoplastic Syndromes

Paraneoplastic syndromes are associated with SCLC but their presence is relatively uncommon. Patients with syndrome of inappropriate antidiuretic hormone present with low serum sodium levels, which may or may not be symptomatic. Cushing syndrome can be caused by adrenocorticotropic hormone production. Several neurologic syndromes also associated with SCLC, including encephalomyelitis and sensory neuropathy from anti-Hu antibodies, and Lambert-Eaton syndrome (usually resulting in proximal muscle weakness) from antibodies against voltage-gated calcium channels and SOX proteins.[7] Anti-Ri, Ma and Ta antibodies, among others, have also been associated with paraneoplastic syndromes. Although treatment of the underlying malignant disease frequently improves the paraneoplastic endocrine syndromes, often the neurologic syndromes remain active even with successful treatment of the malignancy and may require immunosuppression.

LIMITED-STAGE DISEASE

Overview

Long-term cure is possible in patients with LS-SCLC, but only in a small subset of patients: in 1998, the population 5-year survival rate was 10%, up from 4.9% in 1973.[2] In a landmark randomized trial published in 1999,[8] a 5-year overall survival (OS) rate of 25% was achieved. Significant research has been undertaken to prolong survival and increase the cure rate, with modest success in recent years.

The Role of Surgery

Although surgical resection of early-stage disease is the standard treatment of NSCLC, surgery has a more controversial role in the management of SCLC (**Table 1**). Two randomized, prospective trials have examined the use of surgical resection of SCLC, one performed by the British Medical Research Council (BMRC)[9,10] and the other by the Lung Cancer Study Group (LCSG).[11]

The BMRC trial randomized 166 operable patients to resection versus thoracic radiation therapy (TRT). In the surgery arm, 48% of patients had a pneumonectomy with complete resection achieved, 34% underwent a thoracotomy without resection, and 18% did not undergo surgery (because of clinical decline before surgery or patient refusal). In the radiation group, 85% of patients underwent the prescribed course, whereas 11% were given a palliative course and 4% did not receive radiation because of disease deterioration or refusal. Only 20% and 12% of patients in the surgery and radiation arm, respectively, received cytotoxic chemotherapy. The results of this trial favored the radiation arm, with mean survival of 300 days compared with the surgery

Table 1
Summary of selected studies of surgery in LS-SCLC

Study	N	Trial Design	Treatment	Survival Outcome	Note
BMRC[9,10]	166	Prospective, randomized	Surgical resection vs TRT	Mean survival of 199 d vs 300 d (P = .04); 5-y survival of 1% vs 4% (NS)	Only 20% of patients in the surgery arm and 12% in the TRT arm received CT
LCSG[11]	328	Prospective, randomized	CT → surgical resection → TRT vs CT → TRT	Median survival 15.4 mo vs 18.6 mo (NS)	Excluded patients with peripheral nodules as the only site of disease
Rea et al,[13] 1998	104	Prospective, single-arm	Surgical resection	5-y survival (%): stage I 52.2; stage II 30; stage III 15.3	All patients received CT (induction for stage III or adjuvant for stage I or II) followed by TRT
IASLC[5]	339	Retrospective, multicenter database analysis	Complete R0 surgical resection	5-y survival (%): IA 56; IB 57; IIA 38; IIB 40; IIIA 12; IIIB 0	Most patients presumably received platinum-based CT
Brock et al,[12] 2005	82	Retrospective, single-institution analysis	Surgical resection	5-y survival of 42% (62% among those who also received platinum-based CT)	77% of patients received induction or adjuvant CT
Rostad et al,[14] 2004	29	Retrospective, Norway Cancer Registry analysis	Surgical resection	5-y survival of 44.9%	Only stage IA and IB tumors were included (<2% of patients with SCLC); 62% received adjuvant CT

Abbreviations: BMRC, British Medical Research Council; CT, chemotherapy; LCSG, Lung Cancer Study Group; NS, nonsignificant; TRT, thoracic radiotherapy.

group, which had a mean survival of 199 days (P = .04). Although not statistically significant, the 5-year and 10-year survival also favored radiation (4% survival at 5 and 10 years in the radiation group vs 1% at 5 years and 0% at 10 years in the surgery group). Even among the 34 patients who underwent a complete resection, long-term outcomes were poor: only 2 (6%) were alive at 2 years and none was alive at 5 years.

The LCSG trial looked at a different question: whether surgical resection was beneficial after induction chemotherapy compared with chemotherapy alone in LS-SCLC. Three hundred twenty-eight patients with limited-stage disease (excluding supraclavicular lymph nodes) were enrolled; those with peripheral nodules were excluded. All patients received cyclophosphamide, doxorubicin, and vincristine for 5 cycles, and those who achieved an objective response and were considered operable (a total of 146 patients) were randomized to surgery followed by radiation to the chest and brain versus radiation alone. Median survival was 15.4 months in the surgery group and 18.6 months in the nonsurgery group ($P = .78$). Two-year survival for the entire population was 20%. Because of small sample sizes in each of the TNM stages, it was not possible to obtain comparative survival analysis of the surgical versus the nonsurgical group by stage, but among those who underwent surgical resection, there appeared to be a longer median survival in those with T1-2, N0 disease compared with those with T3 disease or nodal involvement.

Although the BMRC and LCSG trials are the only source of prospective randomized data for surgery versus radiation in SCLC, there are several points that shed doubt on applying the results to all patients. The BMRC trial was performed in the 1960s, without advanced imaging such as computed tomography and PET, likely putting many patients with occult metastatic disease into the operable category. In addition, few patients received chemotherapy, whereas currently adjuvant chemotherapy is routinely administered in addition to resection. Thus, patients overall did poorly, with a mean survival of less than 1 year in both groups and few long-term survivors. However, given the statistically significant results of radiation, resulting in a higher mean survival, this trial set the practice standard of avoiding surgery in SCLC for many years. The LCSG study did include treatment with chemotherapy and radiation, but excluded patients with peripheral nodules, which is the patient population that might be expected to benefit from surgical resection.

Since the results of these trials were published, several other retrospective and single-arm prospective studies have emerged that suggest a benefit to surgical resection of early-stage SCLC (many of which have also included induction or adjuvant chemotherapy), with 5-year survival ranging from 27% to 68%.[5,12–14] The benefit to surgery in most of these trials appeared to be in patients without nodal disease (ie, stage I patients). This finding has swayed the practice standard toward resection for select patients (particularly those with small peripheral lesions and no nodal involvement who likely have a different disease biology than those with the more typical SCLC presentation of central, bulky disease), although definitive prospective data confirming the benefit to resection have not been published.

In practice, the question of whether to resect SCLC rarely presents itself. Patients more commonly present with unresectable or advanced disease, or occasionally present with a small nodule that is resected and incidentally is found to be of small cell histology. In the latter situation, adjuvant chemotherapy should be administered when feasible: in 1 retrospective study, adjuvant chemotherapy (plus prophylactic radiation to the brain and mediastinum in a subset of patients) after surgery resulted in a median survival of 20 months, longer than in historic controls of surgery alone.[15] In the rare circumstance that a patient presents with a biopsy-proven SCLC that is amenable to resection, a multidisciplinary approach is crucial, given the various treatment options and the paucity of definitive data.

The Role of Radiation and Chemotherapy

Generally, LS-SCLC is not considered a resectable disease. Therefore, standard of care for these patients is concurrent chemotherapy and TRT, which was shown to be beneficial compared with chemotherapy alone in 2 meta-analyses in the early 1990s (see **Box 1** for details of chemotherapy regimens). The meta-analysis by Pignon and colleagues[16] used data from 13 trials to compare patients with LS-SCLC who were randomized to receive chemotherapy alone or chemotherapy plus TRT. The investigators found a relative risk of death of 0.86 ($P = .001$) and a 5.4% increase in OS at 3 years with the inclusion of radiotherapy (14.3% vs 8.9%). The greatest benefit was found in patients younger than 55 years, with an 8.2% increase in 3-year survival rate with the

Box 1
Chemotherapy regimens for the treatment of LS-SCLC and ES-SCLC

LS-SCLC

- Cisplatin 80 mg/m^2 intravenously (IV) day 1 and etoposide (EP) 100 mg/m^2 IV days 1, 2, 3, every 28 days (with concurrent TRT)
- Cisplatin 60 mg/m^2 IV day 1 and EP 120 mg/m^2 IV days 1, 2, 3, every 28 days (with concurrent TRT)

ES-SCLC (Initial Therapy)

- Cisplatin 75 to 80 mg/m^2 IV day 1 and EP 100 mg/m^2 IV days 1, 2, 3, every 21 days
- Carboplatin area under the curve (AUC) 5 to 6 IV day 1 and EP 100 to 140 mg/m^2 IV days 1, 2, 3, every 21 days
- Cisplatin 60 mg/m^2 IV day 1 and irinotecan 60 mg/m^2 IV days 1, 8, 15, every 28 days
- Cisplatin 30 mg/m^2 IV days 1, 8 and irinotecan 65 mg/m^2 IV days 1, 8 every 21 days
- Carboplatin AUC 5 IV day 1 and irinotecan 50 mg/m^2 IV days 1, 8, 15, every 28 days

ES-SCLC (Second-Line Therapy)

- Sensitive disease (relapse at >6 months)
  - Retreatment with initial regimen
- Sensitive disease (relapse at 3–6 months)
  - Topotecan 2.3 mg/m^2/d by mouth days 1 to 5, every 21 days
  - Topotecan 1.5 mg/m^2/d IV days 1 to 5, every 21 days
  - Irinotecan 100 mg/m^2 IV, weekly
  - Cyclophosphamide 1000 mg/m^2 IV/doxorubicin 45 mg/m^2 IV/vincristine 2 mg IV, every 21 days
  - Paclitaxel 80 mg/m^2 IV, weekly for 6 weeks, every 8 weeks
  - Docetaxel 100 mg/m^2 IV, every 21 days
  - Gemcitabine 1000 mg/m^2 IV, days 1, 8, 15, every 28 days
  - Vinorelbine 30 mg/m^2 IV, weekly
- Refractory disease (relapse at <3 months or no response to initial regimen)
  - Clinical trial
  - Consider other second-line regimen listed above

Note: other dosing and schedules exist for several regimens.

addition of radiation. The other meta-analysis by Warde and Payne[17] included 11 trials that compared chemotherapy with and without radiotherapy in limited-stage disease. This study also showed a benefit with the addition of TRT, with an odds ratio of 1.53 and an overall improvement in 2-year survival of 5.4% (*P*<.05).

There are several limitations inherent in these meta-analyses. Both studies contained trials with significant variability in regards to the chemotherapeutics administered, sequence of chemotherapy and radiation (concurrent or sequential administration), timing of radiation (early or late during chemotherapy), radiation dose and fractionation, and whether prophylactic cranial irradiation (PCI) was given. In addition, neither study included trials that used the current standard-of-care chemotherapy regimen of cisplatin and EP, which is one of the few chemotherapy regimens that can be safely given at full doses along with radiotherapy. However, the studies clearly show that TRT in addition to chemotherapy is an important component in the treatment of fit patients with LS-SCLC, given the small but significant benefit in survival. These survival figures are based on historical radiation techniques and doses, and with modern approaches, the survival difference between chemotherapy alone and combined chemotherapy/radiation is expected to be much larger.

Optimization of TRT

SCLC is a radioresponsive disease, with substantial tumor regression with even low doses of radiation. Historically, this finding has led to the adoption of relatively low doses of radiation (ie, ~45–50 Gy) compared with NSCLC. However, tumor response rate is not a reliable predictor of radiocurability.[18] Locoregional failure rates after 45 to 50 Gy given in once-a-day fractions are high (ie, ~50% or more).[8,19,20] Retrospective data suggest that an increase in dose to 56 to 60 Gy once a day is associated with improved tumor control.[21,22] Although local control rates for doses of 66 to 70 Gy once a day are not yet established, these doses are commonly used in modern randomized phase 3 trials and are recommended by the National Comprehensive Cancer Network guidelines.[23]

The overall duration of a radiation therapy course is an important factor associated with local control in several cancer types, including lung cancer. It is widely accepted that accelerated fractionation (ie, shortening of overall treatment time typically achieved by giving 2 fractions a day) has the potential to reduce the negative impact of accelerated repopulation of tumor stem cells during the course of radiation treatment.[18] In a landmark Intergroup study of 419 patients with LS-SCLC, TRT once a day (45 Gy in 1.8-Gy daily fractions over 5 weeks) was compared with TRT twice a day (45 Gy given twice a day in 1.5-Gy fractions over 3 weeks).[8] All patients received 4 21-day cycles of cisplatin and EP. TRT twice a day resulted in more severe esophagitis (grade 3 or higher) but otherwise had equivalent toxicity to once-a-day treatment. Responses occurred in more than 90% of patients and was not statistically significant between arms. Median survival time and 5-year OS rates were 23 months and 26% for those receiving TRT twice a day, and 19 months and 16% for TRT once a day, respectively ($P = .04$).

Despite these findings, many centers continue to administer radiation once a day, given the concern for increased toxicity and the inconvenience to the patient. In addition, a similar trial did not show a benefit to hyperfractionation in LS-SCLC; however, these results are difficult to interpret because the radiation started with the fourth cycle of chemotherapy.[24] Two large phase 3 randomized trials are ongoing to determine the optimal dose fractionation. CALGB 30610/RTOG 0538, a US Intergroup study, phase III randomized study of three different thoracic radiotherapy regimens in patients with limited-stage small cell lung cancer receiving cisplatin and etoposide is a 3-arm trial comparing TRT 45 Gy twice a day with 70 Gy once a day and 61.2 Gy concomitant boost TRT (NCT00632853). After an interim analysis, the experimental arm with the highest toxicity will be discontinued. Another trial, cisplatin, etoposide, and two different schedules of radiation therapy in treating patients with limited stage small cell lung cancer (CONVERT) is comparing TRT 45 Gy twice a day with 66 Gy once a day (NCT00433563). While these studies are ongoing, reasonable regimens to consider include 45 Gy twice a day or 60 to 70 Gy at 1.8 to 2 Gy once a day.

TRT for LS-SCLC should be delivered concurrently and early with chemotherapy. There have been multiple phase 3 randomized trials and meta-analyses addressing this issue. For example, a trial by the Japan Clinical Oncology Group enrolled 231 patients with LS-SCLC (exclusive of stage I disease) and administered cisplatin and

EP on a 28-day cycle in the concurrent arm and a 21-day cycle in the sequential arm for a total of 4 cycles.[25] TRT (45 Gy twice a day regimen) was started on day 2 of cycle 1 of chemotherapy in the concurrent arm and after completion of cycle 4 of chemotherapy in the sequential arm. Median survival was significantly greater in the concurrent arm (27.2 months vs 19.7 months, adjusted $P = .02$). Five-year survival was also increased from 18.3% to 23.7%. This trial set the standard for concurrent chemotherapy and radiotherapy in treatment of LS-SCLC. Meta-analyses have confirmed the importance of delivering TRT early,[26,27] although whether the start of TRT on day 1 of chemotherapy or within the first 2 chemotherapy cycles is clinically important remains to be determined. However, in individual patients, for example those with poor performance status or large volume disease, delaying TRT until the second half of chemotherapy or until after chemotherapy is completed may be reasonable to reduce toxicity.

PCI in LS-SCLC

The development of brain metastases in LS-SCLC is a source of considerable morbidity and mortality. In the 1970s and 1980s, several trials explored whether PCI could decrease the rate of brain metastases and prolong survival in patients with limited-stage disease after definitive treatment with chemotherapy and TRT. Given the high rate of systemic recurrence, it was believed that any improvement in survival would be in those patients who attained a complete remission, because they were less likely to have systemic relapse. After several trials showed a decrease in the development of brain metastases but no clear improvement in survival, a meta-analysis was performed using the data from 7 clinical trials. This study included trials in which patients who were in complete remission after induction therapy (chemotherapy with or without radiotherapy) were randomized to PCI or no PCI. Total radiation doses varied from 8 Gy to 40 Gy. Among the 987 patients included in the analysis, there was a significant survival benefit in the group who received PCI ($P = .01$), with an absolute increase in survival of 5.4% at 3 years (20.7% in the PCI group and 15.3% in the control group). The incidence of brain metastases was also significantly decreased with PCI, from 58.6% in the control group to 33.3% in the PCI group ($P<.001$). From the results of this study, standard practice now includes PCI for patients with a complete (or good partial) response to induction therapy, given the large decrease in the incidence of brain metastases as well as the small but significant benefit in survival.

A more recent pooled analysis looked at the effect of PCI in patients with at least stable disease after induction therapy to capture a wider population of patients who might benefit from brain radiation. The study found that among the 421 patients with LS-SCLC, median OS was prolonged from 14 to 17 months with PCI ($P = .0045$), with a similar effect among those who achieved complete or partial response or had stable disease.

Increasing the dose of PCI beyond 25 Gy results in no difference in the incidence of brain metastases but is associated with a worse OS[28,29]; therefore the standard PCI dose is 25 Gy at 2.5 Gy once a day. In addition, 30 Gy at 2 Gy once a day, which has not been directly compared against the 25-Gy dose in a prospective clinical trial, may be an acceptable alternative. Controversy remains regarding the long-term neurocognitive effects of PCI, with some studies showing a decline and others showing no change after PCI. Additional data are required to further clarify this issue. **Box 2** summarizes PCI in SCLC.

Smoking Cessation

Because SCLC occurs almost exclusively in association with cigarette smoking, many patients are active smokers at diagnosis. Smoking cessation in limited-stage disease

Box 2
Guidelines on the use of PCI in SCLC

- PCI should be considered in patients who have a complete or partial response (and possibly stable disease as well) to induction therapy.
- PCI is not recommended for patients with poor performance status or impaired mental function.
- The recommended dose for PCI is 25 Gy at 2.5 Gy once a day.
- PCI should not be administered concurrently with chemotherapy because of neurotoxicity.
- PCI should be initiated within 3 to 6 weeks after chemotherapy.
- We recommend brain imaging before initiation of PCI to confirm prophylactic nature of the treatment.

is associated with improved survival. One retrospective study showed that those who quit smoking had a 4.4-month improvement in median survival and a 5% increase in 5-year OS.[30] This finding is of comparable magnitude with other interventions in the treatment of LS-SCLC, including the addition of TRT and PCI. Therefore, clinicians should always encourage smoking cessation to their patients who continue to smoke after a diagnosis of SCLC, using pharmacotherapy and support groups as necessary.

EXTENSIVE-STAGE DISEASE

Overview

Most patients with SCLC have extensive-stage disease at diagnosis because of the aggressive nature of the malignancy and propensity for early metastases. Responses in ES-SCLC are frequent, with 50% to 60% of patients responding to chemotherapy; however, the disease is uniformly fatal, with dismal survival for most patients. Although there has been much research investigating new therapeutics, the 2-year survival for ES-SCLC has improved only from 1.5% in 1973 to 4.6% in 2000.[2] There is great need for improved treatments for this disease.

Initial Treatment of ES-SCLC

Chemotherapy is the mainstay of treatment of extensive-stage SCLC. Cisplatin and EP became the standard-of-care regimen for previously untreated patients in the 1990s after several randomized trials and meta-analyses[31–33] showed equivalent or even superior outcomes compared with other regimens, with a response rate of 60% to 70%, median time to progression of around 4 months, and median OS of approximately 9 months. Specifically, the addition of cisplatin to a regimen increases the probability of survival at 6 months by 2.5% and at 1 year by 4.4%.[32] EP does not seem to be more toxic overall than other active regimens (including cyclophosphamide, doxorubicin, and vincristine), with similar rates of toxic deaths and less neutropenia with the use of EP.[33]

The Japanese Clinical Oncology Group compared EP with cisplatin plus irinotecan (IP) in a phase 3 trial of 154 patients, given the promising results of irinotecan in several phase 2 trials. The trial was closed early because of a difference in OS at an interim analysis; the IP group had a median OS of 12.8 months compared with 9.4 months in the EP group ($P = .002$). In addition, 19.5% of patients who received IP were alive at 2 years versus 5.2% of those who received EP. Response rate was also higher with IP compared with EP (84.4% vs 67.5%, $P = .02$). There was comparable toxicity overall, with the exception of more cytopenias with EP and more diarrhea with IP.

Although there was initially excitement for this combination, the benefit of IP over EP was not confirmed in 2 North American studies.[34,35] One of these studies treated 651 patients with the same dosing as the Japanese study and found no statistically significant difference in response rate, progression-free survival (PFS), or OS,[35] whereas the other used a modified regimen of IP and also found no difference in outcomes compared with EP.[34] Another similar trial from Germany[36] also showed no benefit of a platinum-based regimen containing irinotecan compared with EP (carboplatin was used instead of cisplatin in this study).

It is unclear why the Japanese trial had such dramatically different results from the other similar trials. It may be that the Japanese trial had a small sample size and closed early after an interim analysis, leading to false-positive results. Alternatively, pharmacogenomic differences between the 2 patient populations may account for the varying outcomes. The standard first-line chemotherapy regimen in North America is still EP; however, IP is also a reasonable treatment option, particularly in an Asian population.

The use of cisplatin versus carboplatin is often the subject of debate in the cancer literature. Cisplatin-based regimens were compared with carboplatin-based regimens in a recent meta-analysis that included 4 clinical trials of patients with SCLC.[37] Sixty-eight percent of the 663 patients studied had extensive-stage disease and all were previously untreated. As expected, cisplatin-treated patients had more nausea/vomiting, neurotoxicity, and nephrotoxicity, whereas carpolatin-treated patients had more myelosuppression. Except for this difference in toxicity profile, outcomes were similar for cisplatin and carboplatin, including response rate, PFS, and OS. Subgroup analysis showed a PFS benefit for cisplatin in patients younger than 70 years compared with those older (treatment/age interaction P = .005). Because most of the patients included in this meta-analysis had ES-SCLC and those who had LS-SCLC had bulky or poor prognostic disease, the results can be used to justify either platinum compound for treatment of extensive disease, although it is more controversial whether to extrapolate the data to all patients with limited disease. **Box 1** contains addition detail on chemotherapy regimens for ES-SCLC.

The Role of Radiation Therapy in ES-SCLC

The role of TRT in ES-SCLC is not well defined. In 1 trial from Europe,[38] patients with a complete response outside the thorax and at least partial response in the chest after induction chemotherapy derived benefit from the addition to TRT to additional chemotherapy. Median survival times for added TRT versus chemotherapy alone were 17 months versus 11 months, respectively (P = .041). RTOG 0937 is studying the role of radiation therapy to thorax and metastatic sites in addition to PCI in patients with ES-SCLC (NCT01055197).

Given the physical and psychological detriments and typically short survival time in patients after development of brain metastases even with treatment, investigators have explored whether PCI may be of use in ES-SCLC to prevent the development of central nervous system disease and prolong life. A large randomized phase 3 trial included patients with extensive-stage disease who had any response after 4 to 6 cycles of systemic chemotherapy.[39] Response was determined by the local investigator and did not need to meet specific criteria. The radiation dose was 25 to 39 Gy initiated 4 to 6 weeks after chemotherapy. The incidence of brain metastases was reduced from 41.3% to 16.8% (hazard ratio [HR] 0.27, P<.001). Median survival was increased from 5.4 months in the control group to 6.7 months in the PCI group (HR 0.68, P = .02) and 1-year survival increased from 13.3% to 27.1%. A significant limitation of this trial is that brain scans were not mandated before PCI. Therefore, it is possible that there existed several patients with asymptomatic brain disease for whom PCI was therapeutic rather than prophylactic. Therefore, the magnitude of the benefit of PCI in a setting in which all patients undergo brain imaging before PCI is not defined. Despite this finding, the trial lends support to considering PCI in patients with ES-SCLC who initially respond well to first-line chemotherapy.

The pooled analysis of PCI in patients with at least stable disease that was discussed earlier also included patients with ES-SCLC, who were randomized to PCI or no PCI.[29] Those who received PCI had a median survival of 9.6 months compared with 7.9 months in the no-PCI group ($P = .0282$). This effect was similar across all response categories, implying that there is no difference in the effect of PCI for patients with stable disease compared with those who achieve a response. Therefore, PCI may be a treatment option not only for patients who achieve a response to induction chemotherapy but also for those who have stable disease. Guidelines for PCI are summarized in **Box 2**.

Treatment of Relapsed/Refractory Disease

Even although most patients with ES-SCLC have an excellent response to first-line chemotherapy, all patients eventually relapse, at which time median survival is typically only 4 to 5 months. Sensitive relapsed disease is defined as relapse occurring beyond 3 months after completing initial treatment, whereas refractory disease is defined as relapse within 3 months of initial treatment. Treatment options should be guided by the patient's response to initial therapy.

Occasionally, patients maintain a substantial disease-free period after initial therapy. These patients may benefit from retreatment with the same induction regimen. This approach is supported by 2 trials, one of which retreated patients with cyclophosphamide, doxorubicin, and EP for a response rate of 79% in those who had a first response duration of at least 34 weeks,[40] and the other which showed a response rate of 50% in a few patients who were retreated with the same initial regimen after a median off-therapy time of 30 weeks.[41]

However, for most patients, the duration of response is not long enough to justify retreatment with the same first-line regimen. In this case, second-line agents or clinical trials should be considered. In general, patients with sensitive relapsed disease can have response rates to second-line therapy for up to 20%. For refractory patients, response rates are lower and prognosis is not so good. In all cases, given the relative ineffectiveness of second-line therapies, consideration should be given to clinical trials.

Second-Line Chemotherapy Options

Topotecan is the only agent that is approved by the US Food and Drug Administration for use in relapsed SCLC. In a phase 2 trial, the IV formulation was found to have an overall response rate of 21.7% (37.8% in patients sensitive to and 6.4% in patients refractory or resistant to first-line chemotherapy).[42] Overall median time to progression was 2.8 months and OS was 5.4 months. Myelosuppression was common, with 75% of patients developing grade 3 or 4 neutropenia. A phase 3 trial comparing oral topotecan with best supportive care (BSC) alone found that topotecan significantly prolonged survival, with median survival of 3.5 months in the BSC group and 6.5 months in the topotecan group ($P = .01$).[43] A survival benefit was seen even in patients with a treatment-free interval of less than 60 days and in those with a performance status of 2. Response rate was 7%; however, disease control rate (including those who responded or had confirmed stable disease) was 44%. Although there was some toxicity associated with treatment (in particular myelosuppression), quality-of-life measures favor topotecan over BSC. IV administration was compared with oral administration in another phase 3 trial; outcomes between the 2 groups were comparable, including response rate, time to progression, OS, and toxicity profile.[44] Based on these results, both IV and oral topotecan can be considered for second-line therapy for SCLC.

A related agent, irinotecan, also has activity in relapsed SCLC, with a response rate of 47% and a median survival of about 6 months, as observed in a small single-arm trial.[45] Irinotecan has reasonably good tolerability, with low myelosuppression and controllable diarrhea. Topotecan has not been directly compared with irinotecan; however, irinotecan is another reasonable second-line treatment option in SCLC. Other agents that have some activity in relapsed SCLC but have not been extensively studied include cyclophosphamide/doxorubicin/vincristine, paclitaxel, docetaxel, gemcitabine, and vinorelbine.[46–50] See **Box 1** for details.

Supportive Care

Patients with SCLC are frequently symptomatic with dyspnea, cough, chest pain, bone pain, neurologic compromise, fatigue, anorexia, and weight loss. Because chemotherapy has a high response rate, treatment of the underlying malignancy can palliate many of these symptoms at least temporarily. In addition, focused palliative radiotherapy or orthopedic intervention may be beneficial for very symptomatic sites of disease, particularly those that are chemoresistant. Given the recent data on the benefit of early palliative care in patients with NSCLC in terms of quality of life, mood, and survival,[51] an aggressive, coordinated, early approach to symptom control and psychological distress may also benefit patients with SCLC.

Future Directions

There has yet to be an effective targeted agent in SCLC. Specific agents that have been studied include antiapoptotic pathway agents such as Bcl-2 inhibitors and BH3 mimetics such as navitoclax and obatoclax, antiangiogenic agents including bevacizumab, sorafenib, and sunitib, and mammalian target of rapamycin inhibitors such as everolimus. No targeted agent has shown a benefit in terms of OS, although several trials with these agents are ongoing. Among newer cytotoxic therapies, there was much initial interest in amrubicin, a synthetic 9-amino anthracycline that inhibits topoisomerase II. However a recently reported phase 3 study showed no significant improvement in OS when compared with topotecan, despite better relative risk and PFS with amrubicin.[52] Continued research and clinical trial participation are crucial to make further headway in SCLC treatment.

SUMMARY

SCLC is an aggressive malignancy that most commonly presents as disseminated disease, at which time cure is not possible. Even when disease is discovered at an early stage, treatment is hindered by frequent recurrence and limited survival. Despite decades of research, only marginal progress has been made in the treatment of this disease. Additional insight into the molecular basis of SCLC is critical to be able to identify potential therapeutic targets that offer the promise of improved outcomes with less toxicity.

REFERENCES

1. Siegel R, Naishadham D, Jemal A. Cancer statistics, 2012. CA Cancer J Clin 2012;62:10–29.

2. Govindan R, Page N, Morgensztern D, et al. Changing epidemiology of small-cell lung cancer in the United States over the last 30 years: analysis of the surveillance, epidemiologic, and end results database. J Clin Oncol 2006;24: 4539–44.
3. Zakowski MF. Pathology of small cell carcinoma of the lung. Semin Oncol 2003; 30:3–8.
4. Edge SB, Byrd DR, Compton CC, et al. AJCC cancer staging manual. 7th edition. New York: Springer; 2010.
5. Vallieres E, Shepherd FA, Crowley J, et al. The IASLC Lung Cancer Staging Project: proposals regarding the relevance of TNM in the pathologic staging of small cell lung cancer in the forthcoming (seventh) edition of the TNM classification for lung cancer. J Thorac Oncol 2009;4:1049–59.
6. Bradley JD, Dehdashti F, Mintun MA, et al. Positron emission tomography in limited-stage small-cell lung cancer: a prospective study. J Clin Oncol 2004;22: 3248–54.
7. Kazarian M, Laird-Offringa IA. Small-cell lung cancer-associated autoantibodies: potential applications to cancer diagnosis, early detection, and therapy. Mol Cancer 2011;10:33.
8. Turrisi AT, Kim K, Blum R, et al. Twice-daily compared with once-daily thoracic radiotherapy in limited small-cell lung cancer treated concurrently with cisplatin and etoposide. N Engl J Med 1999;340:265–71.
9. Fox W, Scadding JG. Medical Research Council comparative trial of surgery and radiotherapy for primary treatment of small-celled or oat-celled carcinoma of bronchus: ten-year follow-up. Lancet 1973;302:63–5.
10. Miller AB, Fox W, Tall R. Five-year follow-up of the Medical Research Council comparative trial of surgery and radiotherapy for the primary treatment of small-celled or oat-celled carcinoma of the bronchus: a report to the Medical Research Council Working Party on the evaluation of different methods of therapy in carcinoma of the bronchus. Lancet 1969;294:501–5.
11. Lad T, Piantadosi S, Thomas P, et al. A prospective randomized trial to determine the benefit of surgical resection of residual disease following response of small cell lung cancer to combination chemotherapy. Chest 1994;106:320S–3S.
12. Brock MV, Hooker CM, Syphard JE, et al. Surgical resection of limited disease small cell lung cancer in the new era of platinum chemotherapy: its time has come. J Thorac Cardiovasc Surg 2005;129:64–72.
13. Rea F, Callegaro D, Favaretto A, et al. Long term results of surgery and chemotherapy in small cell lung cancer. Eur J Cardiothorac Surg 1998;14:398–402.
14. Rostad H, Naalsund A, Jacobsen R, et al. Small cell lung cancer in Norway. Should more patients have been offered surgical therapy? Eur J Cardiothorac Surg 2004;26:782–6.
15. Shepherd FA, Evans WK, Feld R, et al. Adjuvant chemotherapy following surgical resection for small-cell carcinoma of the lung. J Clin Oncol 1988;6:832–8.
16. Pignon JP, Arriagada R, Ihde DC, et al. A meta-analysis of thoracic radiotherapy for small-cell lung cancer. N Engl J Med 1992;327:1618–24.
17. Warde P, Payne D. Does thoracic irradiation improve survival and local control in limited-stage small-cell carcinoma of the lung? A meta-analysis. J Clin Oncol 1992;10:890–5.
18. Willers H, Held KD. Introduction to clinical radiation biology. Hematol Oncol Clin North Am 2006;20:1–24.
19. Langer CJ, Swann S, Werner-Wasik M, et al. Phase I study of irinotecan (Ir) and cisplatin (DDP) in combination with thoracic radiotherapy (RT), either twice daily

(45 Gy) or once daily (70 Gy), in patients with limited (Ltd) small cell lung carcinoma (SCLC): early analysis of RTOG 0241. J Clin Oncol 2006;24:7058.
20. Movsas B, Moughan J, Komaki R, et al. Radiotherapy patterns of care study in lung carcinoma. J Clin Oncol 2003;21:4553–9.
21. Miller KL, Marks LB, Sibley GS, et al. Routine use of approximately 60 Gy once-daily thoracic irradiation for patients with limited-stage small-cell lung cancer. Int J Radiat Oncol Biol Phys 2003;56:355–9.
22. Roof KS, Fidias P, Lynch TJ, et al. Radiation dose escalation in limited-stage small-cell lung cancer. Int J Radiat Oncol Biol Phys 2003;57:701–8.
23. National Comprehensive Cancer Network: Small Cell Lung Cancer (version 2). 2012. Available at: http://www.nccn.org/professionals/physician_gls/f_guidelines.asp - site.
24. Bonner JA, Sloan JA, Shanahan TG, et al. Phase III comparison of twice-daily split-course irradiation versus once-daily irradiation for patients with limited stage small-cell lung carcinoma. J Clin Oncol 1999;17:2681–91.
25. Takada M, Fukuoka M, Kawahara M, et al. Phase III study of concurrent versus sequential thoracic radiotherapy in combination with cisplatin and etoposide for limited-stage small-cell lung cancer: results of the Japan Clinical Oncology Group Study 9104. J Clin Oncol 2002;20:3054–60.
26. De Ruysscher D, Pijls-Johannesma M, Bentzen SM, et al. Time between the first day of chemotherapy and the last day of chest radiation is the most important predictor of survival in limited-disease small-cell lung cancer. J Clin Oncol 2006;24:1057–63.
27. Fried DB, Morris DE, Poole C, et al. Systematic review evaluating the timing of thoracic radiation therapy in combined modality therapy for limited-stage small-cell lung cancer. J Clin Oncol 2004;22:4837–45.
28. Le Pechoux C, Dunant A, Senan S, et al. Standard-dose versus higher-dose prophylactic cranial irradiation (PCI) in patients with limited-stage small-cell lung cancer in complete remission after chemotherapy and thoracic radiotherapy (PCI 99-01, EORTC 22003-08004, RTOG 0212, and IFCT 99-01): a randomised clinical trial. Lancet Oncol 2009;10:467–74.
29. Schild SE, Foster NR, Meyers JP, et al. Prophylactic cranial irradiation in small-cell lung cancer: findings from a North Central Cancer Treatment Group Pooled Analysis. Ann Oncol 2012;23:2919–24.
30. Videtic GM, Stitt LW, Dar AR, et al. Continued cigarette smoking by patients receiving concurrent chemoradiotherapy for limited-stage small-cell lung cancer is associated with decreased survival. J Clin Oncol 2003;21:1544–9.
31. Mascaux C, Paesmans M, Berghmans T, et al. A systematic review of the role of etoposide and cisplatin in the chemotherapy of small cell lung cancer with methodology assessment and meta-analysis. Lung Cancer 2000;30:23–36.
32. Pujol JL, Carestia L, Daurès JP. Is there a case for cisplatin in the treatment of small-cell lung cancer? A meta-analysis of randomized trials of a cisplatin-containing regimen versus a regimen without this alkylating agent. Br J Cancer 2000;83:8.
33. Roth BJ, Johnson DH, Einhorn LH, et al. Randomized study of cyclophosphamide, doxorubicin, and vincristine versus etoposide and cisplatin versus alternation of these two regimens in extensive small-cell lung cancer: a phase III trial of the Southeastern Cancer Study Group. J Clin Oncol 1992;10:282–91.
34. Hanna N, Bunn PA Jr, Langer C, et al. Randomized phase III trial comparing irinotecan/cisplatin with etoposide/cisplatin in patients with previously untreated extensive-stage disease small-cell lung cancer. J Clin Oncol 2006;24:2038–43.

35. Lara PN, Natale R, Crowley J, et al. Phase III Trial of irinotecan/cisplatin compared with etoposide/cisplatin in extensive-stage small-cell lung cancer: clinical and pharmacogenomic results from SWOG S0124. J Clin Oncol 2009;27:2530–5.
36. Schmittel A, Sebastian M, Fischer von Weikersthal L, et al. A German multicenter, randomized phase III trial comparing irinotecan-carboplatin with etoposide-carboplatin as first-line therapy for extensive-disease small-cell lung cancer. Ann Oncol 2011;22:1798–804.
37. Rossi A, Di Maio M, Chiodini P, et al. Carboplatin- or cisplatin-based chemotherapy in first-line treatment of small-cell lung cancer: the COCIS meta-analysis of individual patient data. J Clin Oncol 2012;30:1692–8.
38. Jeremic B, Shibamoto Y, Nikolic N, et al. Role of radiation therapy in the combined-modality treatment of patients with extensive disease small-cell lung cancer: a randomized study. J Clin Oncol 1999;17:2092–9.
39. Slotman B, Faivre-Finn C, Kramer G, et al. Prophylactic cranial irradiation in extensive small-cell lung cancer. N Engl J Med 2007;357:664–72.
40. Postmus PE, Berendsen HH, van Zandwijk N, et al. Retreatment with the induction regimen in small cell lung cancer relapsing after an initial response to short term chemotherapy. Eur J Cancer 1987;23:1409–11.
41. Giaccone G, Ferrati P, Donadio M, et al. Reinduction chemotherapy in small cell lung cancer. Eur J Cancer 1987;23:1697–9.
42. Ardizzoni A, Hansen H, Dombernowsky P, et al. Topotecan, a new active drug in the second-line treatment of small-cell lung cancer: a phase II study in patients with refractory and sensitive disease. J Clin Oncol 1997;15:2090–6.
43. O'Brien ME, Ciuleanu TE, Tsekov H, et al. Phase III trial comparing supportive care alone with supportive care with oral topotecan in patients with relapsed small-cell lung cancer. J Clin Oncol 2006;24:5441–7.
44. Eckardt JR, von Pawel J, Pujol JL, et al. Phase III study of oral compared with intravenous topotecan as second-line therapy in small-cell lung cancer. J Clin Oncol 2007;25:2086–92.
45. Masuda N, Fukuoka M, Kusunoki Y, et al. CPT-11: a new derivative of camptothecin for the treatment of refractory or relapsed small-cell lung cancer. J Clin Oncol 1992;10:1225–9.
46. Jassem J, Karnicka-Młodkowska H, van Pottelsberghe C, et al. Phase II study of vinorelbine (Navelbine) in previously treated small cell lung cancer patients. Eur J Cancer 1993;29:1720–2.
47. Masters GA, Declerck L, Blanke C, et al. Phase II trial of gemcitabine in refractory or relapsed small-cell lung cancer: Eastern Cooperative Oncology Group Trial 1597. J Clin Oncol 2003;21:1550–5.
48. Smyth JF, Smith IE, Sessa C, et al. Activity of docetaxel (Taxotere) in small cell lung cancer. Eur J Cancer 1994;30A:1058–60.
49. von Pawel J, Schiller JH, Shepherd FA, et al. Topotecan versus cyclophosphamide, doxorubicin, and vincristine for the treatment of recurrent small-cell lung cancer. J Clin Oncol 1999;17:658.
50. Yamamoto N, Tsurutani J, Yoshimura N, et al. Phase II study of weekly paclitaxel for relapsed and refractory small cell lung cancer. Anticancer Res 2006;26:777–81.
51. Jotte R, Von Pawel J, Spigel DR, et al. Randomized phase III trial of amrubicin versus topotecan as second-line treatment for small cell lung cancer. J Clin Oncol 2011;29 [abstract no. 7000].
52. Temel JS, Greer JA, Muzikansky A, et al. Early palliative care for patients with metastatic non-small-cell lung cancer. N Engl J Med 2010;363:733–42.

Multimodality Treatment of Pleural Mesothelioma

David D. Shersher, MD[a,b], Michael J. Liptay, MD[a,c,*]

KEYWORDS

• Mesothelioma • Biomarkers • Cytoreduction • Pleurectomy
• Extrapleural pneumonectomy

KEY POINTS

- Mesothelioma is mainly linked to asbestos exposure, with a latency period of 20 to 40 years.
- The gold standard for diagnosis is thoracoscopy or thoracotomy. Chest radiograph, computed tomography, positron emission tomography, and serum mesothelin–related protein are useful clinical adjuncts.
- Surgical treatment is preferred for operable candidates—extrapleural pneumonectomy is better for locoregional control compared with pleurectomy/decortication, but both have similar overall rates of survival.
- Acceptable chemotherapy regimens include cisplatin or carboplatin with pemetrexed, with optimal survival seen in patients combining surgery with adjuvant chemotherapy.
- Currently there is no survival advantage with radiation therapy. Benefits include locoregional control of tumor burden and palliation of chest wall pain. Newer modalities are currently in trial.

INTRODUCTION

Malignant mesothelioma is a rare cancer of serosal surfaces with an annual incidence of 3300 new cases in the United States per year.[1] It can affect the pleura, peritoneum, tunica vaginalis, and pericardium and is primarily linked to asbestos exposure. Ionized radiation, exposure to simian virus -40, and an autosomal-dominant gene in Turkish families have also been linked with development of mesothelioma.[2]

Funding Sources: Dr Liptay: Consultant, Covidien; Consultant, Neomend; Dr Shersher: None.
Conflict of Interest: None.

[a] Thoracic Oncology Program, Rush University Medical Center, Rush Professional Office Building, 1725 West Harrison Street, Suite 774, Chicago, IL 60612, USA; [b] Department of General Surgery, Rush University Medical Center, Rush Professional Office Building, 1725 West Harrison Street, Suite 774, Chicago, IL 60612, USA; [c] Division of Thoracic Surgery, Rush University Medical Center, Rush Professional Office Building, 1725 West Harrison Street, Suite 774, Chicago, IL 60612, USA
* Corresponding author. Division of Thoracic Surgery, Rush University Medical Center, Rush Professional Office Building, 1725 West Harrison Street, Suite 774, Chicago, IL 60612.
E-mail address: michael_liptay@rush.edu

Surg Oncol Clin N Am 22 (2013) 345–355
http://dx.doi.org/10.1016/j.soc.2012.12.004
surgonc.theclinics.com
1055-3207/13/$ – see front matter

Epidemiology

The incidence of disease in the United States reached its peak in 2000, consistent with a cancer latency period of 20 to 40 years from time of peak environmental asbestos exposure in the 1930s to 1970s.[2] Epidemiologic studies reveal 3 cohorts of exposed patients. *Immediate exposure* to blue asbestos was demonstrably linked to development of mesothelioma during a large mining disaster in Wittenoom, Australia. *Delayed exposure* was linked to inhalation during the chain of manufacturing of asbestos-containing supplies. In 20% to 30% of cases, there is *no known exposure*, although some of these cases are genetically clustered as in some Turkish families.[1] Interestingly, the remainder of the world did not follow America's fierce reform of workplace asbestos exposure practices in the 1970s, and therefore the incidence of mesothelioma is expected to continue to rise in many developing and undeveloped countries.[1]

Pathogenesis

Pathogenesis of malignant pleural mesothelioma (MPM) is hypothesized to occur in many ways. Blue asbestos fibers can directly irritate pleural surfaces, increasing the risk of malignancy. These fibers can also pierce mitotic spindles of cells and directly disrupt mitosis. Other explanations include DNA damage by production of iron-related reactive oxygen species as well as upregulation of MAP kinases and factors related to proto-oncogenesis. Additionally, simian virus-40 is a potent oncogenic cofactor and contributes greatly to pathogenesis of mesothelioma.[1]

Histology and Staging

There are 3 primary histologic types of malignant mesothelioma: epithelial, sarcomatoid, and biphasic. Sixty percent to 70% of patients have epithelial cancers, demonstrating a best median overall survival of 17 months. These tumors are often confused histologically with adenocarcinoma, which may complicate and delay diagnosis. Twenty percent to 30% of patients have a biphasic histology that carries an intermediate prognosis of 6 to 17 months. Sarcomatoid tumors are rare (~10% of patients) but aggressive with a poor median overall survival of less than 6 months.[2] The 7th edition of the American Joint Committee on Cancer TNM staging does not take into consideration these different histologic patterns but is still used to stage mesothelioma grossly and help partition patients into treatment algorithms and clinical trials (**Table 1**). Other stratification algorithms are also commonly used. The Cancer and Leukemia Group assigns poor performance status, high levels of lactate dehydrogenase, anemia, chest pain, leukocytosis, and age greater than 75 as negative prognostic indicators. The European Organization for Research and Treatment of Cancer prognosticates and stratifies patients into clinical trials using poor performance status, leukocytosis, unclear diagnosis, male gender, and sarcomatoid histology as poor prognostic indicators.[2] Modification has been championed by the International Mesothelioma Interest Group to account for stage-related prognostic variability, combining TNM with important histologic and clinical prognostic factors to partition cohorts of patients better for treatment.

Diagnosis

Most patients initially present for a workup for pleuritic chest pain, dyspnea, constitutional symptoms of fatigue and weight loss, and a finding of pleural fluid on chest radiograph.[2] Additional useful imaging modalities include computed tomography for the evaluation of the intrapleural space, lung parenchyma, and mediastinum, magnetic resonance imaging for involvement of chest wall and soft

Table 1
7th edition TNM staging of mesothelioma

Tumor (T)	
T1	Limited to ipsilateral parietal pleura
a	No involvement of visceral pleura
b	Involvement of visceral pleura
T2	Involvement of ipsilateral parietal, mediastinal, diaphragmatic, and visceral pleura + involvement of at least the diaphragmatic muscle or the pulmonary parenchyma
T3	Advanced but potentially resectable tumor as in T2, with involvement of at least one of the following: endothoracic fascia, mediastinal fat, a solitary focus of soft tissue in chest, or nontransmural extension into pericardium
T4	Unresectable tumor with involvement of chest wall or extension into peritoneum, contralateral pleura, mediastinal organ, or spine
Node (N)	
N1	Ipsilateral bronchopulmonary or hilar nodes
N2	Ipsilateral subcarinal, mediastinal, internal mammary, or paradiaphragmatic nodes
N3	Contralateral nodal involvement or ipsilateral and contralateral supraclavicular nodes
Metastasis (M)	
M0	No distant metastasis
M1	Distant metastasis

Stage	**T**	**N**	**M**
I	T1	N0	M0
a	T1a	N0	M0
b	T1b	N0	M0
II	T1-2	N0	M0
III	T1-2	N1-2	M0
	T3	N0-2	M0
IV	T4	Any N	M0
	Any T	N3	M0
	Any T	Any N	M1

Data from Pleural mesothelioma. In: Edge SB, Byrd DR, Compton CC, et al, editors. AJCC Cancer Staging Manual. 7th edition. New York: Springer; 2010. p. 271–7.

tissue, and positron emission tomography to evaluate for hypermetabolic activity suspicious of metastatic disease. Findings of a mass, interlobular thickening, and an associated pleural effusion (60% of effusions are on the right) on imaging are highly suspicious for malignancy. Conversely, findings of plaques (fibrous sheets) alone may reflect exposure to asbestos (benign asbestosis) but are not predictive of mesothelioma.

Fine-needle aspirate (FNA) is inconclusive in 20% of patients but can provide useful cytologic data. In cases of epithelial histology, FNA may incorrectly suggest adenocarcinoma; high suspicion should lead the clinician to evaluate further by immunohistochemistry staining for epithelial membrane antigen, calretinin, Wilms tumor 1 antigen, cytokeratin 5/6, or mesothelin, which are more commonly found in mesothelioma.[1] When FNA biopsy is inconclusive, most clinicians proceed directly to thoracoscopic biopsy or, in rare cases, thoracotomy.

Fig. 1 illustrates an algorithm for the diagnosis of MPM.

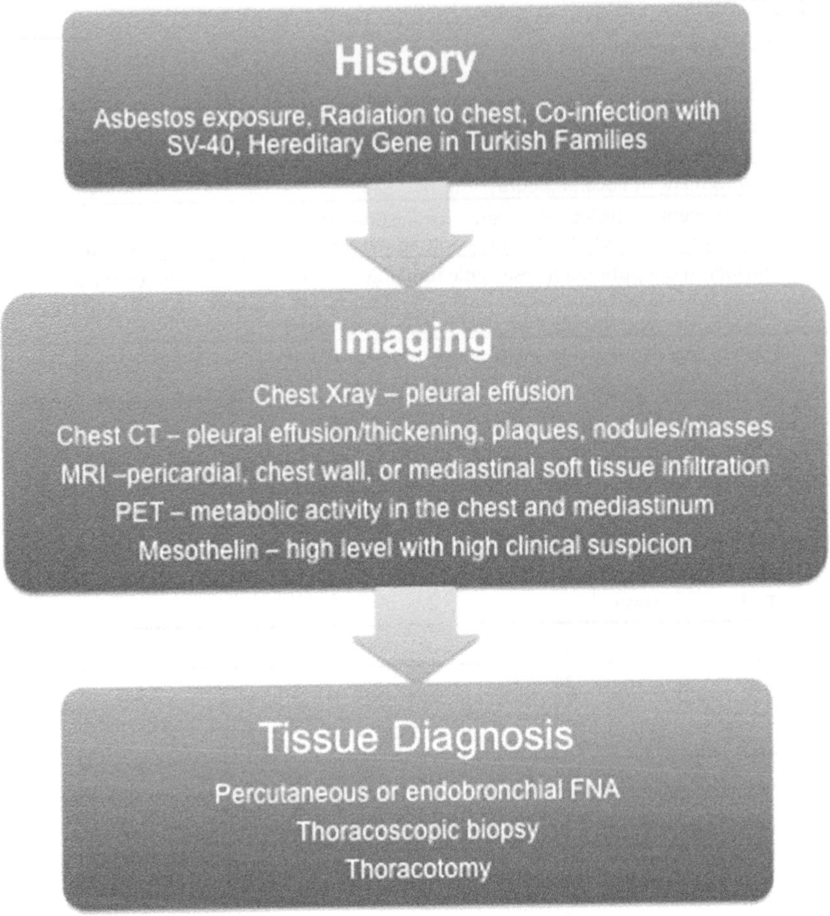

Fig. 1. An algorithm for diagnosis of malignant pleural mesothelioma. CT, computed tomography; MRI, magnetic resonance imaging; PET, positron emission tomography; SV-40, simian virus-40.

MULTIMODALITY THERAPY

Surgery

Surgery remains the gold standard for diagnosis and treatment of mesothelioma but is only performed in 22% of American patients.[2] Thoracoscopic diagnostic biopsy is less invasive and preferred to thoracotomy. Talc pleurodesis can most often be performed to treat dyspnea secondary to pleural effusion simultaneously with obtaining diagnostic tissue. This practice makes it possible to revert to the previous state should resection be contemplated and may provide significant palliation if further surgery is not an option. A technical point of placing as few ports as possible in line of an eventual thoracotomy is prudent. Mesothelioma tends to grow in the port-site tracts, which should be resected at the time of definitive surgery. For patients who meet preoperative criteria (adequate pulmonary function tests and performance status, and potentially resectable tumor), surgical resection is a first-line option.

The 2 options for resection are pleurectomy and decortication (P/D) and extrapleural pneumonectomy (EPP). Both operations now carry a reasonable 4% to 5% operative rate of mortality with a 50% rate of operative morbidity at 30 days, which is a significant improvement from surgical outcomes several decades ago.[3,4] P/D involves resection of parietal and visceral pleura, pericardium, and diaphragm if indicated, leaving behind lung parenchyma. Conversely, EPP involves P/D in addition to en-bloc resection of lung.[4] Although EPP was initially postulated to achieve R0 margins, microscopic disease is often left behind (R1 resection), compared with P/D that may leave behind macronodular disease with an associated higher rate of locoregional recurrence.[3,5] The decision to perform EPP over P/D is infrequently outcomes-data driven, where certain high-volume surgical centers elect to perform the operation with which they have most experience.

Several poorly matched retrospective studies have suggested modest superiority of P/D over EPP with respect to rate of morbidity outcomes for palliation of advanced disease.[6–11] However, randomized control data to suggest superiority of 1 modality over the other *for nonpalliative resection* is lacking. Sugarbaker and colleagues[12] reviewed 636 patients who underwent EPP only and performed a retrospective analysis to explore clinicopathologic factors associated with the 18% of their patients who were 3-year survivors. This cohort of patients was younger consisted of women, had tumors with mainly epithelial histology, and had normal preoperative blood values. The variability of administered neo-adjuvant and adjuvant chemoradiation was noted and excluded from the statistical analysis. The authors concluded that there is a definitive role for EPP for cytoreduction in the context of multimodal therapy.

Flores and colleagues[13] published the most impressive head-to-head comparison of EPP and P/D to date. Their initial single-institution analysis of 945 patients with mesothelioma (22% underwent EPP and 19% underwent P/D) evaluated prognostic factors associated with improved survival. Factors associated with improved survival were surgically resectable disease, no history of smoking, no asbestos history, female gender, absence of pleuritic chest pain, epithelial histology, left-sided tumors, and early-stage disease. In a subgroup analysis, EPP and P/D were statistically similar with respect to overall survival. The greatest survival difference occurred when multimodal therapy (chemoradiation) was added to surgery with a median survival of 20 months, compared with surgery alone with a median survival of 10 months. Follow-up analysis of survival comparing EPP to P/D using a multi-institutional, retrospective data set of 663 patients revealed only modest survival advantage of P/D over EPP (multivariate analysis controlling for stage, histology, gender, and multimodal therapy; hazard ratio 1.4, $P<.01$ for EPP).[5] The author group also noted an increased relapse of locoregional disease after P/D compared with distant disease in EPP.[5] The study suggests that patient selection is critical with respect to choice of operation—complete cytoreduction by EPP is most beneficial for locoregional control but has no overall survival advantage and a higher rate of morbidity than P/D. Until prospective randomized superiority data are demonstrated, the choice of EPP versus P/D should be determined by patient rate of comorbidity, institution experience, and allocation into clinical trials. Additionally, surgery should be performed inclusive of multimodal treatment.

Patients who are not resection candidates can be offered palliative procedures, including single-incision thoracoscopic talc pleurodesis as well as insertion of pleurex catheters to provide convenient conduits of pleural fluid drainage.

Chemotherapy

The role of chemotherapy in the multimodal management of malignant mesothelioma is well described and is currently part of the standard of care. In 2 phase III randomized trials, Vogelzang and colleagues[14] and Van Meerbeeck and colleagues[15] suggested that the addition of an antifolate (premtrexed or raltitrexed) to cisplatin corresponded to a 2.6- to 2.8-month median overall survival improvement compared with using cisplatin alone. Based on the data from these 2 studies, the Food and Drug Administration approved the use of cisplatin-premtrexed as a first-line chemotherapy treatment for MPM. Additionally, for patients who cannot tolerate cisplatin, carboplatin can be substituted. In a head-to-head comparison of carboplatin to cisplatin, Santoro and colleagues[16] demonstrated a statistically similar rate of response, time to progression, and 1-year survival for the 2 regimens, correlating to findings reported in 2 other phase II trials.[17,18]

At this point, there are no definitive recommendations for maintenance therapy, although several studies have demonstrated a progression-free survival benefit when using premtrexed versus supportive care, especially in premtrexed-naïve patients. However, these studies fail to demonstrate an overall survival benefit of using premtrexed for maintenance. An ongoing Cancer and Leukemia Group trial is specifically randomized to answer this question of maintenance.[2]

Current excitement about mesothelioma treatment arises from the following investigational biologic and targeted immunotherapies[19]:

- EGFR—The epidermal growth factor receptor tyrosine kinase is often overexpressed in MPM as well as many other cancers. *Gefitinib* and *erlotinib* are 2 inhibitors that demonstrated no response in patients with mesothelioma in phase II trials. A third inhibitor, *cetuximab*, is being evaluated in a phase II study combined with cisplatin and premtrexed.
- VEGF—The vascular endothelial growth factor (VEGF) is implicated in angiogenesis and also upregulated in many mesotheliomas. In a phase I study of patients with advanced MPM, *bevacizumab*, a monoclonal VEGF-receptor antagonist, was shown to improve progression-free survival, but not demonstrate a difference in overall survival.
- PDGF, c-kit—Platelet-derived growth factor receptors and c-kit antagonists have been studied extensively in many neoplasms and are also upregulated in some patients with mesothelioma as part of a proliferative pathway. *Vatalanib* is a dose-dependent inhibitor of VEGF and platelet-derived growth factor tyrosine kinase receptors as well as c-kit, but did not meet progression-free survival endpoints in a phase II trial of patients with advanced MPM. *Sunitinib* has similar targets with modest activity but was associated with high toxicity in a phase I trial.
- Bcr-abl—A mutation in the bcr-abl tyrosine kinase is also associated with oncogenesis in mesothelioma. *Imatinib* is a potent inhibitor but demonstrates no improvement in survival alone for patients with advanced MPM (phase II studies). However, its synergistic effects with cisplatin and pemetrexed are being investigated.
- m-TOR—The mammalian target of rapamycin has been extensively studied in oncogenesis and is also implicated in MPM. *Rapamycin* analogues have been studied with no effect on tumor response in phase I trials.
- HDAC—Histone deacetylases are also related to oncogenesis in MPM and other cancers by way of morphologic activation and deactivation of histones. Inhibitors of these pathways are promising and show beneficial tumor effect in several small phase I studies. A larger, phase II randomized clinical trial is ongoing to evaluate *vorinostat* against placebo in MPM patients.
- Mesothelin—Mesothelin is overexpressed in nearly all mesotheliomas, as well as in pancreatic, ovarian, and lung adenocarcinomas. *SS1P* is an immunotoxin that

targets the mesothelin and delivers pseudomonas exotoxin to cells that overexpress mesothelin. In phase I studies, it was shown to be safe and its efficacy is being evaluated in a phase II trial, combining it with other chemotherapies. *CRS-207* is a live-attenuated vaccine containing *Listeria monocytogenes* as a genetically modified virulent vector. The targeted utility and safety of this vaccine are being investigated in a phase I trial. *MORAb-009* is a promising chimeric anti-mesothelin monoclonal antibody that blocks the binding of CA (carbohydrate antigen) -125 to mesothelin cell membrane receptors. This binding is a critical step in the pleural and peritoneal metastasis of tumors such as mesothelioma and ovarian cancer. Hassan and colleagues[20,21] demonstrated successful inhibition of CA-125 binding to mesothelin by measuring elevated serum CA-125 in patients given *MORAb-009.* A poorly powered, multicenter phase I trial by the same group demonstrated safety of *MORAb-009* at a maximum tolerated dose of 200 mg/m^2. The drug is undergoing efficacy studies in a larger phase II clinical trial combining it with a cisplatin and pemetrexed regimen, mirroring another study for pancreatic cancer.

Investigational studies in the aforementioned biologicals and vaccine-based treatments of mesothelioma are in their infancy but show promise as combined treatments with currently used chemotherapies. **Table 2** summarizes current chemologic and biologic therapies.

Radiation Therapy

Although radiation treatment is a valuable tool in other malignancies of the chest, its role in MPM is limited secondary to the wide radiation field and the toxic radiation-dose limit to the lungs. Postoperative radiotherapy has shown promise in reducing local rates of recurrence after resection by EPP without any effect on overall survival. Intensity-modulated radiotherapy uses a delivery method of dose-dependent radiation to modulate and minimize radiotherapy to vital peritumoral organs such as the heart and liver. Using this novel technology, radiation can be delivered more effectively to control local recurrence. Phase II trials evaluating intensity-modulated radiotherapy in addition to chemotherapy in a neo-adjuvant and adjuvant setting are ongoing.[19]

Until more data are available from clinical trials, current recommendations for radiation treatment are restricted to palliation of chest wall pain because of tumor recurrence, unless a patient is enrolled in a clinical trial that uses other algorithms for multimodal therapy.

Fig. 2 illustrates an algorithm for treatment of MPM.

BIOMARKERS

The utility of biomarkers in MPM has been evaluated for both diagnostic and prognostic purposes. These tests are noninvasive and are theorized to help diagnose mesothelioma early as well as to stratify patients effectively into clinical trial algorithms. Biomarker panels are likely more effective than individual markers and are being investigated as additions to multimodal trials.

- Mesothelin—Serum mesothelin, formerly known as soluble mesothelin-related protein, is the most commonly assayed and best-described serum biomarker for mesothelioma. It is found in most non–sarcomatoid mesotheliomas as well as in ovarian, pancreatic, and lung cancers. High levels in serum have been associated with poor prognosis and aggressive or bulky disease.[2] In a meta-analysis of 16 diagnostic studies, Hollevoet and colleagues[22] found that at a 95% specificity

Table 2
Current chemotherapeutic and biologic therapies for mesothelioma (see body of text for key)

Therapeutic	Class	Trial	Benefit
Chemotherapy			
Cisplatin	Platinum-based chemotherapy	Phase III	Improved OS and PFS
Carboplatin	Platinum-based chemotherapy	Phase III	Comparable to cisplatin but with less toxicity
Pemetrexed	Alkaloid	Phase III	Improved OS and PFS when combined first line with platinum based treatment. Possible PFS benefit in maintenance therapy
Raltitrexed	Alkaloid	Phase III	Equivalent in efficacy to pemetrexed
Biologics			
Gefitinib, erlotinib, cetuximab	EGFR antagonist	Phase II	No benefit, pending further trial
Bevacizumab	VEGF antagonist	Phase I	Improved PFS, no effect on OS
Vatalanib, sunitinib	VEGF, platelet-derived growth factor receptors, c-kit antagonist	Phase I and II	Did not meet PFS endpoints (vatalanib). Toxicity too high (sunitinib)
Imatinib	Bcr-abl antagonist	Phase II	No benefit alone. Synergism with chemotherapeutics being evaluated
Vorinostat	Histone deacetylases	Phase II	Awaiting result of phase II trial
MORAb-009	Anti-mesothelin monoclonal antibody	Phase II	Safe in small phase I trial. Awaiting efficacy data in phase II trial with cisplatin/pemetrexed
Immunologic vaccines			
SS1P	Mesothelin targeting pseudomonas endotoxin	Phase II	Safe in phase I trial. Efficacy being studied in phase II trials with chemotherapeutics
CRS-207	Mesothelin targeting live attenuated Listeria monocytogenes vector	Phase I	Safety being studied

Abbreviations: EGFR, epidermal growth factor receptor; OS, overall survival; PFS, progression-free survival.

Data from Refs.[2,14–21]

threshold, the sensitivity of mesothelin for detecting mesothelioma is 32% (95% CI, 26%–40%). With such a low sensitivity, mesothelin is not useful alone to detect mesothelioma, but may still be a useful adjunct to other diagnostic modalities. Additionally, its levels of serum seem to parallel disease recurrence, making it an intriguing blood test to follow patients after treatment. The Mesomark

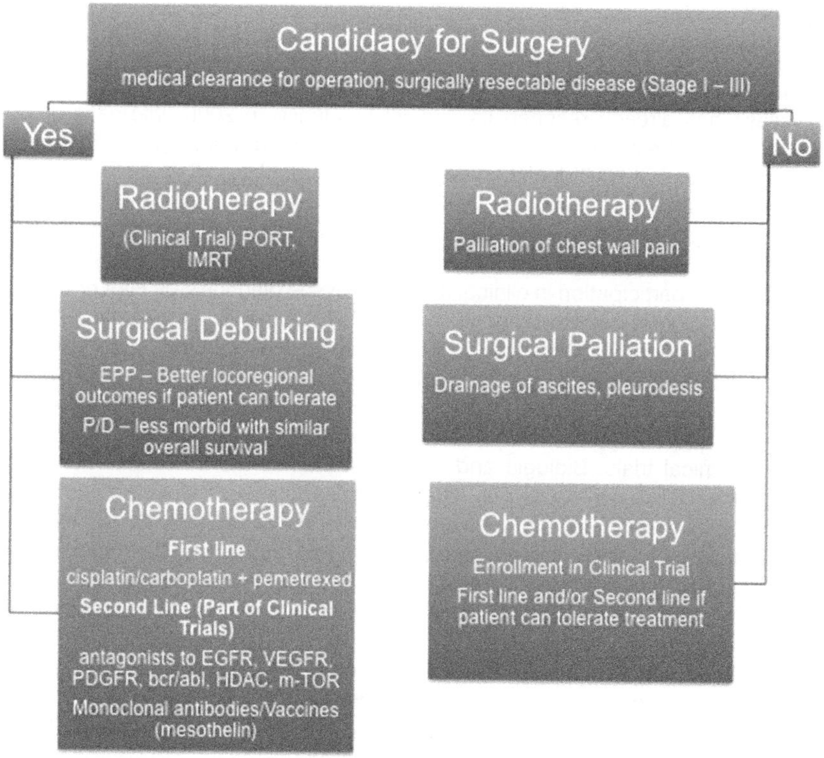

Fig. 2. An algorithm for the treatment of malignant pleural mesothelioma. EGFR, epidermal growth factor receptor; EPP, extrapleural pneumonectomy; HDAC, histone deacetylases; IMRT, intensity modulated radiotherapy; m-TOR, mammalian target of rapamycin; P/D, pleurectomy/decortications; PORT, postoperative radiation treatment.

(Fujirebio Diagnostics, Malvern, PA) assay is currently Food and Drug Administration approved to monitor patients with epithelial and biphasic variants of MPM.

- Osteopontin—Osteopontin is a glycoprotein that mediates cell-cell interactions and is overexpressed in mesothelioma as well as other cancers (lung, breast, colorectal, and ovarian).[2,23] Pass and colleagues[23] demonstrated that levels of serum osteopontin are useful in detecting mesothelioma in a subgroup of patients with known asbestos exposure (sensitivity 77.6, specificity 85.5). This underpowered study compared 3 cohorts of patients—patients with exposure to asbestos without malignant lung disease; patients without exposure to asbestos without mesothelioma; and patients with exposure to asbestos with mesothelioma. Osteopontin is currently being investigated in a panel of biomarkers to improve accuracy in detection of mesothelioma for all patients, irrespective of asbestos exposure.
- Other markers—Van der Bij and colleagues[24] performed a meta-analysis of 82 articles evaluating biomarkers for accurate detection of mesothelioma. The authors concluded that, although soluble mesothelin-related protein, carcinoembryonic antigen, epithelial membrane antigen, calretinin, and Ber-Ep4 antibody were promising biomarkers, there is limited evidence in their utility in detecting mesothelioma. The study compared individual assays only and failed to evaluate the diagnostic value of combining biomarkers.

SUMMARY

The multimodal paradigm for the detection and treatment has changed the quality as well as the length of survival for MPM. Although US epidemiologic data suggest that the disease has already reached its highest incidence in 2000, international data suggest that MPM is on the rise in many undeveloped and developing countries, which corresponds to great multi-institutional interest in optimizing diagnostic and therapeutic modalities.

Patients diagnosed with mesothelioma benefit from receiving care at an institution that specializes in this disease because of advances in surgical and oncologic technique as well as participation in clinical trial. After tissue diagnosis by FNA or thoracoscopic pleural biopsy, treatment should include surgical debulking to attain at least an R1 resection (EPP or P/D, depending on institution experience and patient tolerance) combined with chemotherapy (cisplatin/carboplatin with an antifolate) with or without radiotherapy for local recurrence. The role of maintenance treatment with pemetrexed is questionable but may have utility in pemetrexed-naïve patients or patients enrolled in specific clinical trials. Biologic and vaccine therapies are still experimental and awaiting further clinical trial, but may offer survival advantages when combined with aforementioned multimodal therapy. Finally, although mesothelin and osteopontin have some utility in detecting non–sarcomatoid mesothelioma, their role is likely most beneficial in monitoring disease relapse after treatment. Investigation of biomarker panels to detect subclinical mesothelioma is much needed to improve early detection.

With continued international collaboration and enrollment of patients in clinical trials, the utility of new diagnostic modalities, radiotherapeutics, and novel chemologic and biologic therapies will be optimized as part of a multimodal treatment paradigm to improve mesothelioma outcomes.

REFERENCES

1. Robinson BW, Lake RA. Advances in malignant mesothelioma. N Engl J Med 2005;353:1591–603.
2. Campbell NP, Kindler HL. Update on malignant pleura mesothelioma. Semin Respir Crit Care Med 2011;32:102–10.
3. Sugarbaker DJ. Macroscopic complete resection: the goal of primary surgery in multimodality therapy for pleural mesothelioma. J Thorac Oncol 2006;1:175–6.
4. Opitz I, Kestenholz P, Lardinois D, et al. Incidence and management of complications after neoadjuvant chemotherapy followed by extrapleural pneumonectomy for malignant pleural mesothelioma. Eur J Cardiothorac Surg 2006;29:579–84.
5. Flores RM, Pass HI, Seshan VE, et al. Extrapleural pneumonectomy versus pleurectomy/decortication in the surgical management of malignant pleural mesothelioma: results in 663 patients. J Thorac Cardiovasc Surg 2008;135(3):620–6.
6. Waller DA, Morritt GN, Forty J. Video-assisted thoracoscopic pleurectomy in the management of malignant pleural effusion. Chest 1995;5:1454–6.
7. Soysal O, Karaoğlanoğlu N, Demiracan S, et al. Pleurectomy/decortication for palliation in malignant pleural mesothelioma: results of surgery. Eur J Cardiothorac Surg 1997;11:210–3.
8. Martin-Ucar AE, Edwards JG, Rengajaran A, et al. Palliative and surgical debulking in malignant mesothelioma. Predictors of survival and symptom control. Eur J Cardiothorac Surg 2001;20:1117–21.

9. Halstead JC, Lim E, Venkateswaran RM, et al. Improved survival with VATS pleurectomy-decortication in advanced malignant mesothelioma. Eur J Surg Oncol 2005;31:314–20.
10. Muirhead R, O'Rourke N. Drain site of radiotherapy in malignant pleural mesothemioma: a wasted resource. Eur Respir J 2007;30:1021.
11. Nakas A, Martin Ucar AE, Edwards JG, et al. The role of video assisted thoracoscopic pleurectomy/decortication in the therapeutic management of malignant pleural mesothelioma. Eur J Cardiothorac Surg 2008;33:83–8.
12. Sugarbaker DJ, Wolf AS, Chirieac LR, et al. Clinical and pathological features of three-year survivors of malignant pleural mesothelioma following extrapleural pneumonectomy. Eur J Cardiothorac Surg 2011;40:298–303.
13. Flores RM, Zakowski M, Venkatraman E, et al. Prognostic factors in the treatment of malignant pleural mesothelioma at a large tertiary referral center. J Thorac Oncol 2007;2:957–65.
14. Vogelzang NJ, Rusthoven JJ, Symanowski J, et al. Phase III study of premtrexed in combination with cisplatin versus cisplatin alone in patients with malignant pleural mesothelioma. J Clin Oncol 2003;21:2636–44.
15. Van Meerbeeck JP, Gaafar R, Manegold C, et al. Randomized phase III study of cisplatin with or without raltitrexed in patients with malignant pleural moesothelioma: an intergroup study for Research and Treatment of Cancer Lung Cancer Group and the National Cancer Institute of Canada. J Clin Oncol 2005;23:6881–9.
16. Santoro A, O'Brien ME, Stahel RA, et al. Premtrexed plus cisplatin or premtrexed plus carboplatin for chemonaive patients with malignant pleural mesothelioma: results of the International Expanded Access Program. J Thorac Oncol 2008;7: 756–63.
17. Castagneto B, Botta M, Aitini E, et al. Phase II study of pemtrexed in combination with carboplatin in patient with malignant pleural mesothelioma (MPM). Ann Oncol 2008;19:370–3.
18. Ceresoli GL, Zucali PA, Favaretto AG, et al. Phase II study of pemetrexed plus carboplatin in malignant pleural mesothelioma. J Clin Oncol 2006;24:1443–8.
19. Surmont VF, van Thiel ER, Vermaelen K, et al. Investigational approaches for mesothelioma. Front Oncol 2011;1:22, 1–15.
20. Hassan R, Cohen SJ, Phillips M, et al. Phase I clinical trial of the chimeric anti-mesothelin monoclonal antibody MORAb-009 in patients with mesothelin-expressing cancers. Clin Cancer Res 2010;16:6132–8.
21. Hassan R, Schweizer C, Lu KF, et al. Inhibition of mesothelin-CA-125 interaction in patients with mesothelioma by the anti-mesothelin monoclonal antibody MORAb-009: implications for cancer therapy. Lung Cancer 2010;68(3):455–9.
22. Hollevoet, Reitsma JB, Creaney J, et al. Serum Mesothelin for diagnosing malignant pleural mesothelioma: an individual patient data meta-analysis. J Clin Oncol 2012;30:1541–9.
23. Pass HI, Lott D, Lonardo F, et al. Asbestos exposure, pleural mesothelioma, and serum osteopontin levels. N Engl J Med 2005;353(15):1564–73.
24. Van der Bij S, Schaake E, Koffijberg H, et al. Markers for the non-invasive diagnosis of mesothelioma: a systematic review. Br J Cancer 2011;104(8):1325–33.

Multidisciplinary Management of Patients with Localized Bladder Cancer

Kiranpreet K. Khurana, MD[a], Jorge A. Garcia, MD[b], Rahul D. Tendulkar, MD[b], Andrew J. Stephenson, MD[a,*]

KEYWORDS

- Muscle-invasive bladder cancer • Radical cystectomy
- Pelvic lymph node dissection • Chemotherapy • Chemoradiation

KEY POINTS

- Surgeon-controlled variables including negative surgical margins and extended lymph node dissection are essential to achieve optimal outcomes for patients treated by radical cystectomy.
- Neoadjuvant chemotherapy with methotrexate, vinblastine, doxorubicin, and cisplatin significantly improves the survival of patients undergoing radical cystectomy and represents the optimal treatment approach for patients with muscle-invasive bladder cancer. The use of carboplatin-based regimens is not recommended.
- In addition to insufficient evidence for use of adjuvant chemotherapy, its use and tolerability may be compromised after major surgery because of surgical complications.
- In select patients, bladder-preservation protocols may result in acceptable survival and low toxicity rates, although it has not been widely embraced in the genitourinary oncology community.

INTRODUCTION

Optimal management of invasive bladder cancer involves a multidisciplinary therapeutic approach for improved disease-free and overall survival. Approximately 30% of patients present with muscle-invasive bladder cancer at diagnosis.[1] A total of 50% to 70% of those with high-grade, non–muscle-invasive disease recur and up to 50% progress to muscle-invasive disease.[2] If left untreated, 85% of patients with muscle-invasive bladder cancer die of disease within 2 years of diagnosis.[3] Because of high morbidity and mortality of muscle-invasive bladder cancer, single therapeutic modality may not provide optimal cancer control.

[a] Glickman Urological & Kidney Institute, Cleveland Clinic, 9500 Euclid Avenue, Cleveland, OH 44195, USA; [b] Taussig Cancer Center, Cleveland Clinic, Cleveland, OH, USA
* Corresponding author.
E-mail address: STEPHEA2@ccf.org

Surg Oncol Clin N Am 22 (2013) 357–373
http://dx.doi.org/10.1016/j.soc.2012.12.008 surgonc.theclinics.com

Radical cystectomy plays a pivotal role in the care of patients with invasive bladder cancer and has been the mainstay of treatment for decades. Overall survival for patients with muscle-invasive bladder cancer treated by radical cystectomy ranges from 50% to 60%. Per stage, survival for pT0-2 N0, pT3-4 N0, and pTany N1-3 is 70% to 80%, 45% to 55%, and 25% to 35%, respectively.[4,5] Despite significant advances in the understanding and management of bladder cancer, outcomes have largely remained unchanged in the last 30 years.[6] Bladder-preservation strategies involving a visibly complete transurethral bladder tumor resection followed by radiation therapy and chemotherapy may achieve similar survival rates in select patients. This article reviews different treatment options and discusses possible management strategies to improve outcomes.

SURGICAL ISSUES

Quality of Radical Cystectomy

Radical cystectomy is a critical component in the treatment of invasive bladder cancer. Suboptimal surgery dramatically decreases overall survival. Modifiable surgical factors that can significantly improve survival include surgical margin status and number of lymph nodes removed.[7–11] Analysis of the SWOG 8710 trial showed that positive margins and removal of fewer than 10 nodes were associated with significantly poorer outcomes.[11] The adjusted hazard ratio for death of patients with positive versus negative surgical margin was 2.7 (95% confidence interval, 1.4–2.8). When compared with negative-margin group, local recurrence was 11.2 times greater in the positive-margin group.[11] In a recent paper by Mitra and colleagues,[8] a review of 447 patients showed that positive surgical margin status was significantly associated with worse postrecurrence overall survival.

Number of lymph nodes removed and overall survival have a linear correlation with continuous rise in survival with increasing number of lymph nodes removed.[12] Herr and colleagues[13] showed that disease-specific survival was greater for patients with more than 14 nodes removed as compared with removal of 9 to 14 nodes and 1 to 8 nodes. The quality of surgery may be improved by striving for negative surgical margins and removing adequate number of lymph nodes at the time of surgery.

Another factor that may influence outcomes is surgeon training. In the analysis of the SWOG 8710 study, 106 surgeons were included from 1987 to 1998, of which 38% were fellowship-trained urologic oncologists.[14] No pelvic lymph node dissection (PLND) was done in 9% of the cases and in 50%, less than 10 nodes were removed. Positive surgical margin rate was 10% overall, but 4% for urologic oncologist and 16% for others. Local recurrence rate for urologic oncologist was 6% versus 23% for others. The type of surgeon (fellowship-trained vs others) was a significant predictor of number of nodes removed, local recurrence, and survival. The surgical volume among urologic oncologists does not play a significant role in terms of surgical outcomes.[14] Sixteen surgeons from four centers of excellence with varying experience were compared. Seven surgeons had done fewer than 50 radical cystectomies, whereas four had done more than 100 procedures over a 3-year period. No significant difference was found among urologic oncologists with regards to number of lymph nodes removed and surgical margin status.

To summarize, positive margins are associated with increased local recurrence and worse survival. Surgery by a fellowship-trained urologic oncologist versus others is associated with greater number of nodes removed, lower local recurrence, and higher survival.

Standard Versus Extended PLND

Clinical staging for lymph nodes relies on imaging including computed tomography or magnetic resonance imaging; however, studies have shown that 19% to 28% of those who are N0 preoperatively on imaging are found to have positive nodal disease,[5,15–24] emphasizing the importance of LND. Optimal extent of LND at the time of surgery that provides the best survival is widely debated. "Standard" lymphadenectomy is removal of all tissue within the boundaries of common iliac artery bifurcation where ureter crosses the vessels, internal iliac, external iliac, and obturator fossa.[18,25,26] However, several studies suggest that this may not be sufficient to provide adequate cancer control.[15,16] An "extended" LND is described as dissection up to the aortic bifurcation superiorly, genitofemoral nerve laterally, lymph node of Cloquet inferiorly, obturator fossa posteriorly, and presacral nodes.[27] The concept of extended PLND (EPLND) has come about because of lymph node mapping studies that reveal the high positivity rate of lymph nodes above the bifurcation of the common iliac vessels. Among 336 patients, 19% had lymph node metastasis with 34.4% of those above the bifurcation of the common iliac vessels.[16] In one study, 290 patients were evaluated for lymph node positivity rate in 12 different anatomic locations. The lymph node positivity in each location ranged from 2.9% to 14.1%. Common iliac and presacral nodal involvement was as common as distal nodes.[15] Therefore, if dissection were limited to the obturator fossa, 74% of the positive lymph nodes would not be detected.

Similar results were found in another study of 176 patients undergoing radical cystectomy and PLND, where 24% of the patients were found to have lymph node involvement.[17] The distribution of involved lymph nodes was as follows: 4% in aortic bifurcation, 13.7% in common iliac nodes, 5.1% in presacral nodes, 26% in pelvic nodes, 2.8% in perivesical nodes, and 5.7% in unspecified nodes. Additionally, LND is always bilateral because of bilateral lymph drainage. This is exemplified by a study that showed that 39% of patients with positive lymph nodes had bilateral involvement.[28] Other series have also supported this finding.[5,18,29]

EPLND has several clinical advantages because it allows for more accurate staging, removes occult metastases, and correlates to greater recurrence-free survival.[30,31] It is of value even in those patients with clinically organ-confined, node-negative disease.[32] In one study, 5-year recurrence-free survival was 90% in those who underwent EPLND versus 71% for standard PLND. Another study of 658 patients with N0M0 disease based on preoperative clinical staging also showed greater recurrence-free survival for EPLND. Among those with positive lymph nodes on pathology, patients who underwent limited LND had 7% 5-year recurrence-free survival compared with 35% for EPLND. For those with pT2N0 disease or node-negative disease, the 5-year recurrence-free survival was 67% for limited and 77% for EPLND, and for patients with pT3N0 disease, it was 23% and 57% ($P<.0001$), respectively. EPLND improved survival in node-negative and node-positive invasive bladder cancer.

Morbidity rates of EPLND in contemporary series are comparable with standard LND.[15,33] Although it may prolong operative time, there is no significant difference in perioperative mortality, early complications, need for blood transfusions, and lymphocele formation.[15,32,33] Lymphocele and lymphedema rates were 2% for patients in whom less than 16 lymph nodes were removed and 1% where 16 or more lymph nodes were removed.[15]

The number of lymph nodes involved is an important factor for survival. Recurrence-free and overall survival are directly related to the number of lymph nodes involved, with significantly decreased survival for those with five or more positive lymph nodes when compared with those with less than five positive lymph nodes.[7,16] In a study by Herr,[7] the 5-year overall survival was 38% for patients with less than five positive lymph nodes versus 18% for those with five or more positive lymph nodes.

The concept of lymph node density (LNDt) was designed to include not only the number of lymph nodes involved, but also take into account the extent of LND.

LNDt greater than 20% correlates with worse disease-free survival.[4,5,34] In a study of 1054 patients, Stein and colleagues[5] showed that 10-year recurrence-free survival for patients with LNDt less than or equal to 20% was 43% versus 17% for LNDt greater than 20%. Similarly, another study of 133 patients showed that LNDt was among the most important factors in determining disease-specific survival after cystectomy.[4] Five-year disease-specific survival for patients with LNDt less than or equal to 20% was 54%, whereas it was 0% for LNDt greater than 20%. A study by Herr[35] of 162 patients with lymph node–positive bladder cancer showed 5-year disease-specific survival of 5% for LNDt greater than 20% and 60% for LNDt less than or equal to 20%. This study also compared the use of LNDt with TNM nodal status and showed that LNDt was a better prognostic indicator of recurrence and disease-specific survival. Another study from Memorial Sloan-Kettering Cancer center and M.D. Anderson Cancer Center confirmed this finding.[34] The 5-year disease-specific survival of 134 patients was 55% for patients with LNDt less than or equal to 20% versus 15% for LNDt greater than 20%. Pathologic nodal status and LNDt were important markers of worse disease-specific survival, but in a multivariate model, only LNDt was significantly associated with decreased disease-specific survival.

To summarize:

- Rate of lymph node positivity in clinical negative nodes is approximately 25%.
- Lymph node mapping studies reveal that substantial number of lymph nodes is positive above the bifurcation of the common iliac vessels.
- EPLND improves local recurrence and survival as compared with standard LND in node-positive and node-negative invasive bladder cancer.
- Perioperative morbidity and mortality are similar for standard and EPLND.
- Involvement of greater than five lymph nodes is an indicator of lower recurrence-free and overall survival.
- LNDt greater than or equal to 20% correlates to improved disease-specific survival and may be a better marker of outcomes than number of positive lymph nodes.

Outcomes of Minimally Invasive Surgical Approaches

Minimally invasive surgery plays an increasingly important role in management of invasive bladder cancer. Theoretical benefits of minimally invasive surgery are decreased blood loss and transfusion rate because of better visualization and positive pressure from pneumoperitoneum, smaller incision and resulting improved pain control, decreased morbidity and mortality, better optics to allow aggressive nerve-sparing, higher potency and continence rates, and preservation or improvement in oncologic outcomes.

Recent studies show that some of the benefits of minimally invasive surgery may be improved analgesic requirements and reduced blood loss along with lower transfusion rates.[36] It may also result in quicker recovery, shorter hospital stay, and fewer complications.[37] These results have yet to be definitively proved. In terms of cancer control, surgical margin status and number of lymph nodes removed are similar in retrospective studies.[36,38–40] A single-institution, small, prospective, randomized noninferiority trial was done to compare open versus robotic-assisted radical cystectomy.[41] Robotic-assisted radical cystectomy resulted in significant reduction in estimated blood loss, time to flatus and bowel movement, and use of narcotic pain medication, while resulting in similar complication rate and hospital stay. Operative time was significantly higher in robotic-assisted surgery (4.2 vs 3.5 hours). Positive margin rate and lymph node yield was similar with both techniques. Based on these select studies, oncologic outcomes do not seem to be compromised by use of robotic assistance; however, longer follow-up is needed.

In summary, minimally invasive surgery results in improved pain control, reduced blood loss and transfusion rates, but operative time is higher. Surgical margin rates and extent of LND seem to be similar between minimally invasive and open surgical approaches. Long-term oncologic outcomes with minimally invasive surgery remain to be seen, although shorter-term outcomes do not seem to be compromised.

CHEMOTHERAPY

The main role of perioperative chemotherapy in clinically localized bladder cancer is to deliver effective systemic therapy while the burden of micrometastatic disease is minimal. Theoretically, this should lead to tumor downstaging (ie, pathologic complete response); delay in disease recurrence; and overall survival improvement. The controversy, however, is the timing of its administration (ie, preoperative vs postoperative).

Neoadjuvant Chemotherapy

Neoadjuvant chemotherapy is standard of care for muscle-invasive bladder cancer. During the past two decades, a series of cisplatin-based regimens were evaluated in randomized trials, culminating in two large trials demonstrating a survival impact of chemotherapy administered in the neoadjuvant setting. A randomized, controlled trial (SWOG 8710) comparing three cycles of methotrexate, vinblastine, doxorubicin, and cisplatin (MVAC) plus radical cystectomy versus cystectomy alone increased the survival from a median of 46 months in cystectomy-alone group to 77 months in the combination group.[42] There was a 14% absolute improvement in overall survival at 5 years in the combination group. This was observed in all tumor stages, especially if there were complete pathologic response. Rate of pathologic T0 in patients receiving neoadjuvant chemotherapy is 33% to 40%, whereas it is 6% to 15% for those who undergo radical cystectomy alone.[42]

Alternative treatment regimens have been investigated in several studies. A European Organization for Research and Treatment of Cancer trial randomized 976 patients to definitive local therapy or three cycles of neoadjuvant cisplatin, methotrexate, and vinblastine (CMV).[43] This trial showed a 16% and 23% reduction in all-cause mortality and death or metastasis, respectively, for patients receiving neoadjuvant CMV versus those receiving local therapy alone. The 3-year survival and 10-year survival also increased from 50% to 56% and 30% to 36%, respectively, in the neoadjuvant chemotherapy group. A meta-analysis of 11 phase III randomized, controlled trials that included more than 2600 patients showed a 5% absolute improvement in survival conferred to those patients who received platinum-based neoadjuvant chemotherapy ($P = .016$). The overall survival improvement observed was achieved irrespective of the type of local definitive treatment administered (surgery or radiation).[44]

The use of cisplatin plus gemcitabine (GC) in the perioperative setting has not been prospectively evaluated. Small retrospective series have evaluated the toxicity profile of GC and its ability to lead to tumor down-staging.[45] Four cycles of GC seem to lead to pT0 in 26% of the patients; these data mirror the rate of pT0 disease (28%) observed in the neoadjuvant MVAC trial.[42] Albeit improved side effect profile is the argument often used in the community to favor GC over MVAC, to date no prospective data have compared MVAC with GC in the perioperative setting. Similar to GC, carboplatin-based chemotherapy has not been properly evaluated in the perioperative setting. Carboplatin is an inferior agent to cisplatin and should not be used in the neoadjuvant setting.

Advantages of neoadjuvant chemotherapy include better tolerability of systemic therapy, avoidance of potential delay in delivering systemic therapy while awaiting recovery from surgical treatment, prognostic benefit of monitoring response to chemotherapy,[46] reduction of tumor volume, and treatment of micrometastatic disease. If chemotherapy is deferred until after radical cystectomy, an estimated 30% of the patients may not be able to get adjuvant chemotherapy because of prolonged postoperative convalescence, complications, or compromised renal function.[47]

Despite demonstrable advantages, the use of neoadjuvant chemotherapy has been low. National Cancer Database shows that only 9% of the patients receive neoadjuvant chemotherapy, but the rate has increased from 6% in 2003 to 13% in 2007.[48] A Canadian group revealed a 14% use rate for neoadjuvant chemotherapy after the publication of practice guidelines for muscle-invasive bladder cancer in 2005.[49] Another study evaluated the use of neoadjuvant chemotherapy in a tertiary care center in the United States, and reported that only 17% of eligible patients were administered neoadjuvant chemotherapy.[50]

Potential reasons for underuse of neoadjuvant chemotherapy include inaccurate clinical staging, delay in definitive surgery because of nonresponse, delay in delivery of chemotherapy or definitive local surgery,[51] modest gain in overall survival, and toxicities of chemotherapy rendering patients with higher comorbidities unsuitable for surgery.

To summarize, neoadjuvant chemotherapy with MVAC results in better survival, and is associated with higher pathologic T0 stage. Carboplatin is inferior to cisplatin and should not be used in the neoadjuvant setting. CMV and GC are alternative chemotherapy regimens that have shown significant clinical response, but these regimens have not been compared with MVAC in head-to-head trials. Although neoadjuvant chemotherapy is clearly indicated in patients with muscle-invasive bladder cancer, the use rates are low.

Adjuvant Chemotherapy

Although adjuvant chemotherapy lacks strong evidence for its use, most American clinicians prefer to delay chemotherapy in fear of not being able to complete local definitive therapy, and to provide a perioperative benefit for a more well-defined population.

Arguments in favor of adjuvant chemotherapy are adequate pathologic staging allowing delivery of chemotherapy to only those patients who are at high risk of progression, and avoidance of overtreatment and delay in definitive surgical therapy. The trials for adjuvant chemotherapy, however, suffer from poor accrual, early study terminations, low power, variability in regimens, and lack of long-term follow-up (**Table 1**).

Some of the earlier trials[52–55] comparing cystectomy plus cisplatin-based adjuvant chemotherapy showed mixed results, with two studies showing survival advantage.

Table 1
Adjuvant chemotherapy trials

Author (Year)	No. of Patients	Trial Design	Survival Advantage
Skinner et al,[52] 1991	91	Cystectomy ± CISCA	Yes, OS
Stockle et al,[53] 1995	49	Cystectomy ± MVAC/MVEC	Yes, DFS only
Freiha,[54] 1996	55	Cystectomy ± CMV	No
Studer et al,[55] 1994	77	Cystectomy ± cisplatin	No
Cognetti et al,[92] 2012	194	Cystectomy ± GC	No
Stadler et al,[56] 2011	114	Cystectomy ± MVAC	No

Abbreviations: CISCA, cisplatin, doxorubicin; DFS, disease-free survival; MVEC, methotrexate, cisplatin, epirubicin, cisplatin; OS, overall survival.

However, these trials were underpowered and inconclusive. Studies have been done to incorporate molecular markers to better stratify patients for adjuvant chemotherapy. A phase III trial randomized 114 patients with p53-positive status on cystectomy specimens to adjuvant MVAC versus observation.[56] This trial failed to demonstrate a benefit when p53 status, a known molecular alteration in bladder cancer, was used as a prognostic indicator. This trial also failed to demonstrate an advantage of adjuvant chemotherapy in this p53-positive patient cohort.

A meta-analysis of all the randomized cisplatin-based adjuvant chemotherapy trials including 491 patients revealed a 25% relative risk reduction for all-cause mortality and 9% absolute survival advantage with adjuvant chemotherapy.[57] It also showed a 32% relative increase in disease-free survival and 12% absolute improvement. However, because of poor quality of trials and small number of patients, the Advanced Bladder Cancer Collaboration concluded that there was insufficient evidence for its use. A large retrospective study of 932 patients from 11 institutions treated with adjuvant chemotherapy reported survival benefit for adjuvant chemotherapy, especially in higher-risk patients (≥T3 disease or nodal involvement).[58]

Potential limitations for use of adjuvant chemotherapy are long recovery time after radical cystectomy, possibility of serious perioperative complications leading to difficulty in administering treatment, or decreased ability to tolerate treatment. Approximately 60% of patients have perioperative complications[47,59] and 20% to 27% require readmission within 90 days of surgery,[59,60] which hinders delivery of adjuvant chemotherapy in 30% of eligible patients.[47] The data regarding neoadjuvant and adjuvant chemotherapy must be considered when making a decision regarding choice of appropriate regimen.

To summarize, meta-analysis of all randomized adjuvant chemotherapy trials revealed a 25% relative risk reduction for all-cause mortality and 9% absolute survival but more robust evidence is needed to make definitive recommendations. Because of perioperative complications, 30% of the patients eligible for adjuvant chemotherapy are unable to receive this treatment.

CHEMORADIATION THERAPY

Bladder Preservation

Although robust evidence exists in favor of neoadjuvant chemotherapy and radical cystectomy, some patients with low performance status and high baseline comorbidities may not be able to tolerate surgery. The trimodal approach to selective bladder preservation includes aggressive transurethral resection with goal of complete resection, followed by concomitant radiation and chemotherapy. Chemotherapy serves to radiosensitize the tumor and treats occult metastasis.[61] After these treatments, a cystoscopy is repeated and those with persistent disease proceed to radical cystectomy.

Although no standardized inclusion or exclusion exists, the patients who may be candidates for this approach are those with solitary tumors less than 5 cm, absence of carcinoma in situ, resectable disease, absence of hydronephrosis, normal functioning bladder and bowel, willingness to comply with extensive follow-up schedule, or those who are unfit or unwilling to undergo surgery.[62,63] Generally, accepted exclusion criteria include patients with multifocal tumors or large solitary tumor (>5 cm); unresectable disease or incomplete transurethral resection; prior pelvic radiotherapy; and presence of hydronephrosis or carcinoma in situ.

A multicenter, randomized, phase III trial of 360 patients with T2 to T4a bladder cancer compared radiotherapy alone with radiation and chemotherapy (mitomycin C and fluorouracil).[64] The chemoradiation group had significantly higher locoregional disease-free survival relative to radiotherapy alone at a median follow-up of 70 months. Overall survival at 5-years was similar between the groups. Grade 3 or 4 adverse events were not significantly increased in the chemoradiation group, with preservation of long-term bladder function. Comparison of salvage cystectomy rate was underpowered, but it was 11.4% in the chemoradiation group and 16.8% in the radiotherapy-alone group (P = .07).

Rates of disease-free and overall survival for bladder-preservation protocols have been reported in several studies, but studies directly comparing radical cystectomy with bladder preservation are sparse. Some of the earlier studies reported 3- to 5-year disease-free survival of 62% to 66%,[63,65–68] and overall survival of 49% to 54%.[65,66] One study revealed 10-year overall survival of 36%,[66] which is similar to studies with radical cystectomy for muscle-invasive disease. One-third of the patients ultimately required salvage radical cystectomy for local recurrence, but none because of treatment-related toxicity.[66] Muscle-invasive disease recurrence should prompt treatment with radical cystectomy. Management of non–muscle-invasive disease is controversial. In a study of 190 patients, 26% rate of non–muscle-invasive disease recurrence was noted.[69] The 5- and 8-year survival rates were not significantly different between those with recurrence and those without recurrence. However, 8-year survival with a functional bladder was significantly lower in those with non–muscle-invasive recurrence (34%) compared with recurrence-free patients (61%).

Recent studies have investigated broader chemotherapeutic options including paclitaxel, cisplatin, and gemcitabine in combination with radiotherapy, and revealed 5-year disease-specific survival of 71% and overall survival of 56%.[70] In this study of 80 patients, concomitant cisplatin and paclitaxel with hyperfractionated radiotherapy to 21 Gy were administered, and complete responders received adjuvant gemcitabine with cisplatin with radiotherapy to total 45 Gy. In another study, addition of gemcitabine to cisplatin resulted in 5-year disease-specific survival of 79% and overall survival of 70% at a median follow-up of 74 months.[71]

Challenges with trimodal therapy include lack of standardized chemoradiation protocols, possible need for salvage cystectomy and associated increased morbidity, and lack of phase III randomized trials comparing survival and quality-of-life outcomes between contemporary bladder-preservation protocols and radical cystectomy.

The two main types of radiation schedules used in bladder-sparing therapy are split course and continuous approaches. Split course chemoradiation approaches typically use induction radiotherapy to 40 Gy followed by cystoscopic evaluation and consolidative radiotherapy of 25 Gy to complete responders (**Table 2**).[65,67,68,70,72,73] Five-year overall survival for studies with this approach ranges from 49% to 62%. The continuous scheme includes radiation dose from 50 to 69 Gy, with 5-year overall survival of 39% to 74% (**Table 3**).[62,74–81] Bladder-preservation rate with split course versus continuous course schemes is 36% to 47% and 42% to 61%, respectively.

Surgical therapy after high-dose (>60 Gy) pelvic irradiation results in higher morbidity and mortality than primary radical cystectomy.[82–84] Lower-dose irradiation (40–55 Gy) does not increase postoperative mortality but may have an effect on stomal stenosis, anastomotic stricture, ureteral stricture, wound dehiscence, and wound infection.[83,84]

Pelvic lymph nodes are not surgically addressed by bladder-sparing protocols; however, the pelvic nodes inferior to the common iliac vessels are typically included in the radiation field. The importance of LND at the time of surgery is discussed previously. Including pelvic lymph nodes in the radiation field results in pelvic fracture rates of 8% to 13%.[66,68] A recent study compared response rates, pelvic lymph node recurrence, and overall survival between patients treated with whole-pelvis versus bladder-alone

Table 2
Split-course bladder-preservation protocols

Author (Year)	No. of Patients	NC	Induction CRT	Consolidation CRT	5-y OS	5-y PBS
Housset et al,[67] 1993	54		24 Gy, C/FU	24 Gy, C/FU	59 (3-y)	NA
Tester et al,[68] 1996	91	2 cycles of CMV	39.6 Gy, C	25.2 Gy, C	62 (4-y)	44 (4-y)
Kachnic et al,[73] 1997	106	2 cycles of CMV	39.6 Gy, C	25.2 Gy, C	52	43
Fellin et al,[72] 1997	56	2 cycles of CMV	40 Gy, C	24 Gy, C	55	41
Shipley et al,[65] 1998	123	2 cycles of CMV vs none	39.6 Gy, C	25.2 Gy, C	49 vs 48	36 vs 40
Kaufman et al,[70] 2009	80		40.3 Gy, C/paclitaxel	24 Gy and adjuvant 4–6 cycles of GC	56	47

Abbreviations: C, cisplatin; CRT, chemoradiation therapy; FU, 5-fluorouracil; NC, neoadjuvant chemotherapy; PBS, preserved bladder survival.

radiation.[85] Complete response rates were 93% for both schemes, pelvic lymph node recurrence rates among complete responders were 15.8% versus 17.6%, and 5-year overall survival was 53% and 51%, respectively.

Acute effects from chemoradiation therapy include early self-limited enteritis or cystitis. In an analysis of four prospective Radiation Therapy Oncology Group protocols, 7% of the patients experienced late grade 3 pelvic toxicity with 5.7% genitourinary and 1.9% gastrointestinal, which were usually not persistent.[86] There were no late grade 4 toxicities and no deaths related to treatment. Rate of secondary malignancies in patients treated with such protocols has not been reported, although increased rates are found in other cases of pelvic irradiation.

Quality-of-life outcomes related to bladder, sexual, and bowel function show favorable results. In one study, 75% of the patients with spared bladder had compliant bladders with normal capacity and flow, 50% had normal erectile function, and 80% had normal bowel function.[87] Longer follow-up and studies comparing bladder preservation with radical cystectomy are needed to further elucidate quality-of-life outcomes.

To summarize, survival rates of a chemoradiation approach may be similar to some cystectomy series in highly selected patients. However, in the absence of randomized controlled trials comparing chemoradiation with cystectomy, selective bladder preservation with chemoradiation therapy is typically restricted to those patients with favorable tumors (solitary tumor <5 cm, resectable disease, absence of hydronephrosis, absence of carcinoma in situ) or those who are unfit or unwilling to undergo cystectomy. Prevalence of different chemotherapy protocols, increased morbidity with salvage cystectomy, and lack of phase III randomized trial between contemporary bladder-preservation protocols and radical cystectomy are current challenges for the use of bladder-sparing protocols.

BIOMARKERS AND TARGETED THERAPY

Targeted therapy is playing an important role in other cancer models (renal cell carcinoma, metastatic prostate cancer), and may be a critical area of research for bladder

Table 3
Continuous bladder-preservation protocols

Author (Year)	No. of Patients	NC	CRT	5-y OS	5-y PBS
Given et al,[74] 1995	93	2 or 3 cycles of MVAC or CMV	64.8 Gy, C	39	NA
Rodel et al,[62] 2002	415		50.4–59.4 Gy, C or carboplatin/FU	50	42
Danesi et al,[75] 2004	77	2 cycles CMV	69 Gy, C/FU	58	47
Kragelj et al,[76] 2005	84		64 Gy, vinblastine	25 (9-y)	NA
Dunst et al,[77] 2005	68		50.4–59 Gy, C or paclitaxel	45	NA
Weiss et al,[78] 2007	112		55.8–59.4 Gy, C/FU	74	61
Perdona et al,[79] 2008	121	2 cycles CMV	65 Gy ± C or carboplatin	60 vs 72	47 vs 54
Gamal El-Deen,[80] 2009	186	2 cycles of CMV/MVAC/GC or none	55–64.8 Gy + none vs cisplatin	59.7 vs 68.4	NA
Sabaa et al,[81] 2010	104	3 cycles GC	60–65 Gy, C	54.8	NA
James et al,[64] 2012	360	None or cisplatin-based chemotherapy	55–64 Gy ± FU/mitomycin C	48 vs 35	NA

cancer. Some studies have investigated the mechanism of resistance to chemoradiation therapy and found that expression of Her2 and NFκB are associated with higher resistance rates.[88,89] The chemoradiation therapy resistance rate for tumors with Her2 and NFκB overexpression as compared with tumors without overexpression for both was 89% versus 11%, respectively. A Radiation Therapy Oncology Group trial with trastuzumab, a monoclonal antibody against Her2, along with paclitaxel and radiation in patients with Her2 overexpression is ongoing. Targeting the molecular pathways for Her2 and NFκB in an in vitro model by heat shock protein 90 inhibitor showed that chemoradiation-resistant bladder cancer cells were able to be successfully sensitized. Heat shock protein 90 inhibitors are currently being investigated.[90]

To improve the outcomes of muscle-invasive disease treated by surgery with or without chemotherapy, increased interest in targeted therapies has been generated. Some of the main targeted agents include tyrosine kinase inhibitors (gefitinib, erlotinib, lapatanib, sorafenib, sunitinib, and pazopanib); epidermal growth factor receptor inhibitors (cetuximab, trastuzumab); vascular endothelial growth factor receptor inhibitors (bevacizumab, aflibercept); and TP53 gene therapy (AdCMV-TP53).[91]

FUTURE DIRECTIONS

Refining surgical templates and techniques in open and minimally invasive surgical approaches is needed to decrease the morbidity of definitive surgical interventions. Randomized, controlled trials comparing newer chemotherapeutic agents with MVAC for efficacy and toxicity are imperative in establishing standard regimens. Better imaging, molecular markers, and prognostic factors may assist in further defining appropriate patient cohorts for neoadjuvant versus adjuvant chemotherapy. Further understanding of molecular pathogenesis in development and progression of urothelial carcinoma, leading to development of strategies to alter the molecular mechanisms, will be critical in refining multimodal approaches to muscle-invasive urothelial cancer in the future.

SUMMARY

Muscle-invasive bladder cancer is a heterogeneous spectrum of disease with multimodal therapy playing a key role in management. Radical cystectomy is the mainstay of treatment. However, high quality of surgery is imperative with the goal of negative surgical margins, EPLND, and performance of surgery by trained urologic oncologists. Minimally invasive surgery is an acceptable approach with equivalent complication rates; however, longer-term follow-up is needed to ensure equivalent oncologic outcomes. Neoadjuvant chemotherapy is standard of care, but underused in current clinical practice. The role of adjuvant chemotherapy is unclear with lack of robust evidence. Studies with bladder-preservation protocols of chemoradiation therapy after transurethral resection result in acceptable disease-free and overall survival along with low late toxicity rate; however, there remain no randomized trials directly comparing this approach with radical cystectomy.

REFERENCES

1. Ro JY, Staerkel GA, Ayala AG. Cytologic and histologic features of superficial bladder cancer. Urol Clin North Am 1992;19:435–53.
2. Herr HW, Badalament RA, Amato DA, et al. Superficial bladder cancer treated with bacillus Calmette-Guerin: a multivariate analysis of factors affecting tumor progression. J Urol 1989;141:22–9.

3. Prout GR, Marshall VF. The prognosis with untreated bladder tumors. Cancer 1956;9:551–8.
4. Cheng CW, Ng CF, Chan CK, et al. A fourteen-year review of radical cystectomy for transitional cell carcinoma demonstrating the usefulness of the concept of lymph node density. Int Braz J Urol 2006;32:536–49.
5. Stein JP, Lieskovsky G, Cote R, et al. Radical cystectomy in the treatment of invasive bladder cancer: long-term results in 1,054 patients. J Clin Oncol 2001;19:666–75.
6. Galsky MD, Herr HW, Bajorin DE. The integration of chemotherapy and surgery for bladder cancer. J Natl Compr Canc Netw 2005;3:45–51.
7. Herr HW. Extent of surgery and pathology evaluation has an impact on bladder cancer outcomes after radical cystectomy. Urology 2003;61:105–8.
8. Mitra AP, Quinn DI, Dorff TB, et al. Factors influencing post-recurrence survival in bladder cancer following radical cystectomy. BJU Int 2012;109:846–54.
9. Frazier HA, Robertson JE, Dodge RK, et al. The value of pathologic factors in predicting cancer-specific survival among patients treated with radical cystectomy for transitional cell carcinoma of the bladder and prostate. Cancer 1993;71:3993–4001.
10. Dotan ZA, Kavanagh K, Yossepowitch O, et al. Positive surgical margins in soft tissue following radical cystectomy for bladder cancer and cancer specific survival. J Urol 2007;178:2308–12 [discussion: 13].
11. Herr HW, Faulkner JR, Grossman HB, et al. Surgical factors influence bladder cancer outcomes: a cooperative group report. J Clin Oncol 2004;22:2781–9.
12. Koppie TM, Vickers AJ, Vora K, et al. Standardization of pelvic lymphadenectomy performed at radical cystectomy: can we establish a minimum number of lymph nodes that should be removed? Cancer 2006;107:2368–74.
13. Herr HW, Bochner BH, Dalbagni G, et al. Impact of the number of lymph nodes retrieved on outcome in patients with muscle invasive bladder cancer. J Urol 2002;167:1295–8.
14. Herr H, Lee C, Chang S, et al. Standardization of radical cystectomy and pelvic lymph node dissection for bladder cancer: a collaborative group report. J Urol 2004;171:1823–8 [discussion: 7–8].
15. Leissner J, Ghoneim MA, Abol-Enein H, et al. Extended radical lymphadenectomy in patients with urothelial bladder cancer: results of a prospective multicenter study. J Urol 2004;171:139–44.
16. Steven K, Poulsen AL. Radical cystectomy and extended pelvic lymphadenectomy: survival of patients with lymph node metastasis above the bifurcation of the common iliac vessels treated with surgery only. J Urol 2007;178:1218–23 [discussion: 23–4].
17. Vazina A, Dugi D, Shariat SF, et al. Stage specific lymph node metastasis mapping in radical cystectomy specimens. J Urol 2004;171:1830–4.
18. Mills RD, Turner WH, Fleischmann A, et al. Pelvic lymph node metastases from bladder cancer: outcome in 83 patients after radical cystectomy and pelvic lymphadenectomy. J Urol 2001;166:19–23.
19. Vieweg J, Gschwend JE, Herr HW, et al. The impact of primary stage on survival in patients with lymph node positive bladder cancer. J Urol 1999;161:72–6.
20. Gschwend JE, Dahm P, Fair WR. Disease specific survival as endpoint of outcome for bladder cancer patients following radical cystectomy. Eur Urol 2002;41:440–8.
21. Hautmann RE, de Petriconi R, Volkmer BG. Neobladder formation after pelvic irradiation. World J Urol 2009;27:57–62.

22. Lerner SP, Skinner DG, Lieskovsky G, et al. The rationale for en bloc pelvic lymph node dissection for bladder cancer patients with nodal metastases: long-term results. J Urol 1993;149:758–64 [discussion: 64–5].
23. Madersbacher S, Hochreiter W, Burkhard F, et al. Radical cystectomy for bladder cancer today: a homogeneous series without neoadjuvant therapy. J Clin Oncol 2003;21:690–6.
24. Fleischmann A, Thalmann GN, Markwalder R, et al. Prognostic implications of extracapsular extension of pelvic lymph node metastases in urothelial carcinoma of the bladder. Am J Surg Pathol 2005;29:89–95.
25. Stenzl A, Cowan NC, De Santis M, et al. Treatment of muscle-invasive and metastatic bladder cancer: update of the EAU guidelines. Actas Urol Esp 2012;36(8):449–60.
26. Roth B, Wissmeyer MP, Zehnder P, et al. A new multimodality technique accurately maps the primary lymphatic landing sites of the bladder. Eur Urol 2010; 57:205–11.
27. Stein JP. The role of lymphadenectomy in patients undergoing radical cystectomy for bladder cancer. Curr Oncol Rep 2007;9:213–21.
28. Abol-Enein H, El-Baz M, Abd El-Hameed MA, et al. Lymph node involvement in patients with bladder cancer treated with radical cystectomy: a patho-anatomical study–a single center experience. J Urol 2004;172:1818–21.
29. Leissner J, Hohenfellner R, Thuroff JW, et al. Lymphadenectomy in patients with transitional cell carcinoma of the urinary bladder; significance for staging and prognosis. BJU Int 2000;85:817–23.
30. Karl A, Carroll PR, Gschwend JE, et al. The impact of lymphadenectomy and lymph node metastasis on the outcomes of radical cystectomy for bladder cancer. Eur Urol 2009;55:826–35.
31. Zehnder P, Studer UE, Skinner EC, et al. Super extended versus extended pelvic lymph node dissection in patients undergoing radical cystectomy for bladder cancer: a comparative study. J Urol 2011;186:1261–8.
32. Poulsen AL, Horn T, Steven K. Radical cystectomy: extending the limits of pelvic lymph node dissection improves survival for patients with bladder cancer confined to the bladder wall. J Urol 1998;160:2015–9 [discussion: 20].
33. Brossner C, Pycha A, Toth A, et al. Does extended lymphadenectomy increase the morbidity of radical cystectomy? BJU Int 2004;93:64–6.
34. Kassouf W, Agarwal PK, Herr HW, et al. Lymph node density is superior to TNM nodal status in predicting disease-specific survival after radical cystectomy for bladder cancer: analysis of pooled data from MDACC and MSKCC. J Clin Oncol 2008;26:121–6.
35. Herr HW. Superiority of ratio based lymph node staging for bladder cancer. J Urol 2003;169:943–5.
36. Stephenson AJ, Gill IS. Laparoscopic radical cystectomy for muscle-invasive bladder cancer: pathological and oncological outcomes. BJU Int 2008;102: 1296–301.
37. Challacombe BJ, Bochner BH, Dasgupta P, et al. The role of laparoscopic and robotic cystectomy in the management of muscle-invasive bladder cancer with special emphasis on cancer control and complications. Eur Urol 2011;60:767–75.
38. Hellenthal NJ, Hussain A, Andrews PE, et al. Surgical margin status after robot assisted radical cystectomy: results from the International Robotic Cystectomy Consortium. J Urol 2010;184:87–91.
39. Hellenthal NJ, Hussain A, Andrews PE, et al. Lymphadenectomy at the time of robot-assisted radical cystectomy: results from the International Robotic Cystectomy Consortium. BJU Int 2011;107:642–6.

40. Smith AB, Raynor M, Amling CL, et al. Multi-institutional analysis of robotic radical cystectomy for bladder cancer: perioperative outcomes and complications in 227 patients. J Laparoendosc Adv Surg Tech A 2012;22:17–21.
41. Nix J, Smith A, Kurpad R, et al. Prospective randomized controlled trial of robotic versus open radical cystectomy for bladder cancer: perioperative and pathologic results. Eur Urol 2010;57:196–201.
42. Grossman HB, Natale RB, Tangen CM, et al. Neoadjuvant chemotherapy plus cystectomy compared with cystectomy alone for locally advanced bladder cancer. N Engl J Med 2003;349:859–66.
43. Neoadjuvant cisplatin, methotrexate, and vinblastine chemotherapy for muscle-invasive bladder cancer: a randomised controlled trial. International Collaboration of Trialists. Lancet 1999;354:533–40.
44. Advanced Bladder Cancer Meta-analysis Collaboration. Neoadjuvant chemotherapy in invasive bladder cancer: a systematic review and meta-analysis. Lancet 2003;361:1927–34.
45. Dash A, JA Pettus, Herr HW, et al. A role for neoadjuvant gemcitabine plus cisplatin in muscle-invasive urothelial carcinoma of the bladder: a retrospective experience. Cancer 2008;113:2471–7.
46. Teramukai S, Nishiyama H, Matsui Y, et al. Evaluation for surrogacy of end points by using data from observational studies: tumor downstaging for evaluating neoadjuvant chemotherapy in invasive bladder cancer. Clin Cancer Res 2006;12:139–43.
47. Donat SM, Shabsigh A, Savage C, et al. Potential impact of postoperative early complications on the timing of adjuvant chemotherapy in patients undergoing radical cystectomy: a high-volume tertiary cancer center experience. Eur Urol 2009;55:177–85.
48. Fedeli U, Fedewa SA, Ward EM. Treatment of muscle invasive bladder cancer: evidence from the National Cancer Database, 2003 to 2007. J Urol 2011;185:72–8.
49. Miles BJ, Fairey AS, Eliasziw M, et al. Referral and treatment rates of neoadjuvant chemotherapy in muscle-invasive bladder cancer before and after publication of a clinical practice guideline. Can Urol Assoc J 2010;4:263–7.
50. Raj GV, Karavadia S, Schlomer B, et al. Contemporary use of perioperative cisplatin-based chemotherapy in patients with muscle-invasive bladder cancer. Cancer 2011;117:276–82.
51. Weight CJ, Garcia JA, Hansel DE, et al. Lack of pathologic down-staging with neoadjuvant chemotherapy for muscle-invasive urothelial carcinoma of the bladder: a contemporary series. Cancer 2009;115:792–9.
52. Skinner DG, Daniels JR, Russell CA, et al. The role of adjuvant chemotherapy following cystectomy for invasive bladder cancer: a prospective comparative trial. J Urol 1991;145:459–64 [discussion: 64–7].
53. Stockle M, Meyenburg W, Wellek S, et al. Adjuvant polychemotherapy of nonorgan-confined bladder cancer after radical cystectomy revisited: long-term results of a controlled prospective study and further clinical experience. J Urol 1995;153:47–52.
54. Freiha F, Reese J, Torti FM. A randomized trial of radical cystectomy versus radical cystectomy plus cisplatin, vinblastine and methotrexate chemotherapy for muscle invasive bladder cancer. J Urol 1996;155:495–9 [discussion: 499–500].
55. Studer UE, Bacchi M, Biedermann C, et al. Adjuvant cisplatin chemotherapy following cystectomy for bladder cancer: results of a prospective randomized trial. J Urol 1994;152:81–4.

56. Stadler WM, Lerner SP, Groshen S, et al. Phase III study of molecularly targeted adjuvant therapy in locally advanced urothelial cancer of the bladder based on p53 status. J Clin Oncol 2011;29:3443–9.
57. Advanced Bladder Cancer (ABC) Meta-analysis Collaboration. Adjuvant chemotherapy in invasive bladder cancer: a systematic review and meta-analysis of individual patient data Advanced Bladder Cancer (ABC) Meta-analysis Collaboration. Eur Urol 2005;48:189–99 [discussion: 199–201].
58. Svatek RS, Shariat SF, Lasky RE, et al. The effectiveness of off-protocol adjuvant chemotherapy for patients with urothelial carcinoma of the urinary bladder. Clin Cancer Res 2010;16:4461–7.
59. Styn NR, Montgomery JS, Wood DP, et al. Matched comparison of robotic-assisted and open radical cystectomy. Urology 2012;79:1303–8.
60. Stimson CJ, Chang SS, Barocas DA, et al. Early and late perioperative outcomes following radical cystectomy: 90-day readmissions, morbidity and mortality in a contemporary series. J Urol 2010;184:1296–300.
61. Seiwert TY, Salama JK, Vokes EE. The concurrent chemoradiation paradigm: general principles. Nat Clin Pract Oncol 2007;4:86–100.
62. Rodel C, Grabenbauer GG, Kuhn R, et al. Combined-modality treatment and selective organ preservation in invasive bladder cancer: long-term results. J Clin Oncol 2002;20:3061–71.
63. Koga F, Kihara K. Selective bladder preservation with curative intent for muscle-invasive bladder cancer: a contemporary review. Int J Urol 2012;19:388–401.
64. James ND, Hussain SA, Hall E, et al. Radiotherapy with or without chemotherapy in muscle-invasive bladder cancer. N Engl J Med 2012;366:1477–88.
65. Shipley WU, Winter KA, Kaufman DS, et al. Phase III trial of neoadjuvant chemotherapy in patients with invasive bladder cancer treated with selective bladder preservation by combined radiation therapy and chemotherapy: initial results of Radiation Therapy Oncology Group 89-03. J Clin Oncol 1998;16:3576–83.
66. Shipley WU, Kaufman DS, Zehr E, et al. Selective bladder preservation by combined modality protocol treatment: long-term outcomes of 190 patients with invasive bladder cancer. Urology 2002;60:62–7 [discussion: 7–8].
67. Housset M, Maulard C, Chretien Y, et al. Combined radiation and chemotherapy for invasive transitional-cell carcinoma of the bladder: a prospective study. J Clin Oncol 1993;11:2150–7.
68. Tester W, Caplan R, Heaney J, et al. Neoadjuvant combined modality program with selective organ preservation for invasive bladder cancer: results of Radiation Therapy Oncology Group phase II trial 8802. J Clin Oncol 1996;14:119–26.
69. Zietman AL, Grocela J, Zehr E, et al. Selective bladder conservation using transurethral resection, chemotherapy, and radiation: management and consequences of Ta, T1, and Tis recurrence within the retained bladder. Urology 2001;58:380–5.
70. Kaufman DS, Winter KA, Shipley WU, et al. Phase I-II RTOG study (99-06) of patients with muscle-invasive bladder cancer undergoing transurethral surgery, paclitaxel, cisplatin, and twice-daily radiotherapy followed by selective bladder preservation or radical cystectomy and adjuvant chemotherapy. Urology 2009;73:833–7.
71. Caffo O, Fellin G, Graffer U, et al. Gemcitabine and radiotherapy plus cisplatin after transurethral resection as conservative treatment for infiltrating bladder cancer: long-term cumulative results of 2 prospective single-institution studies. Cancer 2011;117:1190–6.
72. Fellin G, Graffer U, Bolner A, et al. Combined chemotherapy and radiation with selective organ preservation for muscle-invasive bladder carcinoma. A single-institution phase II study. Br J Urol 1997;80:44–9.

73. Kachnic LA, Kaufman DS, Heney NM, et al. Bladder preservation by combined modality therapy for invasive bladder cancer. J Clin Oncol 1997;15:1022–9.
74. Given RW, Parsons JT, McCarley D, et al. Bladder-sparing multimodality treatment of muscle-invasive bladder cancer: a five-year follow-up. Urology 1995; 46:499–504 [discussion 504–5].
75. Danesi DT, Arcangeli G, Cruciani E, et al. Conservative treatment of invasive bladder carcinoma by transurethral resection, protracted intravenous infusion chemotherapy, and hyperfractionated radiotherapy: long term results. Cancer 2004;101:2540–8.
76. Kragelj B, Zaletel-Kragelj L, Sedmak B, et al. Phase II study of radiochemotherapy with vinblastine in invasive bladder cancer. Radiother Oncol 2005;75:44–7.
77. Dunst J, Diestelhorst A, Kuhn R, et al. Organ-sparing treatment in muscle-invasive bladder cancer. Strahlenther Onkol 2005;181:632–7.
78. Weiss C, Engehausen DG, Krause FS, et al. Radiochemotherapy with cisplatin and 5-fluorouracil after transurethral surgery in patients with bladder cancer. Int J Radiat Oncol Biol Phys 2007;68:1072–80.
79. Perdona S, Autorino R, Damiano R, et al. Bladder-sparing, combined-modality approach for muscle-invasive bladder cancer: a multi-institutional, long-term experience. Cancer 2008;112:75–83.
80. Gamal El-Deen H, Elshazly HF, Abo Zeina EA. Clinical experience with radiotherapy alone and radiochemotherapy with platin based regimens in organ-sparing treatment of invasive bladder cancer. J Egypt Natl Canc Inst 2009;21:59–70.
81. Sabaa MA, El-Gamal OM, Abo-Elenen M, et al. Combined modality treatment with bladder preservation for muscle invasive bladder cancer. Urol Oncol 2010;28: 14–20.
82. Eisenberg MS, Dorin RP, Bartsch G, et al. Early complications of cystectomy after high dose pelvic radiation. J Urol 2010;184:2264–9.
83. Ramani VA, Maddineni SB, Grey BR, et al. Differential complication rates following radical cystectomy in the irradiated and nonirradiated pelvis. Eur Urol 2010;57:1058–63.
84. Eswara JR, Efstathiou JA, Heney NM, et al. Complications and long-term results of salvage cystectomy after failed bladder sparing therapy for muscle invasive bladder cancer. J Urol 2012;187:463–8.
85. Tunio MA, Hashmi A, Qayyum A, et al. Whole-pelvis or bladder-only chemoradiation for lymph node-negative invasive bladder cancer: single-institution experience. Int J Radiat Oncol Biol Phys 2012;82:e457–62.
86. Efstathiou JA, Bae K, Shipley WU, et al. Late pelvic toxicity after bladder-sparing therapy in patients with invasive bladder cancer: RTOG 89-03, 95-06, 97-06, 99-06. J Clin Oncol 2009;27:4055–61.
87. Zietman AL, Sacco D, Skowronski U, et al. Organ conservation in invasive bladder cancer by transurethral resection, chemotherapy and radiation: results of a urodynamic and quality of life study on long-term survivors. J Urol 2003;170:1772–6.
88. Chakravarti A, Winter K, Wu CL, et al. Expression of the epidermal growth factor receptor and Her-2 are predictors of favorable outcome and reduced complete response rates, respectively, in patients with muscle-invading bladder cancers treated by concurrent radiation and cisplatin-based chemotherapy: a report from the Radiation Therapy Oncology Group. Int J Radiat Oncol Biol Phys 2005;62:309–17.
89. Koga F, Yoshida S, Tatokoro M, et al. ErbB2 and NFkappaB overexpression as predictors of chemoradiation resistance and putative targets to overcome resistance in muscle-invasive bladder cancer. PLoS One 2011;6:e27616.

90. Trepel J, Mollapour M, Giaccone G, et al. Targeting the dynamic HSP90 complex in cancer. Nat Rev Cancer 2010;10:537–49.
91. Youssef RF, Mitra AP, Bartsch G Jr, et al. Molecular targets and targeted therapies in bladder cancer management. World J Urol 2009;27:9–20.
92. Cognetti F, Ruggeri EM, Felici A, et al. Adjuvant chemotherapy with cisplatin and gemcitabine versus chemotherapy at relapse in patients with muscle-invasive bladder cancer submitted to radical cystectomy: an Italian, multicenter, randomized phase III trial. Ann Oncol 2012;23:695–700.

Advances in the Multimodality Management of High-risk Prostate Cancer

Mark Garzotto, MD[a,b,*], Arthur Y. Hung, MD[b]

KEYWORDS

• Prostate cancer • Adjuvant • Gleason score • Chemotherapy • Radiation
• Prostatectomy • Androgens

KEY POINTS

- Prostate cancer is a disease with a spectrum of clinical outcomes in terms of progression and response to therapy.
- Disease progression may be predicted based on risk stratification using stage, grade, and prostate-specific antigen testing.
- High-risk localized prostate cancer often requires multimodal therapy because of local disease extension and the presence of micrometastases.
- Androgen deprivation therapy improves the results of radiation and surgery in select cases.
- Current studies are focused on adjuvant chemotherapy and biologic agents in combination with surgery and radiation.

INTRODUCTION

Prostate cancer is the most common visceral cancer and the second most lethal malignancy of men in the western hemisphere.[1] In the United States, there are approximately 240,000 new cases detected each year and 28,000 deaths, which account for 9% of all male cancer deaths. Current estimates indicate that a man's lifetime risk of prostate cancer death is about 3%. Since the introduction of prostate-specific antigen (PSA) testing over the last 2 decades, lethality rates have steadily declined, resulting in a 44% overall reduction in rate of prostate cancer mortality.[2,3] During this time period, several technical innovations in local therapies have been introduced that resulted in improved local control with a reduction in treatment morbidity.[4] These initial

[a] Department of Urology, Portland Veterans Administration Medical Center, Oregon Health and Science University, Southwest Veterans Hospital Road, Portland, OR 97239, USA; [b] Department of Radiation Medicine, Oregon Health and Science University, Southwest Sam Jackson Park Road, Portland, OR 97201, USA
* Corresponding author.
E-mail address: garzotto@ohsu.edu

Surg Oncol Clin N Am 22 (2013) 375–394
http://dx.doi.org/10.1016/j.soc.2012.12.012
1055-3207/13/$ – see front matter Published by Elsevier Inc.

successes in patient outcomes from PSA testing fueled an enthusiasm for early prostate cancer screening and treatment as a means to reduce the rate of prostate cancer mortality further. However, due to the often indolent nature of prostate cancer, the rates of diagnosis and treatment of clinically insignificant disease (ie, overdiagnosis and overtreatment) during this time period were calculated to be significant.[5,6] It is estimated that since the introduction of PSA testing, 1.3 million additional men have been diagnosed with prostate cancer, with younger patients experiencing the greatest relative increase compared with the pre-PSA era.[5]

PROSTATE CANCER SCREENING AND DETECTION

The effectiveness of population-based screening for the detection of prostate cancer has been studied in 2 large randomized trials but remains an area of major controversy. A randomized screening trial in Europe enrolling 182,000 men showed a 21% reduction in the rate of prostate cancer mortality at 11 years, increasing to 29% after adjusting for noncompliance.[7] In contrast, a US-based study of 77,000 men showed no survival benefit to PSA screening in comparison to controls.[8] Important limitations of this study that have been cited include a high rate of cross-contamination with frequent PSA screening in the control group and a follow-up period that was too short to assess rate of mortality.[9] A critical limitation of both of these trials was that, of the prostate cancer cases detected, 60% to 65% were low grade and thus had a reduced biologic potential for the development of clinically significant disease.[8,10] Based on the interim results from these trials, the US Preventative Services Task Force currently recommends against the use of PSA screening for prostate cancer detection.[11] Other health policy and professional organizations, including the American Society of Clinical Oncology, the National Comprehensive Cancer Network, and the American Cancer Society, recommend an informed and shared decision process toward prostate cancer screening.[12,13] Given the lack of consensus in this area, a personalized approach seems warranted in which the risks and benefits of screening are each carefully weighed with the individual patient's health concerns in mind.

These studies highlight the need for improved methods of screening, which preferentially identify potentially lethal prostate cancer. Novel strategies such as these would optimize the efficiency of the screening process and ultimately direct the most suitable patients into evidence-based treatment pathways. Several biopsy prediction tools are currently available that demonstrate the capacity for the prediction of high-grade prostate cancer on biopsy (**Table 1**).[14–17] These prediction tools incorporate several readily available clinical biomarkers that can be used to improve risk assessment for the detection of lethal cancer. These strategies help to reduce the number of unnecessary biopsies and reduce the rate of overdiagnosis in men with insignificant cancers. Future studies are likely to incorporate advanced imaging and both serum and urine biomarkers into the risk assessment of patients presenting for prostate cancer screening.[18–21]

RISK FACTORS FOR AGGRESSIVE PROSTATE CANCER

Several clinical and pathologic pretreatment factors are known to predict adverse clinical outcomes in localized prostate cancer. Validated predictors of cancer recurrence and progression that are widely used include Gleason biopsy grade, tumor stage, and level of serum PSA. Tumor stage and level of PSA primarily correlate with extent of tumor burden; however, these are less robust indicators of lethal potential than tumor grade. The effect of tumor grade was clearly demonstrated by Albertsen and colleagues,[22] who showed that the risk of prostate cancer mortality after observation

Table 1
Prostate biopsy prediction tools for the detection of high-grade cancer

Reference	Prediction Tool	Population	Predictors	Accuracy	Validation
Thompson et al,[17] 2006	Logistic regression	Screening trial	Log PSA, DRE, prior biopsy, age, race	AUC = 70%	External
Nam et al,[15] 2007	Logistic regression	Referral cohort	Age, PSA, %fPSA, DRE	NA	Split sample
Ide et al,[14] 2008	Logistic regression	Referral cohort	PSA, testosterone	AUC = 70%	Split sample
Spurgeon et al,[16] 2006	Classification and regression tree analysis	Referral cohort	PSAD, prostate volume, age	Sensitivity = 92% Specificity = 36%	Split sample

Abbreviations: %fPSA, percent-free PSA; AUC, area under curve; DRE, digital rectal examination; NA, not available; PSA, prostate specific antigen; PSAD, PSA density.

alone was 16-fold higher in men with high-grade cancer compared with those with low-grade cancer. Similarly, in a Swedish trial of observation with a mean follow-up of more than 20 years for localized prostate cancer, tumor grade was highly predictive of cancer metastases and mortality.[23] During the follow-up period, 40% of patients experienced clinical progression and nearly half of these developed metastatic disease. In many cases cancer progression accelerated late in the disease course after a long period of nonprogression (10-15 years). In addition to highlighting the effect of Gleason score on cancer progression, this study also showed the need for continued vigilance and close observation in patients with prostate cancer, particularly among those with expected longevity.

A plethora of tissue markers have been studied as predictive biomarkers in prostate cancer.[24,25] These tissue biomarkers include oncogenic molecules involved in cell cycle progression, tissue invasion, metastases, cell survival, and angiogenesis. Although these hold great promise for use in patient management, to date none hae proven to be as effective or cost-efficient as current clinical predictive models. Thus, until further data are available, tissue biomarker analyses should remain the subject of ongoing research studies.

To assess and manage the patient with clinically localized prostate cancer accurately, standardized risk stratification groups have been identified that integrate clinical biomarkers used in routine patient care. These risk stratification groups offer several advantages in patient management, including the following: (1) to serve as standard nomenclature for interdisciplinary teams that comanage patients, (2) to determine the need for staging studies, (3) to compare treatments across similar treatment groups, and (4) to codify patient groups for the development of clinical trials with special target populations in mind.

RISK ASSESSMENT OF PROSTATE CANCER

There are several clinical factors that are predictive of disease recurrence that aid in the designation of patient risk groups. Although many of these variables have been examined individually, newer predictive models capable of combining several factors have resulted in refined tools that are available for routine clinical use. D'amico and colleagues[26] retrospectively developed a widely used strategy based on clinical data from a single institution cohort undergoing either surgery or radiation with curative intent. This straightforward schema is based on biopsy Gleason score, tumor stage, and level of PSA. Rates of relapse in risk groups were as follows (**Box 1**): low-risk: less than 25%, intermediate-risk: 25% to 50%, and high-risk: greater than 50%. Risk factors that predicted a greater than 50% chance of cancer recurrence included the following: clinical stage T3–4, a PSA >20, or a Gleason score ≥8. These predictors have been validated in external datasets and incorporated into routine practice guidelines by the National Comprehensive Cancer Network and the European Association of Urology.[27,28] In addition, tools have been developed that give a more personalized readout in terms of predicting clinical outcomes. Nomograms have been developed that give a numeric value (as opposed to risk grouping) for risk of recurrence. These tools may be of use in informing individual patients of their progression risk in more refined terms than risk groupings provide.[29,30]

IMAGING IN PROSTATE CANCER

Patient risk stratification is the primary means of guiding the need and the type of imaging modality in the workup of newly diagnosed prostate cancer. Prostate cancer has a unique tropism for bone whereby it metastasizes in greater than 80% of patients with systemic disease. Lesions involving bone are typically osteoblastic in nature and are a harbinger of tumor progression and death. Radioisotope bone scans are generally reserved for those with high-risk prostate cancer. In lower risk patients bone scans and other imaging modalities are typically omitted. In these cases patients are subject to a higher rate of false-positive results because of the frequency of benign conditions of the skeleton in elderly men. Newer bone imaging agents such as flourine-18 (^{18}F) and ^{18}F-fluorodeoxyglucose positron emission tomography/computed tomography have shown encouraging preliminary results in terms of improved sensitivity and tumor quantitation; however, these require further study before being incorporated into regular clinical practice.[31,32] Computerized tomogram scans are of limited utility in discerning the primary tumor extent or location,[33] although these are routinely

Box 1
D'amico/National Comprehensive Cancer Network risk stratification in prostate cancer (risk of treatment failure)

Low risk (<25%):

Clinical T1–T2a

Gleason score 2–6

PSA <10 ng/mL

Intermediate risk (25%–50%):

Clinical T2b–T2c, or

Gleason score 7, or

PSA: 10–20 ng/mL

High risk (>50%):

Clinical T3–T4, or

Gleason score 8–10, or

PSA >20 ng/mL

deployed to assess regional lymph node status, especially in high-risk cases considered to be locally advanced (ie, PSA >20 ng/mL or the presence of T3–T4 cancer or if the predicted chance of lymph node disease exceeds 20%).[27,34] In the future, the use of magnetic resonance imaging[35] and ferromagnetic nanoparticles[36] are likely to improve local and regional staging, but further study is needed to bring these promising modalities into the sphere of clinical practice. At the authors' institution, the utility of shutter-speed image analysis for discriminating benign from malignant prostate tissues using shutter-speed modeling is currently being evaluated.[19] This technique has shown encouraging results in early phase testing but requires large-scale prospective testing, which is in the planning stages.

SURGERY IMPROVES SURVIVAL IN PROSTATE CANCER

Radical prostatectomy is considered to be a primary treatment option for appropriate cases of localized prostate cancer.[27,28] This concept is strongly supported by the results of randomized controlled trials demonstrating significant improvements in oncologic outcomes compared with observation alone. The direct impact of curative therapy on the natural history of prostate cancer was first demonstrated in the Scandinavian Prostate Cancer Group Study 4.[37] In this trial, 695 men with localized prostate cancer were randomized to either observation alone or radical prostatectomy. At baseline, the mean PSA was about 13 ng/mL with half of all patients having PSA values greater than 10 ng/mL. With a median follow-up of 12.8 years, significant improvements in cancer outcomes have been reported for men entered onto the surgical intervention arm of the trial (**Table 2**). Surgery resulted in a 38% improvement in disease-specific rate of mortality and a 25% improvement in overall survival. Surgical intervention resulted in a 67% reduction in local progression and a 41% reduction in the spread of metastases. More recently, in a study of 731 men diagnosed primarily through PSA testing, surgery was compared with observation alone.[38] In the Prostate Intervention Versus Observation Trial (PIVOT), the mean PSA was lower at 7.8 ng/mL and greater than 70% of patients had low-grade tumors (Gleason 6 or less). With a median follow-up of 10.0 years, there was no benefit to subjects with Gleason 6 cancer or a preoperative PSA ≤10 ng/mL. However, in patients with a PSA >10 ng/mL, surgery resulted in a 21% improvement in overall survival, a 57% improvement in prostate cancer survival, and a 72% improvement in bone metastases-free survival (see **Table 2**). Similar improvements for these metrics were seen in patients with intermediate-risk and high-risk prostate cancer. Thus, based on these and other studies, surgery is considered a mainstay of therapy in

Table 2
Improvement in clinical outcome over observation in patients treated with surgery in randomized controlled trials

		PIVOT Study	
Outcome	**SPCG-4**	**PSA ≤10 Ng/mL**	**PSA >10 ng/mL**
Overall survival	25%	ns	21%
Prostate cancer survival	38%	ns	57%
Metastases-free survival	41%	ns	72%
Local control	67%	ns	NA

All numerical outcomes statistically significant (*P*<.05).

Abbreviations: NA, not available; ns, nonsignificant; PIVOT, Prostate Cancer Intervention Versus Observation Trial; SPCG, Swedish Prostate Cancer Group.

men with clinically significant, localized prostate cancer. This benefit seems to be greatest for men with higher levels of PSA and higher grade cancers. Because prostate cancer death is a relatively late occurrence among men with Gleason 6 cancer,[23] the PIVOT trial was poorly designed to capture these late events. Because of this, caution must be taken in making data inferences beyond 10 years in patients with a Gleason 6 or less tumor. Thus the long-term effect (>10 years) of surgery on low-grade PSA-detected prostate cancer remains unknown.

SURGERY FOR ADVANCED PROSTATE CANCER

The rate of cancer recurrence measured by PSA testing after radical prostatectomy is reported to be approximately 30% to 40%.[39–41] Data from several contemporary surgery series have shown that the increased D'amico/National Comprehensive Cancer Network (NCCN) category is associated with an increased chance of PSA recurrence and risk of prostate cancer death. In a report by Pound and colleagues[42] of patients with Gleason 8 or higher who were observed at the time of PSA recurrence after surgery, metastases-free survival at 7 years was only 29%. In a single-center experience of a cohort of men treated with either surgery or radiation, the risk of metastatic progression was 6.4-fold higher in D'amico/NCCN high-risk versus intermediate-risk or low-risk patients.[43] In addition, in a large retrospective analysis of US population-based data containing nearly 150,000 prostate cancer cases, 33% were found to be at high risk. With a mean follow-up of 60.7 months, the estimated 10-year cancer-specific rate of mortality after radical prostatectomy was 5.8% for patients less than 60 years old, increasing steadily to 21.1% in patients greater than 80 years of age.[44] Thus, prostate cancer is a fatal disease in high-risk prostate cancer and risk of death increases with advancing age.

Disease recurrence after radical prostatectomy may occur locally in the surgical site or at distant sites such as the axial bones. Imaging is of limited use in locating the anatomic source of PSA recurrences when the levels are low.[45–47] However, recent clinical trial reports show that most of these early recurrences are local within the surgical bed (ie, prostatic fossa).[48] This finding clearly highlights the need for technical improvements in the surgical procedure along with the need for effective combination therapy when indicated.

Improvements in our comprehension of prostatic anatomy and its surrounding structures as well as the pathways of disease extension have resulted in technical advancements in the surgical procedure.[49] Surgery may be performed through a standard open technique or by robotic-assisted laparoscopy. These procedural modifications must include a precise and thorough apical dissection along with the wide local excision of the neurovascular bundles in advanced disease.[50,51] Currently it is unclear which of these 2 methods is superior, because limited comparative data are available for high-risk cases.

Further improvements in the tumor staging and clinical outcomes result from the performance of an extended pelvic lymph node dissection versus a more limited pelvic dissection.[33,52] Long-term PSA-free survival is possible in 10% to 20% of patients with positive lymph nodes treated with an extended (vs limited) pelvic lymph node dissection.[33,53] Extended pelvic lymph node dissection should be performed in all patients with intermediate-risk or high-risk prostate cancer. In low-risk patients a lymph node dissection is generally omitted but should be considered on a case-by-case basis, particularly if other adverse features are present. Long-term cancer control in these node-positive cases is achievable but may require the addition adjuvant and salvage therapies.

Contemporary modifications to standard treatment have resulted in improved cancer-free rates in patients undergoing either surgery or radiation. These contemporary modifications are considered effective treatment options for low-risk to intermediate–risk prostate cancer; however, satisfactory therapeutic approaches have yet to be developed for patients with clinically localized, high-risk disease.[54]

ADJUVANT AND SALVAGE RADIATION THERAPY

Disease recurrence after radical prostatectomy or radiation therapy may occur locally in the surgical site or at distant sites. Existing or suspected subclinical, microscopic disease is below the threshold of detection of any imaging modality and may forever be.[46,47] However, recent scientific data support the concept that, despite technically adequate dissections, residual disease in the surgical bed can progress to metastases and death unless eradicated.

The benefit of maximizing local control in high-risk prostate cancer is strongly supported by controlled prospective trials of adjuvant radiotherapy after prostatectomy (**Table 3**).[55–57] In a phase III trial of adjuvant pelvic radiation versus observation after surgery for high-risk disease, postoperative radiation resulted in improved disease control.[55] The European Organization for Research and Treatment of Cancer (EORTC) reported the results of 1005 men who were randomized to receive postoperative radiation if they had 1 of 3 well-known prognostic factors for disease recurrence after radical prostatectomy: positive margins, extracapsular extension, or seminal vesicle invasion. After a median follow-up of 5.0 years, the group treated with adjuvant radiotherapy after prostatectomy had a 52% reduction (74% vs 53%) in either biochemical or clinical progression compared with control subjects.[55] In this study, follow-up is ongoing to assess the effects on cancer-specific and overall survival.

Accordingly, the Southwest Oncology Group (SWOG) has reported the mature results of a phase III trial of postsurgery adjuvant radiotherapy. Entry criteria in this trial are identical to the aforementioned EORTC trial, with patients requiring a minimum of 1 of 3 poor prognostic factors. The study showed that adjuvant radiation after prostatectomy resulted in a 25% reduction in metastases or death.[56,58] The SWOG trial differed from the EORTC trial mainly in that although only 431 men were accrued, they were followed for a median of 10.6 years. Localized radiation reduced the risk of PSA recurrence by 57% and increased the time to PSA failure from 2.2 to 9.2 years.[56,58] In a subsequent analysis using updated trial data with an additional 2 years of median follow-up, Thompson and colleagues[56] showed that adjuvant radiation resulted in a statistically significant increase in metastasis-free survival (12.9 vs 14.7 years) and overall survival (13.3 vs 15.2 years) in the group receiving early postoperative radiation therapy. In a third phase III trial reported by Wiegel and colleagues[57] in 2009, 307 patients with pathologic T3 disease or positive margins disease after radical prostatectomy were also randomized to undergo postoperative radiation or observation. The unique feature of this trial is that all patients were required to have an undetectable PSA postprostatectomy. After only a median follow-up period of 53.7 months, they demonstrated a roughly 50% reduction in biochemical recurrence (hazard ratio = 0.53, P = .0015) and this was despite the fact that greater than 20% of the patients assigned to adjuvant radiation refused immediate radiation therapy.

Three separate phase III trials have now demonstrated significant reduction in biochemical recurrence for adjuvant radiation for patients with high-risk features after radical prostatectomy. All 3 trials meticulously captured toxicity data and demonstrated very little short-term toxicity and no significant long-term toxicity or impact

Table 3
Results of adjuvant localized radiotherapy versus observation after surgery for high-risk prostate cancer

Study	No. Subjects (Follow-up, Years)	Main Entry Criteria	Primary Endpoint	Treatment	Main Results
Thompson et al,[58] 2006	431 (10.6)	Extracapsular extension, positive surgical margin, *or* seminal vesicle invasion	Metastases-free survival	60–64 Gy to prostate fossa	Metastases or death improved in RT group (HR 0.75, 95% CI, 0.55–1.02; *P* = .06). Improved PSA-free survival.
Bolla et al,[55]	1005 (5.0)	Extracapsular extension, positive surgical margin, *or* seminal vesicle invasion	PSA recurrence-free survival	60 Gy treatment within 16 wk of surgery to prostate fossa	RT reduced PSA recurrence by 52% (HR 0.48, 98% CI 0.37–0.62; *P* <.0001). Improved locoregional control but no difference in metastases or overall survival
Wiegel et al,[57]	307 (4.5)	Pathologic T3–T4, N0 Undetectable PSA	PSA recurrence-free survival	60 Gy treatment within 6–12 wk of surgery to prostate fossa	RT reduced PSA recurrence (HR = 0.53; 95% CI, 0.37 to 0.79; *P* = .0015). No difference in metastases or overall survival

Abbreviations: CI, confidence interval; Gy, Gray; HR, hazard ratio; PSA, prostate-specific antigen.

on quality-of-life measures.[59] With the body of evidence favoring adjuvant radiation, patients with high-risk features after prostatectomy should be considered for this treatment.

An alternative approach to adjuvant therapy that has been advocated by some experts is to implement early salvage radiation for a rising PSA after prostatectomy. Prostate cancer is unique from other tumor types in that a serum marker of early recurrence is readily available for assessment (ie, PSA). In untreated prostate cancer, the detection of PSA precedes the development of metastases and other clinical symptoms by many years.[42,45] Thus, close monitoring of the PSA with early treatment of recurrent disease may present an opportunity to improve the risk-benefit ratio of postoperative radiation. An important caveat of the use of early salvage therapy is that all published studies in this area are retrospective analyses of either single institution or pooled multi-institutional cohort samples. Thus, the published data reflect the wide variance in the selection characteristics for patients undergoing treatment as well as the interinstitutional treatment techniques for salvage therapy.

The largest of study to date was reported by Stephenson and colleagues[60] on 1540 patients undergoing salvage radiation therapy to the prostatic fossa for PSA-only recurrence. A complete PSA response was achieved in 55% of patients with radiotherapy alone and in 59% of those receiving androgen deprivation in combination with radiation. The benefit of salvage radiation was observed across all risk groups including those with high-risk pathologic features such as Gleason 8–10 and seminal vesicle invasion. The presence of positive surgical margins, which is a predictor of poor local control in prostate cancer and other tumor types, paradoxically predicted a better response to local radiotherapy than did the absence of surgical margins.

The 6-year PSA progression-free survival was 32% for the cohort, but improved to 48% for those with a starting PSA of 0.5 ng/mL or less. The authors of this study make the case that this reduction in PSA recurrence is similar to the proportional decrease seen with adjuvant radiation (≈50%).[57,58,61] Based on these findings, some authorities advocate for determining the need for adjuvant versus planned early salvage on a case-by-case basis using a shared decision approach with the patient.[62]

Until further studies are completed, the debate between the choices of adjuvant versus salvage therapy will continue for patients with high-risk features after prostate surgery. Currently there are 2 ongoing phase III trials comparing the efficacy and safety of adjuvant versus salvage radiotherapy. The Medical Research Council is conducting a phase III trial entitled Radiotherapy and Androgen Deprivation in Combination After Local Surgery Trial, which has 2 main substudies. The first compares adjuvant to salvage radiotherapy in men who may or may not be ideal candidates for local radiation. The second substudy compares the length of androgen deprivation (0, 6, or 24 months) in men designated to have radiation (adjuvant or salvage). The primary endpoint of this study is prostate cancer–specific survival. Trial accrual is targeted for 3000 subjects and enrollment is ongoing in Europe and Canada. A second study is the Radiotherapy Adjuvant Versus Early Salvage Following Radical Prostatectomy, which is being performed by the Tasmanian Radiation Oncology Group. Men in the adjuvant radiation arm will initiate radiation within 4 months of surgery, whereas in the delayed treatment arm, radiation will begin if the PSA exceeds 0.2 ng/mL. The primary endpoint is 5-year biochemical recurrence-free survival. Accrual of 470 men with high-risk features is ongoing in Australia and New Zealand. It is hoped that these 2 studies will provide the much-needed insight as to the optimal approach for men with high-risk features after surgery.

ADJUVANT AND NEOADJUVANT ANDROGEN DEPRIVATION WITH SURGERY

The antitumoral effects of androgen deprivation on prostate cancer are well known to clinicians. However, recent studies have shown the androgen receptor (AR) to be the most important molecular target in the treatment of lethal prostate cancer.[63] It is a primary mediator of the development of prostate cancer as well as pan-resistance to multiple lines of treatment.[64,65] Many novel therapies incorporate AR targeting as a basis for improving treatment outcomes in combination with other treatments. Androgen deprivation has been studied extensively in combination with surgery in both preoperative and postoperative settings. The addition of androgen deprivation to surgery for lymph node–positive disease results in a significant improvement in cancer-specific and overall survival compared with surgery alone. In a randomized trial of early versus delayed androgen deprivation for node-positive disease, the use of early androgen deprivation resulted in a 4–fold improvement in prostate cancer–specific survival and a 2-fold improvement in overall survival.[66] In contrast, in a study of androgen deprivation alone for advanced nonoperable patients, the administration of early androgen deprivation failed to show an improvement in cancer-specific survival over delayed treatment, suggesting the potential need for surgical debulking.[67] Short-term neoadjuvant (preoperative) treatment with standard androgen deprivation has been studied in several clinical trials in Europe and North America. These trials have shown a uniform reduction in positive surgical margins and other histologic changes. Unfortunately, these studies have failed to show an effect on PSA recurrence or long-term survival.[68–72] Despite these shortcomings, newer more effective agents for AR targeting have shown promise in this area. Recently, Taplin[73] presented the results of a phase II trial of combined AR targeting with standard androgen deprivation plus the androgen biosynthesis inhibitor, abiraterone, before prostatectomy. This drug combination resulted in a 34% rate of either complete or near complete response in the prostatectomy specimens. Future studies of this and other AR targeting agents are warranted in the perioperative setting.

ANDROGEN DEPRIVATION WITH RADIOTHERAPY

Radiation is a mainstay in the treatment of prostate cancer, especially when used in conjunction with androgen deprivation. The rationale for this combination includes reducing cellular resistance to radiotherapy by reducing AR signaling and through the early treatment of micrometastatic disease. Androgen deprivation was initially combined cautiously with radiation because of concerns that testosterone suppression would induce treatment antagonism. Thus the original trial combining androgen suppression and radiation, Radiation Therapy Oncology Group (RTOG) 85-31, randomized patients to observation or androgen suppression immediately after the radiation concluded. The trial demonstrated an overall survival advantage at 10 years for patients with higher grade tumors, Gleason 7–10.[74] A contemporary trial, RTOG 86-10, asked the question directly of whether the androgen suppression would engender radiation resistance by randomizing patients to radiation alone or radiation with 4 months of hormone therapy, 2 months before the radiation and 2 months concurrent.[75] Although RTOG 86-10 did demonstrate an improvement in overall survival, it was not statistically significant. The 10-year prostate cancer–specific rate of mortality was statistically significant, however. These results were the basis for the subsequent trials testing the overall benefit of concurrent radiation and androgen deprivation (**Table 4**).[74,76–85]

One of the first trials to demonstrate a difference in overall survival as a primary endpoint was an EORTC trial of radiation alone versus radiation and concurrent

Table 4
Data summary of randomized trials demonstrating the oncologic benefits of androgen deprivation to radiotherapy in intermediate-risk and high-risk prostate cancer patients

Study	Eligibility Criteria	Years	No. of Patients	Androgen Deprivation	Radiation Dose	Significant Results
Long-term hormones vs RT alone						
RTOG 85-31[74]	cT3, pT3, or N1 M0	1987–1992	977	Adjuvant indefinite LHRH	65–70 Gy	With median f/u 7.6 all, 11 for living patients, 10-y overall survival was 49% vs 39% (*P* = .002) Gleason 7–10 10 prostate cancer-specific rate of mortality was 16% vs 22% (*P* = .0052) Gleason 8–10
Umea University[80]	T3 N0-1 M0	1986–1991	91	Orchiectomy	65 Gy	Mean f/u 9.7 y all patients, 16.5 y for survivors Overall survival advantage for androgen therapy in N1 patients No significant difference for patients with N0
EORTC 22863[77]	T1–T2 WHO grade 3, or T3–T4	1987–1995	415	Concurrent and adjuvant × 3 y	70 Gy	Median f/u was 9.1 y 10-y overall survival was 39.8% vs 58.1% (*P* = .0004) 10-y prostate cancer rate of mortality was 30.4% vs 10.3% (*P*<.0001)

(*continued on next page*)

Table 4
(continued)

Study	Eligibility Criteria	Years	No. of Patients	Androgen Deprivation	Radiation Dose	Significant Results
Short-term hormones vs RT alone						
RTOG 86-10[83]	Bulky T2–T4	1987–1991	456	Neoadjuvant 2 mo and concurrent	65–70 Gy	Median f/u for survivors between 11.9 and 13.2 y 10-y overall survival was 43% vs 34% (P = .12) 10-y prostate cancer-specific rate of mortality was 23% vs 36% (P = .01)
TROG 96-01[79]	T2b–T4 N0	1996–2000	818	Neoadjuvant 2 mo and concurrent vs Neoadjuvant 5 mo and concurrent vs RT alone	66 Gy	Median f/u 10.6 y 10-y prostate cancer-specific rate of mortality was 22% vs 18.9% vs 11.4% (P = .0008) for 0, 3, 6 mo of ADT 10-y all-cause rate of mortality was 42.5% vs 36.7% vs 29.2% (P = .0008) for 0, 3, 6 mo ADT In summary, only 6 mo of ADT, 5 neo and 1 concurrent, showed significant improvement
D'amico Trial[78]	T1b–T2b and 1 of 3 factors: PSA >10 ng/mL, <40 ng/mL, Gleason 7–10 or MRI T3	1995–2001	206	Neoadjuvant 2 mo and concurrent 4 mo	70 Gy	Median f/u 7.6 y 8-y overall survival 74% vs 61% (P = .01) 8-y prostate cancer-specific rate of mortality HR 4.1 (P = .01)
RTOG 94-08[82]	T1b–T2b, PSA <20	1994–2001	1979	Neoadjuvant 2 mo and concurrent 2 mo	66.6 Gy	Median f/u 9.1 y 10-y overall survival was 62% vs 57% (P = .03) 10-y prostate cancer-specific rate of mortality 8% vs 4% (P = .001)

Short-term vs long-term androgen deprivation with concurrent RT						
RTOG 92-02[81]	T2c–T4 N0	1992–1995	1554	Neoadjuvant 2 mo and concurrent 2 mo vs Neoadjuvant 2 mo and concurrent 24 mo	65–70 Gy	Median f/u survivors 11.31 and 11.27 y 10-y overall survival 51.6% vs 53.9% (P = .36) 10-y prostate cancer-specific survival 83.9% vs 88.7% (P = .0042) 10-y overall survival Gleason 8–10 31.9% vs 45.1% (P = .0061)
EORTC 22961[76]	T1c–T2b pN+ or T2c–cT4 N0–N1	1997–2001	970	Concurrent 6 mo vs Concurrent 36 mo	70 Gy	Median f/u 6.4 y 5-y overall rate of mortality 19.0% vs 15.2% (P = .65 noninferiority test) 5-y prostate cancer-specific rate of mortality 4.7% vs 3.2% (P = .002)
RT and long-term hormones vs long-term hormones alone						
SPCGF-7/SFUO-3[85]	T1b–T2 WHO G2–G3 M0 T3 M0	1996–2002	875	Lifelong ADT vs Neoadjuvant 3 mo, concurrent, and lifelong	70 Gy	Median f/u 7.6 y 10-y overall rate of mortality 39.4% in ADT alone vs 11.9% in ADT and RT (P = .004 at 7 y) 10-y prostate cancer-specific rate of mortality was 23.9% in ADT alone and 11.9% in ADT and RT (P<.0001 at 7 y)
NCIC CTG PR3/MRC PR07/SWOG[84]	T3–T4 or T2 PSA >40 ng/mL or PSA >20 Gleason ≥8	1995–2005	1205	Lifelong ADT	65–69 Gy	Median f/u 6 y 7-y overall survival 74% vs 66% (P = .03) 7-y prostate cancer-specific rate of mortality 9% vs 19% (P = .01)

androgen-deprivation therapy (ADT) for 3 years. The 10-year results demonstrated a doubling in disease-free survival, 22.7% versus 47.7%, along with an improvement in overall survival from 39.8% to 58.1%.[77,86] The use of concurrent androgen deprivation has been demonstrated to improve overall survival with only 6 months of therapy.[82,87] An RTOG study, 92-02, demonstrated an overall survival difference for patients with Gleason 8–10 cancers when subjects received more than 2 years of androgen deprivation therapy versus only 4 months.[81] An independent EORTC study demonstrated 3 years of ADT to be superior to 6 months of androgen deprivation for all patients with high-risk disease.[76] In conclusion, these trials demonstrated a significant improvement in all outcomes with androgen deprivation when added to radiation treatment. Underlying these positive results was a growing appreciation for the significance of the androgen suppression in prostate cancer and a nagging concern about whether the same benefits were achievable without the radiation.

In the last few years, 2 additional trials have been reported that asked the question of whether radiation could improve on continuous ADT alone. These 2 separate, large, randomized trials have demonstrated a large and very significant overall survival advantage for patients with high-risk disease when they receive ADT and radiation over receiving indefinite ADT by itself. Both of these trials emphatically demonstrate the synergy of multimodality therapy in prostate cancer.

INTEGRATION OF CHEMOTHERAPY INTO PRIMARY THERAPY

Disease recurrence after primary treatment may occur in the local treatment site or in distant areas such as bone or regional lymph nodes. In other cancer types the use of systemic therapies are commonly used to treat both the local tumor and the micrometastatic disease not removed with surgery. Several treatment combinations are currently under study for prostate cancer.

Adjuvant Chemotherapy

Taxane-based chemotherapies have been shown to improve overall survival in advanced prostate cancer. In phase III trials of men with metastatic castration–resistant prostate cancer, taxanes demonstrated a survival advantage over controls in both the first-line and the second-line settings.[88–90] These encouraging studies have led investigators to study these drugs after standard treatment with either surgery or radiation. Postprostatectomy docetaxel was studied in a phase II trial of 77 men with high-risk prostate cancer. For the group, the predicted time to PSA progression was 10.0 months based on tumor characteristics; however, observed time to progression was 15.7 months. The RTOG is examining the effect of radiation with androgen deprivation plus or minus docetaxel chemotherapy on overall survival in high-risk prostate cancer.[91] This trial has fully accrued its planned 600 patients and is awaiting completed follow-up. The Veterans Administration is studying the effect of docetaxel plus prednisone after prostatectomy versus surgery alone on PSA recurrence and metastases-free survival.[92] For this trial accrual is complete and follow-up is ongoing. These important studies will offer the first insights into the effect of active chemotherapy on the progression of prostate cancer in the posttreatment setting.

Neoadjuvant Chemotherapy

Taxane-based chemotherapies have been studied by several investigative groups including the authors' group in the neoadjuvant setting for high-risk prostate cancer.[54] These trials have shown that in the castration-sensitive setting, taxanes have antineoplastic activity as demonstrated by PSA changes and histologic findings in prostate specimens; however, the effects are limited and have not met treatment thresholds to justify larger scale trials.[93–97] The use of docetaxel in combination with androgen deprivation has been studied with more promising results.[98] In a phase II study of docetaxel and androgen deprivation before prostatectomy, a complete tumor response was observed in 3% of subjects.[98] One limitation of the study was that because there was no control arm, it is unknown if these effects are due to the drug combination or to the androgen deprivation itself. Currently the effectiveness of this combination is being studied in a phase III trial comparing this regimen with surgery to surgery alone. The accrual target for this trial is 750 subjects and the primary endpoint is progression-free survival. As advanced treatments that harness the knowledge of specific molecular targets expand, the need for large-scale neoadjuvant trials will increase.

SUMMARY

In summary, numerous developments in the fields of surgery and radiation have improved treatment outcomes in high-risk prostate cancer. However, continued advancements in these monotherapies are limited by prevalence of subclinical metastases and microscopic local tumor extension. The selective addition of adjuvant treatment significantly improves survival over standard treatment. These options should be presented to the patient in a balanced manner that considers risks and benefits. Future developments in the treatment of advanced prostate cancer therapy will likely be guided by advances in the understanding of prostate cancer biology.

REFERENCES

1. Siegel R, Naishadham D, Jemal A. Cancer statistics, 2012. CA Cancer J Clin 2012;62(1):10–29.
2. Thompson IM Jr, Tangen CM. Prostate cancer–uncertainty and a way forward. N Engl J Med 2012;367(3):270–1.
3. Etzioni R, Tsodikov A, Mariotto A, et al. Quantifying the role of PSA screening in the US prostate cancer mortality decline. Cancer Causes Control 2008;19(2):175–81.
4. Walsh PC, DeWeese TL, Eisenberger MA. Clinical practice. Localized prostate cancer. N Engl J Med 2007;357(26):2696–705.
5. Welch HG, Albertsen PC. Prostate cancer diagnosis and treatment after the introduction of prostate-specific antigen screening: 1986-2005. J Natl Cancer Inst 2009;101(19):1325–9.
6. Cooperberg MR, Broering JM, Carroll PR. Time trends and local variation in primary treatment of localized prostate cancer. J Clin Oncol 2010;28(7):1117–23.
7. Schroder FH, Hugosson J, Roobol MJ, et al. Prostate-cancer mortality at 11 years of follow-up. N Engl J Med 2012;366(11):981–90.
8. Andriole GL, Crawford ED, Grubb RL 3rd, et al. Mortality results from a randomized prostate-cancer screening trial. N Engl J Med 2009;360(13):1310–9.
9. Barry MJ. Screening for prostate cancer–the controversy that refuses to die. N Engl J Med 2009;360(13):1351–4.
10. Schroder FH, Hugosson J, Roobol MJ, et al. Screening and prostate-cancer mortality in a randomized European study. N Engl J Med 2009;360(13):1320–8.
11. Moyer VA. Screening for prostate cancer: U.S. Preventive Services Task Force recommendation statement. Ann Intern Med 2012;157(2):120–34.
12. Basch E, Oliver TK, Vickers A, et al. Screening for prostate cancer with prostate-specific antigen testing: American Society of Clinical Oncology provisional clinical opinion. J Clin Oncol 2012;30(24):3020–5.

13. Brawley OW. Prostate cancer screening: what we know, don't know, and believe. Ann Intern Med 2012;157(2):135–6.
14. Ide H, Yasuda M, Nishio K, et al. Development of a nomogram for predicting high-grade prostate cancer on biopsy: the significance of serum testosterone levels. Anticancer Res 2008;28(4C):2487–92.
15. Nam RK, Toi A, Klotz LH, et al. Assessing individual risk for prostate cancer. J Clin Oncol 2007;25(24):3582–8.
16. Spurgeon SE, Hsieh YC, Rivadinera A, et al. Classification and regression tree analysis for the prediction of aggressive prostate cancer on biopsy. J Urol 2006;175(3 Pt 1):918–22.
17. Thompson IM, Ankerst DP, Chi C, et al. Assessing prostate cancer risk: results from the Prostate Cancer Prevention Trial. J Natl Cancer Inst 2006;98(8):529–34.
18. Hansen J, Auprich M, Ahyai SA, et al. Initial prostate biopsy: development and internal validation of a biopsy-specific nomogram based on the prostate cancer antigen 3 assay. Eur Urol 2013;63(2):201–9.
19. Li X, Priest RA, Woodward WJ, et al. Feasibility of shutter-speed DCE-MRI for improved prostate cancer detection. Magn Reson Med 2013;69(1):171–8.
20. Litjens GJ, Hambrock T, Hulsbergen-van de Kaa C, et al. Interpatient variation in normal peripheral zone apparent diffusion coefficient: effect on the prediction of prostate cancer aggressiveness. Radiology 2012;265(1):260–6.
21. Tosoian JJ, Loeb S, Feng Z, et al. Association of [-2]proPSA with biopsy reclassification during active surveillance for prostate cancer. J Urol 2012;188(4): 1131–6.
22. Albertsen PC, Hanley JA, Fine J. 20-year outcomes following conservative management of clinically localized prostate cancer. JAMA 2005;293(17):2095–101.
23. Johansson JE, Andren O, Andersson SO, et al. Natural history of early, localized prostate cancer. JAMA 2004;291(22):2713–9.
24. Bjartell A, Montironi R, Berney DM, et al. Tumour markers in prostate cancer II: diagnostic and prognostic cellular biomarkers. Acta Oncol 2011;50(Suppl 1):76–84.
25. Shariat SF, Scherr DS, Gupta A, et al. Emerging biomarkers for prostate cancer diagnosis, staging, and prognosis. Arch Esp Urol 2011;64(8):681–94.
26. D'Amico AV, Whittington R, Malkowicz SB, et al. Biochemical outcome after radical prostatectomy, external beam radiation therapy, or interstitial radiation therapy for clinically localized prostate cancer. JAMA 1998;280(11):969–74.
27. Mohler JL. The 2010 NCCN clinical practice guidelines in oncology on prostate cancer. J Natl Compr Canc Netw 2010;8(2):145.
28. Heidenreich A, Aus G, Bolla M, et al. EAU guidelines on prostate cancer. Eur Urol 2008;53(1):68–80.
29. Stephenson AJ, Scardino PT, Eastham JA, et al. Postoperative nomogram predicting the 10-year probability of prostate cancer recurrence after radical prostatectomy. J Clin Oncol 2005;23(28):7005–12.
30. Cooperberg MR, Hilton JF, Carroll PR. The CAPRA-S score: a straightforward tool for improved prediction of outcomes after radical prostatectomy. Cancer 2011; 117(22):5039–46.
31. Even-Sapir E, Metser U, Mishani E, et al. The detection of bone metastases in patients with high-risk prostate cancer: 99mTc-MDP Planar bone scintigraphy, single- and multi-field-of-view SPECT, 18F-fluoride PET, and 18F-fluoride PET/CT. J Nucl Med 2006;47(2):287–97.
32. Jadvar H, Desai B, Ji L, et al. Prospective evaluation of 18F-NaF and 18F-FDG PET/CT in detection of occult metastatic disease in biochemical recurrence of prostate cancer. Clin Nucl Med 2012;37(7):637–43.

33. Briganti A, Blute ML, Eastham JH, et al. Pelvic lymph node dissection in prostate cancer. Eur Urol 2009;55(6):1251–65.
34. Greene KL, Albertsen PC, Babaian RJ, et al. Prostate specific antigen best practice statement: 2009 update. J Urol 2009;182(5):2232–41.
35. Fuchsjager M, Akin O, Shukla-Dave A, et al. The role of MRI and MRSI in diagnosis, treatment selection, and post-treatment follow-up for prostate cancer. Clin Adv Hematol Oncol 2009;7(3):193–202.
36. Harisinghani MG, Barentsz J, Hahn PF, et al. Noninvasive detection of clinically occult lymph-node metastases in prostate cancer. N Engl J Med 2003;348(25): 2491–9.
37. Bill-Axelson A, Holmberg L, Ruutu M, et al. Radical prostatectomy versus watchful waiting in early prostate cancer. N Engl J Med 2011;364(18):1708–17.
38. Wilt TJ, Brawer MK, Jones KM, et al. Radical prostatectomy versus observation for localized prostate cancer. N Engl J Med 2012;367(3):203–13.
39. Freedland SJ, Humphreys EB, Mangold LA, et al. Risk of prostate cancer-specific mortality following biochemical recurrence after radical prostatectomy. JAMA 2005;294(4):433–9.
40. Han M, Partin AW, Pound CR, et al. Long-term biochemical disease-free and cancer-specific survival following anatomic radical retropubic prostatectomy. The 15-year Johns Hopkins experience. Urol Clin North Am 2001;28(3):555–65.
41. Stephenson AJ, Shariat SF, Zelefsky MJ, et al. Salvage radiotherapy for recurrent prostate cancer after radical prostatectomy. JAMA 2004;291(11):1325–32.
42. Pound CR, Partin AW, Eisenberger MA, et al. Natural history of progression after PSA elevation following radical prostatectomy. JAMA 1999;281(17):1591–7.
43. Zelefsky MJ, Eastham JA, Cronin AM, et al. Metastasis after radical prostatectomy or external beam radiotherapy for patients with clinically localized prostate cancer: a comparison of clinical cohorts adjusted for case mix. J Clin Oncol 2010; 28(9):1508–13.
44. Abdollah F, Sun M, Thuret R, et al. A competing-risks analysis of survival after alternative treatment modalities for prostate cancer patients: 1988-2006. Eur Urol 2011;59(1):88–95.
45. Antonarakis ES, Feng Z, Trock BJ, et al. The natural history of metastatic progression in men with prostate-specific antigen recurrence after radical prostatectomy: long-term follow-up. BJU Int 2012;109(1):32–9.
46. Hricak H, Schoder H, Pucar D, et al. Advances in imaging in the postoperative patient with a rising prostate-specific antigen level. Semin Oncol 2003;30(5): 616–34.
47. Scattoni V, Montorsi F, Picchio M, et al. Diagnosis of local recurrence after radical prostatectomy. BJU Int 2004;93(5):680–8.
48. Swanson GP, Hussey MA, Tangen CM, et al. Predominant treatment failure in postprostatectomy patients is local: analysis of patterns of treatment failure in SWOG 8794. J Clin Oncol 2007;25(16):2225–9.
49. Walsh PC. 2008 Whitmore Lecture: Radical prostatectomy–where we were and where we are going. Urol Oncol 2009;27(3):246–50.
50. Hull GW, Rabbani F, Abbas F, et al. Cancer control with radical prostatectomy alone in 1,000 consecutive patients. J Urol 2002;167(2 Pt 1):528–34.
51. Ward JF, Zincke H, Bergstralh EJ, et al. The impact of surgical approach (nerve bundle preservation versus wide local excision) on surgical margins and biochemical recurrence following radical prostatectomy. J Urol 2004;172(4 Pt 1):1328–32.
52. Wagner M, Sokoloff M, Daneshmand S. The role of pelvic lymphadenectomy for prostate cancer–therapeutic? J Urol 2008;179(2):408–13.

53. La Rochelle JC, Amling CL. Role of lymphadenectomy for prostate cancer: indications and controversies. Urol Clin North Am 2011;38(4):387–95, v.
54. Sonpavde G, Chi KN, Powles T, et al. Neoadjuvant therapy followed by prostatectomy for clinically localized prostate cancer. Cancer 2007;110(12): 2628–39.
55. Bolla M, van Poppel H, Collette L, et al. Postoperative radiotherapy after radical prostatectomy: a randomised controlled trial (EORTC trial 22911). Lancet 2005; 366(9485):572–8.
56. Thompson IM, Tangen CM, Paradelo J, et al. Adjuvant radiotherapy for pathological T3N0M0 prostate cancer significantly reduces risk of metastases and improves survival: long-term followup of a randomized clinical trial. J Urol 2009; 181(3):956–62.
57. Wiegel T, Bottke D, Steiner U, et al. Phase III postoperative adjuvant radiotherapy after radical prostatectomy compared with radical prostatectomy alone in pT3 prostate cancer with postoperative undetectable prostate-specific antigen: ARO 96-02/AUO AP 09/95. J Clin Oncol 2009;27(18):2924–30.
58. Thompson IM Jr, Tangen CM, Paradelo J, et al. Adjuvant radiotherapy for pathologically advanced prostate cancer: a randomized clinical trial. JAMA 2006; 296(19):2329–35.
59. Moinpour CM, Hayden KA, Unger JM, et al. Health-related quality of life results in pathologic stage C prostate cancer from a Southwest Oncology Group trial comparing radical prostatectomy alone with radical prostatectomy plus radiation therapy. J Clin Oncol 2008;26(1):112–20.
60. Stephenson AJ, Scardino PT, Kattan MW, et al. Predicting the outcome of salvage radiation therapy for recurrent prostate cancer after radical prostatectomy. J Clin Oncol 2007;25(15):2035–41.
61. Bolla M. Does adjuvant androgen suppression after radiotherapy for prostate cancer improve long-term outcomes? Nat Clin Pract Urol 2005;2(11):536–7.
62. Stephenson AJ, Bolla M, Briganti A, et al. Postoperative radiation therapy for pathologically advanced prostate cancer after radical prostatectomy. Eur Urol 2012;61(3):443–51.
63. Attard G, Richards J, de Bono JS. New strategies in metastatic prostate cancer: targeting the androgen receptor signaling pathway. Clin Cancer Res 2011;17(7): 1649–57.
64. Mostaghel EA, Page ST, Lin DW, et al. Intraprostatic androgens and androgen-regulated gene expression persist after testosterone suppression: therapeutic implications for castration-resistant prostate cancer. Cancer Res 2007;67(10): 5033–41.
65. Scher HI, Sawyers CL. Biology of progressive, castration-resistant prostate cancer: directed therapies targeting the androgen-receptor signaling axis. J Clin Oncol 2005;23(32):8253–61.
66. Messing EM, Manola J, Yao J, et al. Immediate versus deferred androgen deprivation treatment in patients with node-positive prostate cancer after radical prostatectomy and pelvic lymphadenectomy. Lancet Oncol 2006;7(6):472–9.
67. Studer UE, Whelan P, Albrecht W, et al. Immediate or deferred androgen deprivation for patients with prostate cancer not suitable for local treatment with curative intent: European Organisation for Research and Treatment of Cancer (EORTC) Trial 30891. J Clin Oncol 2006;24(12):1868–76.
68. Aus G, Abrahamsson PA, Ahlgren G, et al. Three-month neoadjuvant hormonal therapy before radical prostatectomy: a 7-year follow-up of a randomized controlled trial. BJU Int 2002;90(6):561–6.

69. Gleave ME, Goldenberg SL, Chin JL, et al. Randomized comparative study of 3 versus 8-month neoadjuvant hormonal therapy before radical prostatectomy: biochemical and pathological effects. J Urol 2001;166(2):500–6 [discussion: 506–7].
70. Hurtado-coll A, Goldenberg SL, Klotz L, et al. Preoperative neoadjuvant androgen withdrawal therapy in prostate cancer: the Canadian experience. Urology 2002;60(3 Suppl 1):45–51 [discussion: 51].
71. Rabbani F, Perrotti M, Bastar A, et al. Prostate specific antigen doubling time after radical prostatectomy: effect of neoadjuvant androgen deprivation therapy. J Urol 1999;161(3):847–52.
72. Soloway MS, Pareek K, Sharifi R, et al. Neoadjuvant androgen ablation before radical prostatectomy in cT2bNxMo prostate cancer: 5-year results. J Urol 2002;167(1):112–6.
73. Taplin EA. Effect of neoadjuvant abiraterone acetate (AA) plus leuprolide acetate (LHRHa) on PSA, pathological complete response (pCR), and near pCR in localized high-risk prostate cancer (LHRPC): Results of a randomized phase II study. Paper presented at: American Society of Clinical Oncology. Chicago, June 1-5, 2012.
74. Pilepich MV, Winter K, Lawton CA, et al. Androgen suppression adjuvant to definitive radiotherapy in prostate carcinoma–long-term results of phase III RTOG 85-31. Int J Radiat Oncol Biol Phys 2005;61(5):1285–90.
75. Pilepich MV, Winter K, John MJ, et al. Phase III radiation therapy oncology group (RTOG) trial 86-10 of androgen deprivation adjuvant to definitive radiotherapy in locally advanced carcinoma of the prostate. Int J Radiat Oncol Biol Phys 2001; 50(5):1243–52.
76. Bolla M, de Reijke TM, Van Tienhoven G, et al. Duration of androgen suppression in the treatment of prostate cancer. N Engl J Med 2009;360(24):2516–27.
77. Bolla M, Van Tienhoven G, Warde P, et al. External irradiation with or without long-term androgen suppression for prostate cancer with high metastatic risk: 10-year results of an EORTC randomised study. Lancet Oncol 2010;11(11):1066–73.
78. D'Amico AV, Chen MH, Renshaw AA, et al. Androgen suppression and radiation vs radiation alone for prostate cancer: a randomized trial. JAMA 2008;299(3): 289–95.
79. Denham JW, Steigler A, Lamb DS, et al. Short-term neoadjuvant androgen deprivation and radiotherapy for locally advanced prostate cancer: 10-year data from the TROG 96.01 randomised trial. Lancet Oncol 2011;12(5):451–9.
80. Granfors T, Modig H, Damber JE, et al. Long-term followup of a randomized study of locally advanced prostate cancer treated with combined orchiectomy and external radiotherapy versus radiotherapy alone. J Urol 2006;176(2):544–7.
81. Horwitz EM, Bae K, Hanks GE, et al. Ten-year follow-up of radiation therapy oncology group protocol 92-02: a phase III trial of the duration of elective androgen deprivation in locally advanced prostate cancer. J Clin Oncol 2008; 26(15):2497–504.
82. Jones CU, Hunt D, McGowan DG, et al. Radiotherapy and short-term androgen deprivation for localized prostate cancer. N Engl J Med 2011;365(2):107–18.
83. Roach M 3rd, Bae K, Speight J, et al. Short-term neoadjuvant androgen deprivation therapy and external-beam radiotherapy for locally advanced prostate cancer: long-term results of RTOG 8610. J Clin Oncol 2008;26(4):585–91.
84. Warde P, Mason M, Ding K, et al. Combined androgen deprivation therapy and radiation therapy for locally advanced prostate cancer: a randomised, phase 3 trial. Lancet 2011;378(9809):2104–11.

85. Widmark A, Klepp O, Solberg A, et al. Endocrine treatment, with or without radiotherapy, in locally advanced prostate cancer (SPCG-7/SFUO-3): an open randomised phase III trial. Lancet 2009;373(9660):301–8.
86. Bolla M, Gonzalez D, Warde P, et al. Improved survival in patients with locally advanced prostate cancer treated with radiotherapy and goserelin. N Engl J Med 1997;337(5):295–300.
87. D'Amico AV, Manola J, Loffredo M, et al. 6-month androgen suppression plus radiation therapy vs radiation therapy alone for patients with clinically localized prostate cancer: a randomized controlled trial. JAMA 2004;292(7):821–7.
88. Petrylak DP, Tangen CM, Hussain MH, et al. Docetaxel and estramustine compared with mitoxantrone and prednisone for advanced refractory prostate cancer. N Engl J Med 2004;351(15):1513–20.
89. Tannock IF, de Wit R, Berry WR, et al. Docetaxel plus prednisone or mitoxantrone plus prednisone for advanced prostate cancer. N Engl J Med 2004;351(15): 1502–12.
90. de Bono JS, Oudard S, Ozguroglu M, et al. Prednisone plus cabazitaxel or mitoxantrone for metastatic castration-resistant prostate cancer progressing after docetaxel treatment: a randomised open-label trial. Lancet 2010;376(9747): 1147–54.
91. Patel AR, Sandler HM, Pienta KJ. Radiation Therapy Oncology Group 0521: a phase III randomized trial of androgen suppression and radiation therapy versus androgen suppression and radiation therapy followed by chemotherapy with docetaxel/prednisone for localized, high-risk prostate cancer. Clin Genitourin Cancer 2005;4(3):212–4.
92. Montgomery B, Lavori P, Garzotto M, et al. Veterans Affairs Cooperative Studies Program study 553: chemotherapy after prostatectomy, a phase III randomized study of prostatectomy versus prostatectomy with adjuvant docetaxel for patients with high-risk, localized prostate cancer. Urology 2008;72(3):474–80.
93. Garzotto M, Higano CS, O'Brien C, et al. Phase 1/2 study of preoperative docetaxel and mitoxantrone for high-risk prostate cancer. Cancer 2010;116(7): 1699–708.
94. Gleave M, Kelly WK. High-risk localized prostate cancer: a case for early chemotherapy. J Clin Oncol 2005;23(32):8186–91.
95. Hussain M, Smith DC, El-Rayes BF, et al. Neoadjuvant docetaxel and estramustine chemotherapy in high-risk/locallyadvanced prostate cancer. Urology 2003; 61(4):774–80.
96. Konety BR, Eastham JA, Reuter VE, et al. Feasibility of radical prostatectomy after neoadjuvant chemohormonal therapy for patients with high risk or locally advanced prostate cancer: results of a phase I/II study. J Urol 2004;171(2 Pt 1): 709–13.
97. Dreicer R, Magi-Galluzzi C, Zhou M, et al. Phase II trial of neoadjuvant docetaxel before radical prostatectomy for locally advanced prostate cancer. Urology 2004; 63(6):1138–42.
98. Chi KN, Chin JL, Winquist E, et al. Multicenter phase II study of combined neoadjuvant docetaxel and hormone therapy before radical prostatectomy for patients with high risk localized prostate cancer. J Urol 2008;180(2):565–70 [discussion: 570].

Index

Note: Page numbers of article titles are in **boldface** type.

Surg Oncol Clin N Am 22 (2013) 395–404
http://dx.doi.org/10.1016/S1055-3207(13)00011-2

E

R

S